HEART&™ STROKE FOUNDATION OF CANADA

Pediatric Advanced Life Support

PROVIDER MANUAL

Editors

Leon Chameides, MD, *Content Consultant*
Ricardo A. Samson, MD, *Associate Science Editor*
Stephen M. Schexnayder, MD, *Associate Science Editor*
Mary Fran Hazinski, RN, MSN, *Senior Science Editor*

Senior Managing Editor

Jennifer Ashcraft, RN, BSN

Special Contributors

Marc D. Berg, MD
Jeffrey M. Berman, MD
Laura Conley, BS, RRT, RCP, NPS
Allan R. de Caen, MD
Aaron Donoghue, MD, MSCE
Melinda L. Fiedor Hamilton, MD, MSc
Monica E. Kleinman, MD
Mary Ann McNeil, MA, NREMT-P
Brenda Schoolfield, *PALS Writer*
Cindy Tuttle, RN, BSN
Sallie Young, PharmD, BCPS, *Pharmacotherapy Editor*

Pediatric Subcommittee 2010-2011

Marc D. Berg, MD, *Chair*
Monica E. Kleinman, MD, *Immediate Past Chair, 2007-2009*
Dianne L. Atkins, MD
Kathleen Brown, MD
Adam Cheng, MD
Laura Conley, BS, RRT, RCP, NPS
Allan R. de Caen, MD
Aaron Donoghue, MD, MSCE
Melinda L. Fiedor Hamilton, MD, MSc
Ericka L. Fink, MD
Eugene B. Freid, MD
Cheryl K. Gooden, MD
Kelly Kadlec, MD
Sharon E. Mace, MD
Bradley S. Marino, MD, MPP, MSCE
Reylon Meeks, RN, BSN, MS, MSN, EMT, PhD
Jeffrey M. Perlman, MB, ChB
Lester Proctor, MD
Faiqa A. Qureshi, MD
Kennith Hans Sartorelli, MD
Wendy Simon, MA
Mark A. Terry, MPA, NREMT-P
Alexis Topjian, MD
Elise W. van der Jagt, MD, MPH

© 2011 American Heart Association
ISBN 978-1-926969-24-4
Printed in Canada

First Heart and Stroke Foundation of Canada Printing March 2012
10 9 8 7 6 5 4 3 2 1

i

Pediatric Subcommittee 2009-2010

Marc D. Berg, MD, *Chair*

Monica E. Kleinman, MD, *Immediate Past Chair, 2007-2009*

Dianne L. Atkins, MD

Jeffrey M. Berman, MD

Kathleen Brown, MD

Adam Cheng, MD

Laura Conley, BS, RRT, RCP, NPS

Allan R. de Caen, MD

Aaron Donoghue, MD, MSCE

Melinda L. Fiedor Hamilton, MD, MSc

Ericka L. Fink, MD

Eugene B. Freid, MD

Cheryl K. Gooden, MD

John Gosford, BS, EMT-P

Patricia Howard

Kelly Kadlec, MD

Sharon E. Mace, MD

Bradley S. Marino, MD, MPP, MSCE

Reylon Meeks, RN, BSN, MS, MSN, EMT, PhD

Vinay Nadkarni, MD

Jeffrey M. Perlman, MB, ChB

Lester Proctor, MD

Faiqa A. Qureshi, MD

Kennith Hans Sartorelli, MD

Wendy Simon, MA

Mark A. Terry, MPA, NREMT-P

Alexis Topjian, MD

Elise W. van der Jagt, MD, MPH

Arno Zaritsky, MD

American Academy of Pediatrics Reviewer

Susan Fuchs, MD

Contents

Contents

Contents

Contents

Part 1

Course Overview

Course Objectives

The Pediatric Advanced Life Support (PALS) Provider Course is designed for healthcare providers who initiate and direct basic through advanced life support. Course concepts are designed to be used throughout the stabilization and transport phases for both in-hospital and out-of-hospital pediatric emergencies. In this course you will enhance your skills in the evaluation and management of an infant or child with respiratory compromise, circulatory compromise, or cardiac arrest.

During the course you will actively participate in a series of simulated core cases. These simulations are designed to reinforce important concepts, including

- Identification and treatment of problems that place the child at risk for cardiac arrest
- Application of a systematic approach to pediatric assessment
- Use of the "evaluate-identify-intervene" sequence
- Use of PALS algorithms and flowcharts
- Demonstration of effective resuscitation team dynamics

Cognitive Course Objectives

Upon successful completion of this course, you should be able to do the following, independently, when presented with a scenario of a critically ill or injured pediatric patient:

- Describe the timely recognition and interventions required to prevent respiratory and cardiac arrest in any pediatric patient

- Describe the systematic approach to pediatric assessment by using the initial impression, primary and secondary assessments, and diagnostic tests
- Describe priorities and specific interventions for infants and children with respiratory and/or circulatory emergencies
- Explain the importance of effective team dynamics, including individual roles and responsibilities, during a pediatric resuscitation
- Describe the key elements of postresuscitation management

Psychomotor Course Objectives

Upon successful completion of this course, you should be able to do the following, independently, when presented with a scenario of a critically ill or injured pediatric patient:

- Perform effective, high-quality cardiopulmonary resuscitation (CPR) when appropriate
- Perform effective respiratory management within your scope of practice
- Select and apply appropriate cardiorespiratory monitoring
- Select and administer the appropriate medications and electrical therapies when presented with an arrhythmia scenario
- Establish rapid vascular access to administer fluid and medications
- Demonstrate effective communication and team dynamics both as a team member and as a team leader

Goal of the PALS Provider Course	The goal of the PALS Provider Course is to improve the quality of care provided to seriously ill or injured children, resulting in improved outcomes.

Course Description

To help you achieve these objectives the PALS Provider Course includes:

- Basic life support (BLS) competency testing
- Skills stations
- Core case discussions and simulations
- Core case testing stations
- A written exam

BLS Competency Testing

You must pass 2 BLS tests to receive a Heart and Stroke Foundation of Canada (HSFC) PALS Provider course completion card.

BLS Skills Testing Requirements
• Pass 1- and 2-Rescuer Child BLS With AED Skills Test
• Pass 1- and 2-Rescuer Infant BLS Skills Test

The PALS Provider Course does not include detailed instruction on how to perform basic CPR or how to use an automated external defibrillator (AED). You must know this in advance. Consider taking a BLS for Healthcare Providers course if necessary. Before taking the PALS Course, review the student BLS practice sheets and BLS skills testing sheets in the Appendix. Also see Table 1: Summary of Key BLS Components for Adults, Children, and Infants and the Pediatric Cardiac Arrest Algorithm in Part 10: "Recognition and Management of Cardiac Arrest."

Skills Stations

The course includes the following skills stations:

- Management of Respiratory Emergencies
- Rhythm Disturbances/Electrical Therapy
- Vascular Access

During the skills stations you will have an opportunity to practice specific skills and then demonstrate competency. Below is a brief description of each station. During the course you will use the skills stations competency checklists while practicing the skills. Your instructor will evaluate your skills based on the criteria specified in these checklists. See the Appendix for the skills station checklists, which list detailed steps for performing each skill.

Management of Respiratory Emergencies Skills Station

In the Management of Respiratory Emergencies Skills Station you will need to demonstrate your understanding of oxygen (O_2) delivery systems and airway adjuncts. You will have an opportunity to practice and demonstrate competency in airway management skills, including:

- Insertion of an oropharyngeal airway (OPA)
- Effective bag-mask ventilation
- OPA and endotracheal (ET) tube suctioning
- Confirmation of advanced airway device placement by physical examination and an exhaled carbon dioxide (CO_2) detector device
- Securing the ET tube

If it is within your scope of practice, you may be asked to demonstrate advanced airway skills, including correct insertion of an ET tube.

Rhythm Disturbances/Electrical Therapy Skills Station

In the Rhythm Disturbances/Electrical Therapy Skills Station you will have an opportunity to practice and demonstrate competency in rhythm identification and operation of a cardiac monitor and manual defibrillator. Skills include:

- Correct placement of electrocardiographic (ECG) leads
- Correct paddle/electrode pad selection and placement/positioning
- Identification of rhythms that require defibrillation
- Identification of rhythms that require synchronized cardioversion
- Operation of a cardiac monitor
- Safe performance of manual defibrillation and synchronized cardioversion

Vascular Access Skills Station

In the Vascular Access Skills Station you will have an opportunity to practice and demonstrate competency in intraosseous (IO) access and other related skills. In this skills station you will:

- Insert an IO needle
- Summarize how to confirm that the needle has entered the marrow cavity
- Summarize/demonstrate the method of giving an intravenous (IV)/IO bolus
- Use a colour-coded length-based resuscitation tape to calculate correct drug doses

PALS Core Case Discussions and Simulations

In the learning stations you will actively participate in a variety of learning activities, including:

- Core case discussions using a systematic approach for evaluation and decision making
- Core case simulations

In the learning stations you will apply your knowledge and practice essential skills both individually and as part of a team. This course emphasizes effective team skills as a vital part of the resuscitative effort. You will receive training in effective team behavior and have the opportunity to practice as a team member and a team leader.

PALS Core Case Testing Stations

At the end of the course you will participate as a team leader in 2 core case testing stations to validate your achievement of the course objectives. You will be permitted to use the PALS pocket reference card and the *2010 Handbook of Emergency Cardiovascular Care for Healthcare Providers*. These simulated clinical scenarios will test the following:

- Ability to evaluate and identify specific medical problems covered in the course
- Recognition and management of respiratory and shock emergencies
- Interpretation of core arrhythmias and management using appropriate medications and electrical therapy
- Performance as an effective team leader

A major emphasis of this evaluation will be your ability to direct the integration of BLS and PALS skills by your team members according to their scope of practice. Review Part 3: "Effective Resuscitation Team Dynamics" before the course.

Written Exam

The written exam evaluates your mastery of the cognitive objectives. The written exam is closed-book; no resources or aids are permitted. You must score 84% or higher on the written exam.

Precourse Preparation

To successfully pass the PALS Provider Course, *you must prepare before the course.* Do the following:

- Make sure you are proficient in BLS skills.
- Practice identifying and interpreting core ECG rhythms.
- Study basic pharmacology and know *when* to use *which* drug.
- Practice applying your knowledge to clinical scenarios.

Because the PALS Provider Course does not teach algorithms, ECG recognition, pharmacology, or BLS skills, you will need to review these topics and identify any deficiencies in your knowledge. Increase your knowledge by studying the applicable content in the *PALS Provider Manual* or other supplementary resources.

BLS Skills

Strong BLS skills are the foundation of advanced life support. Everyone involved in the care of pediatric patients must be able to perform high-quality CPR. Without high-quality CPR, PALS interventions will fail. For this reason, each student must pass the 1- and 2-Rescuer Child BLS With AED and 1- and 2-Rescuer Infant BLS Skills Tests in the PALS Provider Course. *Make sure that you are proficient in BLS skills before attending the course.*

See the section "BLS Competency Testing" in the Appendix for testing requirements and resources.

ECG Rhythm Identification

You must be able to identify and interpret the following core rhythms during case simulations and core case tests:

- Normal sinus rhythm
- Sinus bradycardia
- Sinus tachycardia
- Supraventricular tachycardia
- Ventricular tachycardia
- Ventricular fibrillation
- Asystole

If you have difficulty with pediatric rhythm identification, improve your knowledge by studying the section "Rhythm Recognition Review" in the Appendix.

Basic Pharmacology

You must know basic information about drugs used in the PALS algorithms and flowcharts. Basic pharmacology information includes the indications, contraindications, and methods of administration. You will need to know *when* to use *which* drug based on the clinical situation.

If you have difficulty with basic pharmacology, improve your knowledge by studying the *PALS Provider Manual* and the *2010 Handbook of Emergency Cardiovascular Care for Healthcare Providers*.

Practical Application of Knowledge to Clinical Scenarios

Practical application will help you evaluate your ability to apply your knowledge when presented with a clinical scenario. You will need to make decisions based on:

- The PALS Systematic Approach Algorithm and the evaluate-identify-intervene sequence
- Identification of core rhythms
- Knowledge of core medications
- Knowledge of PALS flowcharts and algorithms

Be sure that you understand the PALS Systematic Approach Algorithm and the evaluate-identify-intervene sequence. Review the core rhythms and medications. Be familiar with the PALS algorithms and flowcharts so that you can apply them to clinical scenarios. Note that the PALS Course does not teach the details of each algorithm.

The manual is organized into the following parts:

Sources of information are the *PALS Provider Manual,* and *2010 Handbook of Emergency Cardiovascular Care for Healthcare Providers.*

Course Materials
PALS Provider Manual

The *PALS Provider Manual* contains material that you will use *before, during, and after the course.* It contains important information that you need to know to effectively participate in the course, so *please read and study the manual before the course.* This important material includes concepts of pediatric evaluation and the recognition and management of respiratory, shock, and cardiac emergencies. Some students may already know much of this information; others may need extensive study before the course.

Part		Read to Learn More About...
1	**Course Overview**	What you need to know before the course, how to prepare for the course, and what to expect during the course
2	**Systematic Approach to the Seriously Ill or Injured Child**	The PALS systematic approach, initial impression, evaluate-identify-intervene sequence, including the primary assessment, secondary assessment, and diagnostic tests
3	**Effective Resuscitation Team Dynamics**	Roles of team leader and team members; how to effectively communicate as a team leader or team member
4	**Recognition of Respiratory Distress and Failure**	Basic concepts of respiratory distress and failure; how to identify respiratory problems according to type and severity
5	**Management of Respiratory Distress and Failure**	Intervention options for respiratory problems and emergencies
6	**Recognition of Shock**	Basic concepts of shock; shock identification according to type and severity
7	**Management of Shock**	Intervention options for shock according to etiology
8	**Recognition and Management of Bradycardia**	Clinical and ECG characteristics of bradyarrhythmias; medical and electrical therapies
9	**Recognition and Management of Tachycardia**	Clinical and ECG characteristics of tachyarrhythmias; medical and electrical therapies
10	**Recognition and Management of Cardiac Arrest**	Signs of cardiac arrest and terminal cardiac rhythms; resuscitation and electrical therapy
11	**Postresuscitation Management**	Postresuscitation evaluation and management; postresuscitation transport
12	**Pharmacology**	Details about common medications used in pediatric emergencies
	Appendix	Checklists for BLS competency testing, skills stations competencies, and core case simulations; a brief rhythm recognition review

Throughout the *PALS Provider Manual* you will find specific information in the following types of boxes:

Type of Box	Contains
Fundamental Fact	Basic information that every PALS provider should know
Critical Concept	Important core concepts that are key to caring for critically ill or injured children
Identify and Intervene	An important evaluation or an immediate lifesaving intervention
FYI	Advanced information that you can use to increase your knowledge but that is not required for successful course participation

Remember to take this manual with you to the course.

Course Completion Requirements

To successfully complete the PALS Provider Course and obtain your course completion card, you must do the following:

- Actively participate in, practice, and complete all skills stations and learning stations
- Pass the 1- and 2-Rescuer Child BLS With AED and 1- and 2-Rescuer Infant BLS Skills Tests
- Pass a written exam with a minimum score of 84%
- Pass 2 PALS core case tests as a team leader

Suggested Reading List

Donoghue A, Nishisaki A, Sutton R, Hales R, Boulet J. Reliability and validity of a scoring instrument for clinical performance during Pediatric Advanced Life Support simulation scenarios. *Resuscitation*. 2010;81:331-336.

Hunt EA, Vera K, Diener-West M, Haggerty JA, Nelson KL, Shaffner DH, Pronovost PJ. Delays and errors in cardiopulmonary resuscitation and defibrillation by pediatric residents during simulated cardiopulmonary arrests. *Resuscitation*. 2009;80:819-825.

Niles D, Sutton RM, Donoghue A, Kalsi MS, Roberts K, Boyle L, Nishisaki A, Arbogast KB, Helfaer M, Nadkarni V. "Rolling Refreshers": a novel approach to maintain CPR psychomotor skill competence. *Resuscitation*. 2009;80:909-912.

Roy KM, Miller MP, Schmidt K, Sagy M. Pediatric residents experience a significant decline in their response capabilities to simulated life-threatening events as their training frequency in cardiopulmonary resuscitation decreases
[published online ahead of print October 1, 2010]. *Pediatr Crit Care Med*. doi:10.1097/PCC.0b013e3181f3a0d1.

Sutton RM, Niles D, Meaney PA, Aplenc R, French B, Abella BS, Lengetti EL, Berg RA, Helfaer MA, Nadkarni V. "Booster" training: evaluation of instructor-led bedside

cardiopulmonary resuscitation skill training and automated corrective feedback to improve cardiopulmonary resuscitation compliance of Pediatric Basic Life Support providers during simulated cardiac arrest [published online ahead of print July 9, 2010]. *Pediatr Crit Care Med*. doi:10.1097/PCC.0b013e3181e91271.

Part 2

Systematic Approach to the Seriously Ill or Injured Child

Overview

The PALS provider should use a systematic approach when caring for a seriously ill or injured child. The purpose of this organized approach is to enable you to quickly recognize signs of respiratory distress, respiratory failure, and shock and immediately provide lifesaving interventions. If not appropriately treated, children with respiratory failure and shock can quickly develop cardiopulmonary failure and even cardiac arrest (Figure 1).

Rapid Intervention to Prevent Cardiac Arrest

In infants and children, most cardiac arrests result from progressive respiratory failure, shock, or both. Less commonly, pediatric cardiac arrests can occur without warning (i.e., with sudden collapse) secondary to an arrhythmia (ventricular fibrillation [VF] or ventricular tachycardia [VT]).

Once cardiac arrest occurs, even with optimal resuscitation efforts, the outcome is generally poor. In the out-of-hospital setting only 4% to 13% of children who experience cardiac arrest survive to hospital discharge. The outcome is better for children who experience cardiac arrest in the hospital, although only about 33% of those children survive to hospital discharge. For this reason it is important to learn the concepts presented in the PALS Provider Course so that

you can identify signs of respiratory failure and shock and rapidly intervene to prevent progression to cardiac arrest.

Learning Objectives

After completing this Part you should be able to:

- Discuss the evaluate-identify-intervene sequence
- Explain the purpose and components of the initial impression
- Describe the ABCDE components of the primary assessment
- Interpret the clinical findings during the primary assessment
- Evaluate respiratory or circulatory problems by using the ABCDE model in the primary assessment
- Describe the components of the secondary assessment
- List diagnostic and laboratory tests used to identify respiratory and circulatory problems

Preparation for the Course

You need to know all of the concepts presented in this Part to be able to identify respiratory or circulatory problems and target appropriate management in case simulations. The ongoing process of evaluate-identify-intervene is a core component of systematic evaluation and care of a seriously ill or injured child.

Identify and Intervene Rapid, Systematic Intervention Is Key	Rapid, systematic intervention for seriously ill or injured infants and children is key to preventing progression to cardiac arrest. Such rapid intervention can save lives.

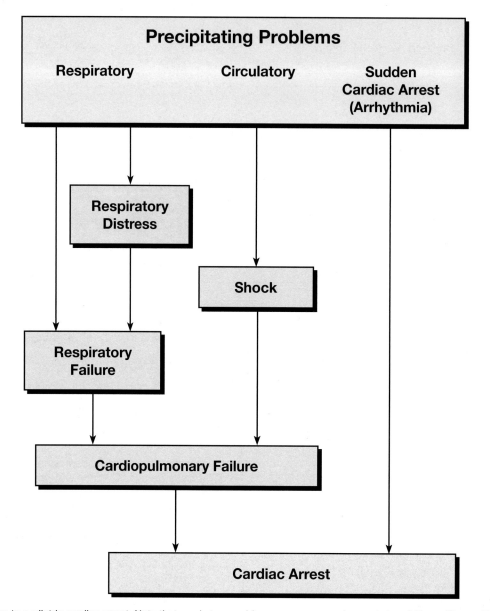

Figure 1. Pathways to pediatric cardiac arrest. Note that respiratory problems may progress to respiratory failure with or without signs of respiratory distress. Respiratory failure without respiratory distress occurs when the child fails to maintain an open airway or adequate respiratory effort and is typically associated with a decreased level of consciousness. Sudden cardiac arrest in children is less common than in adults and typically results from arrhythmias such as VF or VT. During sports activities, sudden cardiac arrest can occur in children with underlying cardiac problems that may or may not have been previously recognized.

PALS Systematic Approach Algorithm

The PALS Systematic Approach Algorithm (Figure 2) outlines the approach to caring for a critically ill or injured child.

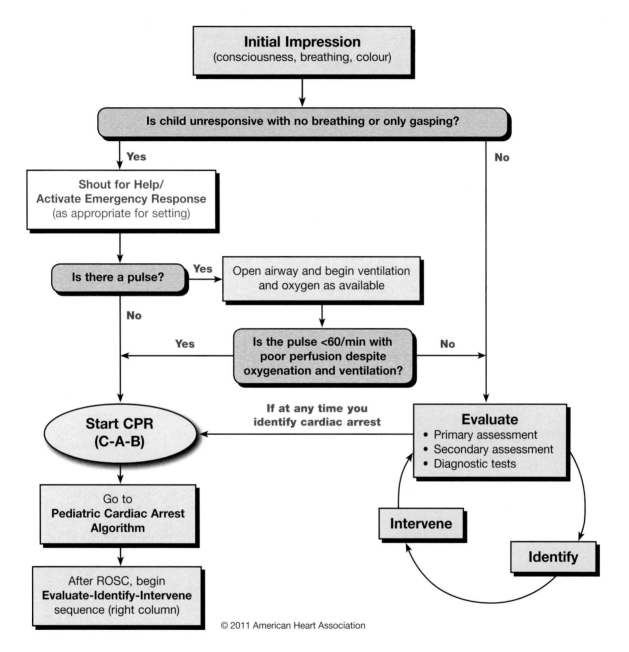

© 2011 American Heart Association

Figure 2. PALS Systematic Approach Algorithm.

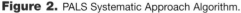

Identify and Intervene **If You Identify a Life-Threatening Problem**	If at any time you identify a life-threatening problem, immediately begin appropriate interventions. Activate emergency response as indicated in your practice setting.

Initial Impression

The initial impression (Figure 2) is your first quick "from the doorway" observation. This initial visual and auditory observation of the child's consciousness, breathing, and colour is accomplished within seconds of encountering the child.

	Initial Impression
Consciousness	Level of consciousness (e.g., unresponsive, irritable, alert)
Breathing	Increased work of breathing, absent or decreased respiratory effort, or abnormal sounds heard without auscultation
Colour	Abnormal skin colour, such as cyanosis, pallor, or mottling

The level of consciousness may be characterized as unresponsive, irritable, or alert. Decreased level of consciousness may result from inadequate O_2 or substrate delivery or brain trauma/dysfunction. Abnormal breathing includes use of accessory muscles, extra sounds of breathing, or abnormal breathing patterns. Pale, mottled, or bluish/gray skin colour suggests poor perfusion, poor oxygenation, or both. A flushed appearance suggests fever or the presence of a toxin.

Use your initial impression to determine the next best steps:

- If the child is *unresponsive and not breathing or only gasping*, shout for help or activate emergency response (as appropriate for your practice setting). Check to see if there is a pulse.
  - If there is *no pulse,* start CPR, beginning with chest compressions. Proceed according to the Pediatric Cardiac Arrest Algorithm. After return of spontaneous circulation (ROSC), begin the evaluate-identify-intervene sequence.
  - If a pulse is present, *provide rescue breathing.*
    - *If, despite adequate oxygenation and ventilation, the heart rate is <60/min with signs of poor perfusion,*

provide compressions and ventilations. Proceed according to the Pediatric Cardiac Arrest Algorithm.
    - If the heart rate is ≥*60/min,* begin the evaluate-identify-intervene sequence. Be prepared to intervene according to the Pediatric Cardiac Arrest Algorithm if needed.
- If the child is breathing adequately, proceed with the evaluate-identify-intervene sequence. If at any time you identify cardiac arrest, begin CPR and proceed according to the Pediatric Cardiac Arrest Algorithm.

Evaluate-Identify-Intervene

Use the evaluate-identify-intervene sequence (Figure 3) when caring for a seriously ill or injured child. This will help you to determine the best treatment or intervention at any point. From the information gathered during your evaluation, identify the child's problem by type and severity. Intervene with appropriate actions. Then repeat the sequence. This process is ongoing.

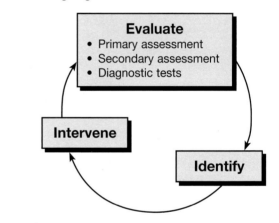

Evaluate
- Primary assessment
- Secondary assessment
- Diagnostic tests

Intervene

Identify

Figure 3. Evaluate-identify-intervene sequence.

Always be alert to a life-threatening problem. If at any point you identify a life-threatening problem, immediately activate emergency response (or send someone to do so) while you begin lifesaving interventions.

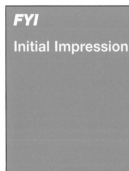

FYI

Initial Impression

The initial impression used in this version of the PALS Provider Course is a modification of the Pediatric Assessment Triangle (PAT)[1] that was used in the 2006 PALS Provider Course.[2] The PAT, like the rapid cardiopulmonary assessment (which was taught in all of the PALS courses before 2006),[3] is part of a systematic approach to assessing an ill or injured child. These slightly different assessment approaches use many of the same common terms. The goal of all of these approaches is to help the provider quickly recognize a child at risk for deterioration and prioritize actions and interventions.

[1]Dieckmann RD, Brownstein DR, Gausche-Hill M, eds. *Pediatric Education for Prehospital Professionals Instructor Toolkit.* Sudbury, MA: American Academy of Pediatrics and Jones & Bartlett Publishers; 2000. [2]Ralston M, Hazinski MF, Zaritsky AL, Schexnayder SM, Kleinman ME, eds. *Pediatric Advanced Life Support Provider Manual.* Dallas, TX: American Heart Association; 2006. [3]Hazinski MF, Zaritsky AL, Nadkarni VM, Hickey RW, Schexnayder SM, Berg RA, eds. *Pediatric Advanced Life Support Provider Manual.* Dallas, TX: American Heart Association; 2002.

Evaluate

If no life-threatening problem is present, evaluate the child's condition by using the clinical assessment tools described below.

Clinical Assessment	Brief Description
Primary assessment	A rapid, hands-on ABCDE approach to evaluate respiratory, cardiac, and neurologic function; this step includes assessment of vital signs and pulse oximetry
Secondary assessment	A focused medical history and a focused physical exam
Diagnostic tests	Laboratory, radiographic, and other advanced tests that help to identify the child's physiologic condition and diagnosis

Note: Providers should be aware of potential environmental dangers when providing care. In out-of-hospital settings, always assess the scene before you evaluate the child.

Identify

Try to identify the type and severity of the child's problem.

	Type	Severity
Respiratory	• Upper airway obstruction • Lower airway obstruction • Lung tissue disease • Disordered control of breathing	• Respiratory distress • Respiratory failure
Circulatory	• Hypovolemic shock • Distributive shock • Cardiogenic shock • Obstructive shock	• Compensated shock • Hypotensive shock
Cardiopulmonary Failure		
Cardiac Arrest		

The child's clinical condition can result from a combination of respiratory and circulatory problems. As a seriously ill or injured child deteriorates, one problem may lead to others.

Note that in the initial phase of your identification you may be uncertain about the type or severity of problems.

Identifying the problem will help you determine the best initial interventions. Recognition and management are discussed in detail later in this manual.

Intervene

On the basis of your identification of the child's problem, intervene with appropriate actions within your scope of practice. PALS interventions may include:

- Positioning the child to maintain a patent airway
- Activating emergency response
- Starting CPR
- Obtaining the code cart and monitor
- Placing the child on a cardiac monitor and pulse oximeter
- Administering O_2
- Supporting ventilation
- Starting medications and fluids (e.g., nebulizer treatment, IV/IO fluid bolus)

Continuous Sequence

The sequence of evaluate-identify-intervene continues until the child is stable. Use this sequence before and after each intervention to look for trends in the child's condition. For example, after you give O_2, reevaluate the child. Is the child breathing a little easier? Are colour and mental status improving? After you give a fluid bolus to a child in hypovolemic shock, do heart rate and perfusion improve? Is another bolus needed? Use the evaluate-identify-intervene sequence whenever the child's condition changes.

Determine If Problem Is Life Threatening

On the basis of the initial impression and throughout care, determine if the child's problem is:

- Life threatening
- Not life threatening

Life-threatening problems include absent or agonal respirations, respiratory distress, cyanosis, or decreased level of consciousness (see the section "Life-Threatening Problems" later in this Part). If the problem is life threatening, immediately begin appropriate interventions. Activate emergency response as indicated in your practice setting. If the problem is not life threatening, continue with the systematic approach.

Critical Concept The Evaluate-Identify-Intervene Sequence Is Continuous	Remember to repeat the evaluate-identify-intervene sequence until the child is stable • After each intervention • When the child's condition changes or deteriorates

Sometimes a child's condition may seem stable despite the presence of a life-threatening problem. An example is a child who has ingested a toxin but is not yet showing effects. Another example is a trauma victim with internal bleeding who may initially maintain blood pressure by increasing heart rate and systemic vascular resistance (SVR).

Primary Assessment

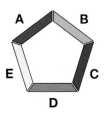

The primary assessment uses an ABCDE model:

- **A**irway
- **B**reathing
- **C**irculation
- **D**isability
- **E**xposure

The primary assessment is a *hands-on* evaluation of respiratory, cardiac, and neurologic function. This assessment includes evaluation of vital signs and O$_2$ saturation by pulse oximetry.

Airway

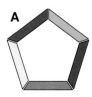

When you assess the airway, you determine if it is patent (open). To assess upper airway patency:

- Look for movement of the chest or abdomen
- Listen for air movement and breath sounds

Decide if the upper airway is clear, maintainable, or not maintainable as described in the following table:

Status	Description
Clear	Airway is open and unobstructed for normal breathing
Maintainable	Airway is obstructed but can be maintained by *simple measures* (e.g., head tilt–chin lift)
Not maintainable	Airway is obstructed and cannot be maintained without *advanced interventions (e.g., intubation)*

The following signs suggest that the upper airway is obstructed:

- Increased inspiratory effort with retractions
- Abnormal inspiratory sounds (snoring or high-pitched stridor)
- Episodes where no airway or breath sounds are present despite respiratory effort (i.e., complete upper airway obstruction)

If the upper airway is obstructed, determine if you can open and maintain the airway with *simple measures* or if you need *advanced interventions*.

Simple Measures

Simple measures to open and maintain a patent upper airway may include one or more of the following:

- Allow the child to assume a position of comfort or position the child to improve airway patency.
- Use head tilt–chin lift or jaw thrust to open the airway.
  - Use the head tilt–chin lift maneuver to open the airway unless you suspect cervical spine injury. Avoid overextending the head/neck in infants because this may occlude the airway.
  - If you suspect cervical spine injury (e.g., the child has head or neck injury), open the airway by using a jaw thrust without neck extension. If this maneuver does not open the airway, use a head tilt–chin lift or jaw thrust with neck extension because opening the airway is a priority. During CPR stabilize the head and neck manually rather than with immobilization devices.

If at any time you identify a life-threatening problem, immediately begin appropriate interventions. Activate emergency response as indicated in your practice setting.

– Note that the jaw thrust may be used in children without trauma as well.

- Avoid overextending the head/neck in infants because this may occlude the airway. Suction the nose and oropharynx.
- Perform foreign-body airway obstruction (FBAO) relief techniques if you suspect that the child has aspirated a foreign body, has complete airway obstruction (is unable to make any sound), and is still responsive. Repeat the following as needed:
  – <1 year of age: Give 5 back slaps and 5 chest thrusts
  – ≥1 year of age: Give abdominal thrusts
- Use airway adjuncts (e.g., nasopharyngeal airway [NPA] or oropharyngeal airway [OPA]) to keep the tongue from falling back and obstructing the airway.

Advanced Interventions

Advanced interventions to maintain airway patency may include one or more of the following:

- Endotracheal intubation or placement of a laryngeal mask airway
- Application of continuous positive airway pressure (CPAP) or noninvasive ventilation
- Removal of a foreign body; this intervention may require direct laryngoscopy (i.e., visualizing the larynx with a laryngoscope)
- Cricothyrotomy (a needle puncture or surgical opening through the skin and cricothyroid membrane and into the trachea below the vocal cords)

Breathing

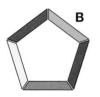

Assessment of breathing includes evaluation of:

- Respiratory rate
- Respiratory effort
- Chest expansion and air movement
- Lung and airway sounds
- O_2 saturation by pulse oximetry

Normal Respiratory Rate

Normal spontaneous breathing is accomplished with minimal work, resulting in quiet breathing with unlabored inspiration and passive expiration. The normal respiratory rate is inversely related to age (see Table 1); it is rapid in the neonate and decreases as the child gets older.

Table 1. Normal Respiratory Rates by Age

Age	Breaths/min
Infant (<1 year)	30 to 60
Toddler (1 to 3 years)	24 to 40
Preschooler (4 to 5 years)	22 to 34
School age (6 to 12 years)	18 to 30
Adolescent (13 to 18 years)	12 to 16

Respiratory rate is often best evaluated before your hands-on assessment because anxiety and agitation commonly alter the baseline rate. If the child has any condition that causes an increase in metabolic demand (e.g., excitement, anxiety, exercise, pain, or fever), it is appropriate for the respiratory rate to be higher than normal.

Determine the respiratory rate by counting the number of times the chest rises in 30 seconds and multiplying by 2. Be aware that normal sleeping infants may have irregular (periodic) breathing with pauses lasting up to 10 or even 15 seconds. If you count the number of times the chest rises for <30 seconds, you may estimate the respiratory rate inaccurately. Count the respiratory rate several times as you assess and reassess the child to detect changes. Alternatively, the respiratory rate may be displayed continuously on a monitor.

A decrease in respiratory rate from a rapid to a more "normal" rate may indicate overall improvement if it is

Identify and Intervene **Don't Rely on an Adjunct Alone to Maintain an Open Airway**	An airway adjunct will help to maintain an open airway, but you may still need to use a head tilt–chin lift. Don't rely only on an adjunct alone. Assess the patient!

Critical Concept **Very Slow or Very Fast Respiratory Rate Is a Warning Sign**	A consistent respiratory rate of less than 10 or more than 60 breaths/min in a child of any age is abnormal and suggests the presence of a potentially serious problem.

associated with an improved level of consciousness and reduced signs of air hunger and work of breathing. A decreasing or irregular respiratory rate in a child with a deteriorating level of consciousness, however, often indicates a worsening of the child's clinical condition.

Abnormal Respiratory Rate

Abnormal respiratory rates are classified as:

- Tachypnea
- Bradypnea
- Apnea

Tachypnea

Tachypnea is a breathing rate that is more rapid than normal for age. It is often the first sign of respiratory distress in infants. Tachypnea also can be a physiologic (appropriate) response to stress.

Tachypnea with respiratory distress is, by definition, associated with other signs of increased respiratory effort. "Quiet tachypnea" is the term used if tachypnea is present without signs of increased respiratory effort (i.e., without respiratory distress). This often results from an attempt to maintain near-normal blood pH by increasing the amount of air moving in and out of the lungs (ventilation); this decreases CO_2 levels in the blood and increases blood pH.

Quiet tachypnea commonly results from nonpulmonary problems, including:

- High fever
- Pain
- Mild metabolic acidosis associated with dehydration or diabetic ketoacidosis (DKA)
- Sepsis (without pneumonia)
- Congestive heart failure (early)
- Severe anemia
- Some cyanotic congenital heart defects (e.g., transposition of the great arteries)

Bradypnea

Bradypnea is a breathing rate that is slower than normal for age. Frequently the breathing is both slow and irregular. Possible causes are respiratory muscle fatigue, central nervous system injury or infection, hypothermia, or medications that depress respiratory drive.

Apnea

Apnea is the cessation of breathing for 20 seconds or cessation for less than 20 seconds if accompanied by bradycardia, cyanosis, or pallor.

Agonal gasps are common in adults after sudden cardiac arrest and may be confused with normal breathing. Agonal gasps will not produce effective oxygenation and ventilation.

Respiratory Effort

Increased respiratory effort results from conditions that increase resistance to airflow (e.g., asthma or bronchiolitis) or that cause the lungs to be stiffer and difficult to inflate (e.g., pneumonia, pulmonary edema, or pleural effusion). Nonpulmonary conditions that result in severe metabolic acidosis (e.g., DKA, salicylate ingestion, inborn errors of metabolism) can also cause increased respiratory rate and effort. Signs of increased respiratory effort reflect the child's attempt to improve oxygenation, ventilation, or both. Use the presence or absence of these signs to assess the severity of the condition and the urgency for intervention. Signs of increased respiratory effort include:

- Nasal flaring
- Retractions
- Head bobbing or seesaw respirations

Other signs of increased respiratory effort are prolonged inspiratory or expiratory times, open-mouth breathing, gasping, and use of accessory muscles. Grunting is a serious sign and may indicate respiratory distress or respiratory failure. (See "Grunting" later in this Part.)

Critical Concept **Bradypnea or Irregular Respiratory Rate Often Signals Impending Arrest**	Bradypnea or an irregular respiratory rate in an acutely ill infant or child is an ominous clinical sign and often signals impending arrest.
FYI **3 Types of Apnea**	Apnea is classified into 3 types, depending on whether inspiratory muscle activity is present: - In *central apnea* there is no respiratory effort because of an abnormality or suppression of the brain or spinal cord. - In *obstructive apnea* there is inspiratory effort without airflow (i.e., airflow is partially or completely blocked). - In *mixed apnea* there are periods of obstructive apnea and periods of central apnea.

Nasal Flaring

Nasal flaring is dilation of the nostrils with each inhalation. The nostrils open more widely to maximize airflow. Nasal flaring is most commonly observed in infants and younger children and is usually a sign of respiratory distress.

Retractions

Retractions are inward movements of the chest wall or tissues, neck, or sternum during inspiration. Chest retractions are a sign that the child is trying to move air into the lungs by using the chest muscles, but air movement is impaired by increased airway resistance or stiff lungs. Retractions may occur in several areas of the chest. The severity of the retractions generally corresponds with the severity of the child's breathing difficulty.

The following table describes the location of retractions commonly associated with each level of breathing difficulty:

Breathing Difficulty	Location of Retraction	Description
Mild to moderate	Subcostal	Retraction of the abdomen, just below the rib cage
	Substernal	Retraction of the abdomen at the bottom of the breastbone
	Intercostal	Retraction between the ribs

(continued)

(continued)

Breathing Difficulty	Location of Retraction	Description
Severe (may include the same retractions as seen with mild to moderate breathing difficulty)	Supraclavicular	Retraction in the neck, just above the collarbone
	Suprasternal	Retraction in the chest, just above the breastbone
	Sternal	Retraction of the sternum toward the spine

Head Bobbing or Seesaw Respirations

Head bobbing and seesaw respirations often indicate that the child has increased risk for deterioration.

- *Head bobbing* is caused by the use of neck muscles to assist breathing. The child lifts the chin and extends the neck during inspiration and allows the chin to fall forward during expiration. Head bobbing is most frequently seen in infants and can be a sign of respiratory failure.
- *Seesaw respirations* are present when the chest retracts and the abdomen expands during inspiration. During expiration the movement reverses: the chest expands and the abdomen moves inward. Seesaw respirations usually indicate upper airway obstruction. They also may be observed in severe lower airway obstruction, lung tissue disease, and disordered control of breathing. Seesaw respirations are characteristic of infants and children with neuromuscular weakness. This inefficient form of ventilation can quickly lead to fatigue.

FYI **Combination of Retractions and Other Signs to Identify Type of Respiratory Problem**	Retractions accompanied by stridor or an inspiratory snoring sound suggest upper airway obstruction. Retractions accompanied by expiratory wheezing suggest marked lower airway obstruction (asthma or bronchiolitis), causing obstruction during both inspiration and expiration. Retractions accompanied by grunting or labored respirations suggest lung tissue disease. Severe retractions also may be accompanied by head bobbing or seesaw respirations.

Fundamental Fact **Cause of Seesaw Breathing**	The cause of seesaw breathing in most children with neuromuscular disease is weakness of the abdominal and chest wall muscles. Seesaw breathing is caused by strong contraction of the diaphragm that dominates the weaker abdominal and chest wall muscles. The result is retraction of the chest and expansion of the abdomen during inspiration.

Chest Expansion and Air Movement

Evaluate magnitude of chest wall expansion and air movement to assess adequacy of the child's tidal volume. Tidal volume is the volume of air inspired with each breath. Normal tidal volume is approximately 5 to 7 mL/kg of body weight and remains fairly constant throughout life. Tidal volume is difficult to measure unless a child is mechanically ventilated, so your clinical assessment is very important.

Chest Wall Expansion

Chest expansion (chest rise) during inspiration should be symmetric. Expansion may be subtle during spontaneous quiet breathing, especially when clothing covers the chest. But chest expansion should be readily visible when the chest is uncovered. In normal infants the abdomen may move more than the chest. Decreased or asymmetric chest expansion may result from inadequate effort, airway obstruction, atelectasis, pneumothorax, hemothorax, pleural effusion, mucous plug, or foreign-body aspiration.

Air Movement

Auscultation for air movement is critical. Listen for the intensity of breath sounds and quality of air movement, particularly in the distal lung fields. To evaluate distal air entry, listen below both axillae. Because these areas are farthest from the larger conducting airways, upper airway sounds are less likely to be transmitted. Typical inspiratory sounds can be heard distally as soft, quiet noises occurring simultaneously with observed inspiratory effort. Normal expiratory breath sounds are often short and quieter. Sometimes you may not hear normal expiratory breath sounds.

You should also auscultate for lung and airway sounds over the anterior and posterior chest. Because the chest is small and the chest wall is thin in infants or children, breath sounds are readily transmitted from one side of the chest to the other. Breath sounds also may be transmitted from the upper airway.

Decreased chest excursion or decreased air movement observed during auscultation often accompanies poor respiratory effort. In the child with apparently normal or increased respiratory effort, diminished distal air entry suggests airflow obstruction or lung tissue disease. If the child's work of breathing and coughing suggest lower airway obstruction but no wheezes are heard, the amount and rate of airflow may be insufficient to cause wheezing.

Distal air entry may be difficult to hear in the obese child. As a result, it may be difficult to identify significant airway abnormalities in this population.

Lung and Airway Sounds

During the primary assessment, listen for lung and airway sounds. Abnormal sounds include stridor, grunting, gurgling, wheezing, and crackles.

Stridor

Stridor is a coarse, usually higher-pitched breathing sound typically heard on inspiration. It also may be heard during both inspiration and expiration. Stridor is a sign of upper airway (extrathoracic) obstruction and may indicate that the obstruction is critical and requires immediate intervention.

There are many causes of stridor, such as FBAO and infection (e.g., croup). Congenital airway abnormalities (e.g., laryngomalacia) and acquired airway abnormalities (e.g., tumor or cyst) also can cause stridor. Upper airway edema (e.g., allergic reaction or swelling after a medical procedure) is another cause of this abnormal breathing sound.

Grunting

Grunting is typically a short, low-pitched sound heard during expiration. Sometimes it can be misinterpreted as a soft cry. Grunting occurs as the child exhales against a partially closed glottis. Although grunting may accompany the response to pain or fever, infants and children often grunt to help keep the small airways and alveolar sacs in the lungs open. This is an attempt to optimize oxygenation and ventilation.

Grunting is often a sign of lung tissue disease resulting from small airway collapse, alveolar collapse, or both. Grunting may indicate progression of respiratory distress

FYI **Minute Ventilation**	Minute ventilation is the volume of air that moves into or out of the lungs each minute. It is the product of the number of breaths per minute (respiratory rate) and the volume of each breath (tidal volume). **Minute Ventilation = Respiratory Rate × Tidal Volume** Low minute ventilation (hypoventilation) may result from • Slow respiratory rate • Small tidal volume (i.e., shallow breathing, high airway resistance, stiff lungs) • Extremely rapid respiratory rate (if tidal volumes are very small)

Identify and Intervene **Grunting Is a Sign of Severe Respiratory Distress or Failure**	Grunting is typically a sign of severe respiratory distress or failure from lung tissue disease. Identify and treat the cause as quickly as possible. Be prepared to quickly intervene if the child's condition worsens.

to respiratory failure. Pulmonary conditions that cause grunting include pneumonia, pulmonary contusion, and acute respiratory distress syndrome (ARDS). It may be caused by cardiac conditions, such as congestive heart failure, that result in pulmonary edema. Grunting may be a sign of pain resulting from abdominal pathology (e.g., bowel obstruction, perforated viscus, appendicitis, or peritonitis).

Gurgling

Gurgling is a bubbling sound heard during inspiration or expiration. It results from upper airway obstruction due to airway secretions, vomit, or blood.

Wheezing

Wheezing is a high-pitched or low-pitched whistling or sighing sound heard most often during expiration. It is heard less frequently during inspiration. This sound typically indicates lower (intrathoracic) airway obstruction, especially of the smaller airways. Common causes of wheezing are bronchiolitis and asthma. Isolated inspiratory wheezing suggests a foreign body or other cause of partial obstruction of the trachea or upper airway.

Crackles

Crackles, also known as *rales*, are sharp, crackling inspiratory sounds. The sound of dry crackles can be described as the sound made when you rub several hairs together close to your ear. Crackles may be described as moist or dry. Moist crackles indicate accumulation of alveolar fluid. They are typically associated with lung tissue disease (e.g., pneumonia and pulmonary edema) or interstitial lung

disease. Dry crackles are more often heard with atelectasis (small airway collapse) and interstitial lung disease. Note that you may not hear crackles despite the presence of pulmonary edema.

Oxygen Saturation by Pulse Oximetry

Pulse oximetry is a tool to monitor the percentage of the child's hemoglobin that is saturated with O_2 (SpO_2). The pulse oximeter consists of a probe linked to a monitor. The probe is attached to the child's finger, toe, or earlobe. The unit displays the calculated percentage of oxygenated hemoglobin. Most units make an audible sound for each pulse beat and display the heart rate. Some models display the quality of the pulse signal as a waveform or with bars.

Pulse oximetry can indicate low O_2 saturation (hypoxemia) before it causes cyanosis or bradycardia. Providers can use pulse oximetry to monitor trends in O_2 saturation in response to treatment. If available, continuously monitor pulse oximetry for a child in respiratory distress or failure during stabilization, transport, and postresuscitation care.

Caution in Interpreting Pulse Oximetry Readings

Be careful to interpret pulse oximetry readings in conjunction with your clinical assessment and other signs, such as respiratory rate, respiratory effort, and level of consciousness. A child may be in respiratory distress yet maintain normal O_2 saturation by increasing respiratory rate and effort, especially if supplementary O_2 is administered. If the heart rate displayed by the pulse oximeter is not the same as the heart rate determined by ECG monitoring,

Fundamental Fact **O_2 Saturation**	The O_2 saturation is the percent of total hemoglobin that is saturated with O_2. This saturation does not indicate the amount of O_2 delivered to the tissues. O_2 delivery is the product of arterial O_2 content (oxygen bound to hemoglobin plus dissolved O_2) and cardiac output. It is also important to note that O_2 saturation does not provide information about effectiveness of ventilation (CO_2 elimination).

Rapid Response Intervention **Need for O_2 Administration or Additional Intervention**	An O_2 saturation (SpO_2) ≥94% while a child is breathing room air usually indicates that oxygenation is adequate. Consider administration of supplementary O_2 if the O_2 saturation is below this value in a critically ill or injured child. An SpO_2 of <90% in a child receiving 100% O_2 is usually an indication for additional intervention.

the O₂ saturation reading is not reliable. *When the pulse oximeter does not detect a consistent pulse or there is an irregular or poor waveform, the child may have poor distal perfusion and the pulse oximeter reading may not be accurate—check the child and intervene as needed.* The pulse oximeter may not be accurate if the child develops severe shock and won't be accurate during cardiac arrest. As noted above, pulse oximetry only indicates O₂ saturation and does not indicate O₂ delivery. For example, if the child is profoundly anemic (hemoglobin is very low), the saturation may be 100%, but O₂ content in the blood and O₂ delivery may be low.

The pulse oximeter does not accurately recognize methemoglobin or carboxyhemoglobin (hemoglobin bound to carbon monoxide). If carboxyhemoglobin (from carbon monoxide poisoning) is present, the pulse oximeter will reflect a falsely high O₂ saturation. If methemoglobin concentrations are above 5%, the pulse oximeter will read approximately 85% regardless of the degree of methemoglobinemia. If you suspect either of these conditions, obtain a blood gas with O₂ saturation measurement by using a co-oximeter.

Circulation

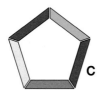

Circulation is assessed by the evaluation of:

- Heart rate and rhythm
- Pulses (both peripheral and central)
- Capillary refill time
- Skin colour and temperature
- Blood pressure

Urine output and level of consciousness also reflect adequacy of circulation. See the Fundamental Fact box "Assessment of Urine Output" at the end of this section. For more information on assessing level of consciousness, see the section "Disability" later in this Part.

Heart Rate and Rhythm

To determine heart rate, check the pulse rate, listen to the heart, or view a monitor display of the electrocardiogram (ECG) or pulse oximeter waveform. The heart rate should be appropriate for the child's age, level of activity, and clinical condition (Table 2). Note that there is a wide range for normal heart rates. For example, a child who is sleeping or is athletic may have a heart rate lower than the normal range for age.

Table 2. Normal Heart Rates (per Minute) by Age

Age	Awake Rate	Mean	Sleeping Rate
Newborn to 3 months	85 to 205	140	80 to 160
3 months to 2 years	100 to 190	130	75 to 160
2 years to 10 years	60 to 140	80	60 to 90
>10 years	60 to 100	75	50 to 90

Modified from Gillette PC, Garson A Jr, Crawford F, Ross B, Ziegler V, Buckles D. Dysrhythmias. In: Adams FH, Emmanouilides GC, Reimenschneider TA, eds. *Moss' Heart Disease in Infants, Children, and Adolescents*. 4th ed. Baltimore, MD: Williams & Wilkins; 1989:925-939.

The heart rhythm is typically regular with only small fluctuations in rate. When checking the heart rate, assess for abnormalities in the monitored ECG. Cardiac rhythm disturbances (arrhythmias) result from abnormalities in, or insults to, the cardiac conduction system or heart tissue. Arrhythmias also can result from shock or hypoxia. In the advanced life support setting, an arrhythmia in a child can be broadly classified according to the observed heart rate or effect on perfusion:

Heart Rate	Classification
Slow	Bradycardia
Fast	Tachycardia
Absent	Cardiac arrest

Bradycardia is a heart rate slower than normal for a child's age. Slight bradycardia may be normal in athletic children, but a very slow rate in a child with other symptoms is a worrisome sign and may indicate that cardiac arrest is imminent. Hypoxia is the most common cause of bradycardia in children. If a child with bradycardia has signs of poor perfusion (decreased responsiveness, weak peripheral pulses, cool mottled skin), immediately support ventilation with a bag and mask and administer supplementary O₂. If the child with bradycardia is alert and has no signs of poor perfusion, consider other causes of a slow heart rate, such as heart block or drug overdose.

Tachycardia is a resting heart rate that is faster than the normal range for a child's age. Sinus tachycardia is a common, nonspecific response to a variety of conditions. It is often appropriate when the child is seriously ill or injured. To determine if the tachycardia is a sinus tachycardia or represents a cardiac rhythm disturbance, evaluate the child's history, clinical condition, and ECG.

| *Fundamental Fact* **Evaluating Heart Rate and Rhythm** | Consider the following when evaluating the heart rate and rhythm in any seriously ill or injured child:

• The child's typical heart rate and baseline rhythm
• The child's level of activity and clinical condition (including baseline cardiac function)

Children with congenital heart disease may have conduction abnormalities. Consider the child's baseline ECG when interpreting heart rate and rhythm. Children with poor cardiac function are more likely to be symptomatic from arrhythmias than are children with good cardiac function. |

| *Fundamental Fact* **Relationship of Breathing to Heart Rhythm** | In healthy children the heart rate may fluctuate with the respiratory cycle, increasing with inspiration and slowing down with expiration. This condition is called *sinus arrhythmia*. Note if the child has an irregular rhythm that is not related to breathing. An irregular rhythm may indicate an underlying rhythm disturbance, such as premature ventricular or atrial contractions or an atrioventricular (AV) block. |

For more information, see Part 8: "Recognition and Management of Bradycardia," Part 9: "Recognition and Management of Tachycardia," and Part 10: "Recognition and Management of Cardiac Arrest."

Pulses

Evaluation of pulses is critical to the assessment of systemic perfusion in an ill or injured child. Palpate both central and peripheral pulses. Central pulses are ordinarily stronger than peripheral pulses because they are present in vessels of larger size that are located closer to the heart. Exaggeration of the difference in quality between central and peripheral pulses occurs when peripheral vasoconstriction is associated with shock. The following pulses are easily palpable in healthy infants and children (unless the child is obese or the ambient temperature is cold).

Central Pulses	Peripheral Pulses
• Femoral • Brachial (in infants) • Carotid (in older children) • Axillary	• Radial • Dorsalis pedis • Posterior tibial

Weak central pulses are worrisome and indicate the need for very rapid intervention to prevent cardiac arrest.

Beat-to-beat fluctuation in pulse volume may occur in children with arrhythmias (e.g., premature atrial or ventricular contractions). Fluctuation in pulse volume with the respiratory cycle (pulsus paradoxus) can occur in children with severe asthma and pericardial tamponade. In an intubated child receiving positive-pressure ventilatory support, a reduction in pulse volume with each positive-pressure breath may indicate hypovolemia.

Capillary Refill Time

Capillary refill time is the time it takes for blood to return to tissue blanched by pressure. Capillary refill time increases as skin perfusion decreases. A prolonged capillary refill time may indicate low cardiac output. Normal capillary refill time is ≤2 seconds.

It is best to evaluate capillary refill in a neutral thermal environment (i.e., room temperature). To evaluate capillary refill time, lift the extremity slightly above the level of the heart, press on the skin, and rapidly release the pressure. Note how many seconds it takes for the area to return to its baseline colour.

| *Critical Concept* **Weakening of Pulses as Perfusion Decreases** | As cardiac output decreases in shock, systemic perfusion decreases incrementally. The decrease in perfusion starts in the extremities with a decrease in intensity of pulses and then an absence of peripheral pulses. As cardiac output and perfusion decrease further, there is eventual weakening of central pulses.

A cold environment can cause vasoconstriction and a discrepancy between peripheral and central pulses. However, if cardiac output remains adequate, central pulses should remain strong. |

Common causes of sluggish, delayed, or prolonged capillary refill (a refill time >2 seconds) are dehydration, shock, and hypothermia. Note that shock can be present despite a normal (or even brisk) capillary refill time. Children with "warm" septic shock (see Part 6: "Recognition of Shock") may have excellent (i.e., <2 seconds) capillary refill time despite the presence of shock.

Skin Colour and Temperature

Monitor changes in skin colour, temperature, and capillary refill time to assess a child's perfusion and response to therapy. Normal skin colour and temperature should be consistent over the trunk and extremities. The mucous membranes, nail beds, palms of the hands, and soles of the feet should be pink. When perfusion deteriorates and O_2 delivery to the tissues becomes inadequate, the hands and feet are typically affected first. They may become cool, pale, dusky, or mottled. If perfusion becomes worse, the skin over the trunk and extremities may undergo similar changes.

Carefully monitor for the following skin findings, which may indicate inadequate O_2 delivery to the tissues:

- Pallor
- Mottling
- Cyanosis

Pallor, or paleness, is a lack of normal colour in the skin or mucous membrane. Pallor may be caused by

- Decreased blood supply to the skin (cold, stress, shock, especially hypovolemic and cardiogenic)
- A decreased number of red blood cells (anemia)
- Decreased skin pigmentation

Pallor must be interpreted within the context of other signs and symptoms. It is not necessarily abnormal and can result from lack of exposure to sunlight or inherited paleness. Pallor is often difficult to detect in a child with dark skin. Thick skin and variation in the vascularity of subcutaneous tissue also can make detection of pallor difficult. Family members often can tell you if a child's colour is abnormal. Central pallor (i.e.,

pale colour of the lips and mucous membranes) strongly suggests anemia or poor perfusion. Pallor of the mucous membranes (the lips, lining of the mouth, tongue, lining of the eyes) and pale palms and soles are more likely to be clinically significant.

Mottling is an irregular or patchy discolouration of the skin. Areas may appear as an uneven combination of pink, bluish gray, or pale skin tones. Mottling may occur due to variations in distribution of skin melanin and may be normal. Serious conditions, such as hypoxemia, hypovolemia, or shock, may cause intense vasoconstriction from an irregular supply of oxygenated blood to the skin, leading to mottling.

Cyanosis is a blue discolouration of the skin and mucous membranes. Blood saturated with O_2 is bright red, whereas unoxygenated blood is dark bluish-red. The location of cyanosis is important.

Acrocyanosis is a bluish discolouration of the hands and feet. It is a common normal finding during the newborn period.

Peripheral cyanosis (i.e., bluish discolouration of the hands and feet seen beyond the newborn period) can be caused by diminished O_2 delivery to the tissues. It may be seen in conditions such as shock, congestive heart failure, or peripheral vascular disease, or conditions causing venous stasis.

Central cyanosis is a blue colour of the lips and other mucous membranes. Cyanosis is not apparent until at least 5 g/dL of hemoglobin are desaturated (not bound to O_2). The O_2 saturation at which a child will appear cyanotic depends on the child's hemoglobin concentration. For example, in a child with a hemoglobin concentration of 16 g/dL, cyanosis will appear at an O_2 saturation of approximately 70% (i.e., 30% of the hemoglobin, or 4.8 g/dL, is desaturated). If the hemoglobin concentration is low (e.g., 8 g/dL), a very low arterial O_2 saturation (e.g., <40%) is required to produce cyanosis. Thus, cyanosis may be apparent with a milder degree of hypoxemia in a child

---

Fundamental Fact

Evaluating Skin Temperature

Consider the temperature of the child's surroundings (i.e., ambient temperature) when evaluating skin colour and temperature. If the ambient temperature is cool, peripheral vasoconstriction may produce mottling or pallor with cool skin and delayed capillary refill, particularly in the extremities. These changes develop despite normal cardiovascular function.

To assess skin temperature, use the back of your hand. The back of the hand is more sensitive to temperature changes than the palm, which has thicker skin. Slide the back of your hand up the extremity to determine if there is a point where the skin changes from cool to warm. Monitor this line of demarcation between warm and cool skin over time to determine the child's response to therapy. The line should move distally as the child improves.

with cyanotic congenital heart disease and polycythemia (increased amount of hemoglobin and red blood cells) but may not be apparent despite significant hypoxemia if the child is anemic.

The causes of central cyanosis include:

- Low ambient O_2 tension (e.g., high altitude)
- Alveolar hypoventilation (e.g., traumatic brain injury, drug overdose)
- Diffusion defect (e.g., pneumonia)
- Ventilation/perfusion imbalance (e.g., asthma, bronchiolitis, ARDS)
- Intracardiac shunt (e.g., cyanotic congenital heart disease)

Cyanosis may be more obvious in the mucous membranes and nail beds than in the skin, particularly if the skin is dark. It also can be seen on the soles of the feet, tip of the nose, and earlobes. As noted above, children with different hemoglobin levels will be cyanotic at different levels of O_2 saturation; cyanosis is more readily detected at higher O_2 saturations if the hemoglobin level is high. The development of central cyanosis typically indicates the need for emergency intervention, such as O_2 administration and ventilatory support.

Blood Pressure

Accurate blood pressure measurement requires a properly sized cuff. The cuff bladder should cover about 40% of the mid–upper arm circumference. The blood pressure cuff should extend at least 50% to 75% of the length of the upper arm (from the axilla to the antecubital fossa). For more details see *The Fourth Report on the Diagnosis, Evaluation, and Treatment of High Blood Pressure in Children and Adolescents*, 2005 (full reference in the Suggested Reading List at the end of this Part).

Normal Blood Pressures

Table 3 lists normal blood pressures by age. This table summarizes the range of systolic and diastolic blood pressures according to age and gender from 1 standard deviation below to 1 standard deviation above the mean in the first year of life and from the 50th to 95th percentile (assuming the 50th percentile for height) for children ≥1 year of age. Like heart rate, there is a wide range of values within the normal range.

Table 3. Normal Blood Pressures in Children by Age

Age	Systolic Blood Pressure (mm Hg)		Diastolic Blood Pressure (mm Hg)	
	Female	Male	Female	Male
Neonate (1 day)	60 to 76	60 to 74	31 to 45	30 to 44
Neonate (4 days)	67 to 83	68 to 84	37 to 53	35 to 53
Infant (1 month)	73 to 91	74 to 94	36 to 56	37 to 55
Infant (3 months)	78 to 100	81 to 103	44 to 64	45 to 65
Infant (6 months)	82 to 102	87 to 105	46 to 66	48 to 68
Infant (1 year)	86 to 104	85 to 103	40 to 58	37 to 56
Child (2 years)	88 to 105	88 to 106	45 to 63	42 to 61
Child (7 years)	96 to 113	97 to 115	57 to 75	57 to 76
Adolescent (15 years)	110 to 127	113 to 131	65 to 83	64 to 83

Blood pressure ranges for neonate and infant (1 to 6 months) are from Gemelli M, Manganaro R, Mamì C, De Luca F. Longitudinal study of blood pressure during the 1st year of life. *Eur J Pediatr.* 1990;149:318-320.

Blood pressure ranges for infant (1 year), child, and adolescent are from National High Blood Pressure Education Program Working Group on High Blood Pressure in Children and Adolescents. *The Fourth Report on the Diagnosis, Evaluation, and Treatment of High Blood Pressure in Children and Adolescents.* Bethesda, MD: National Heart, Lung, and Blood Institute; 2005. NIH publication 05-5267.

Hypotension

Hypotension is defined by the thresholds of systolic blood pressure in Table 4.

Table 4. Definition of Hypotension by Systolic Blood Pressure and Age

Age	Systolic Blood Pressure (mm Hg)
Term neonates (0 to 28 days)	<60
Infants (1 to 12 months)	<70
Children 1 to 10 years (5th blood pressure percentile)	<70 + (age in years × 2)
Children >10 years	<90

Note that these blood pressure thresholds approximate just above the 5th percentile systolic blood pressures for age, so they will overlap with normal blood pressure values for 5% of healthy children. An observed decrease in systolic blood pressure of 10 mm Hg from baseline should prompt serial evaluations for additional signs of shock. In addition, remember that these threshold values were established in normal, resting children. Children with injury and stress typically have increased blood pressure. A blood pressure in the low-normal range may be abnormal in a seriously ill child.

Disability

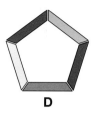

D

The disability assessment is a quick evaluation of neurologic function. Rapid assessment can use one of several tools to evaluate responsiveness and level of consciousness. Perform this evaluation at the end of the primary assessment. Repeat it during the secondary assessment to monitor for changes in the child's neurologic status.

Clinical signs of brain perfusion are important indicators of circulatory function in the ill or injured pediatric patient. These signs include level of consciousness, muscle tone, and pupil responses. Signs of inadequate O_2 delivery to the brain correlate with the severity and duration of cerebral hypoxia.

Sudden and severe cerebral hypoxia may present with the following neurologic signs:

- Decreased level of consciousness
- Loss of muscular tone
- Generalized seizures
- Pupil dilation

Fundamental Fact **Hypotension: An Ominous Sign of Impending Arrest**	When hypotension develops in a child with shock, physiologic compensatory mechanisms (e.g., tachycardia and vasoconstriction) have failed. Hypotension with hemorrhage is thought to be consistent with an acute loss of 20% to 25% of circulating blood volume. Hypotension may be a sign of septic shock, where there is inappropriate vasodilation rather than loss of intravascular volume. The development of bradycardia in a child with tachycardia and hypotension is an ominous sign. Management of airway and breathing and aggressive fluid resuscitation are needed to prevent cardiac arrest.

Fundamental Fact **Assessment of Urine Output**	Urine output is an indirect indication of kidney perfusion. Children with shock typically have decreased urine output. Measure urine output in all critically ill or injured children with an indwelling catheter. Initial urine output is not a reliable indicator of the child's clinical condition because much of the urine may have been produced before the onset of symptoms. An increase in urine output is a good indicator of positive response to therapy.

You may observe other neurologic signs when cerebral hypoxia develops gradually. These signs can be subtle and are best detected with repeated measurements over time:

- Decreased level of consciousness with confusion
- Irritability
- Lethargy
- Agitation alternating with lethargy

Standard evaluations include:

- AVPU (Alert, Responsive to Voice, Responsive to Pain, Unresponsive) Pediatric Response Scale
- Glasgow Coma Scale (GCS)
- Pupil response to light

AVPU Pediatric Response Scale

To rapidly evaluate cerebral cortex function, use the AVPU Pediatric Response Scale. This scale is a system for rating a child's level of consciousness, an indicator of cerebral cortex function. The scale consists of 4 ratings:

Alert	The child is awake, active, and appropriately responsive to parents and external stimuli. "Appropriate response" is assessed in terms of the anticipated response based on the child's age and the setting or situation.
Voice	The child responds only to voice (e.g., calling the child's name or speaking loudly).
Painful	The child responds only to a painful stimulus, such as pinching the nail bed.
Unresponsive	The child does not respond to any stimulus.

Causes of decreased level of consciousness in children include:

- Poor cerebral perfusion
- Traumatic brain injury
- Encephalitis, meningitis
- Hypoglycemia
- Drugs
- Hypoxemia
- Hypercarbia

Glasgow Coma Scale Overview

The GCS is the most widely used method of evaluating a child's level of consciousness and neurologic status. The child's *best* eye opening (E), verbal (V), and motor (M) responses are individually scored (Table 5). The individual scores are then added together to produce the GCS score.

For example: A child who has spontaneous eye opening (E = 4), is fully oriented (V = 5), and is able to follow commands (M = 6) is assigned a GCS score of 15, the highest possible score. A child with no eye opening (E = 1), no verbal response (V = 1), and no motor response (M = 1) to a painful stimulus is assigned a GCS score of 3, the lowest possible score.

Severity of head injury is categorized into 3 levels based on GCS score after initial resuscitation:

- Mild head injury: GCS score 13 to 15
- Moderate head injury: GCS score 9 to 12
- Severe head injury: GCS score 3 to 8

Glasgow Coma Scale Scoring

The GCS has been modified for preverbal or nonverbal children (Table 5). Scores for eye opening are essentially the same as for the standard GCS. The best motor response score (of a possible 6) requires that a child follow commands, so this section was adapted to accommodate the preverbal or nonverbal child. The verbal score was also adapted to assess age-appropriate responses.

Important: When using the GCS or its pediatric modification, record the individual components of the score. If the patient is intubated, unconscious, or preverbal, the most important part of this scale is motor response. Providers should carefully evaluate this component.

Rapid Response Intervention **Decreased Responsiveness**	If an ill or injured child has decreased responsiveness, immediately assess oxygenation, ventilation, and perfusion.

Table 5. Glasgow Coma Scale* for Adults and Modified Glasgow Coma Scale for Infants and Children†

Response	Adult	Child	Infant	Coded Value
Eye opening	Spontaneous	Spontaneous	Spontaneous	4
	To speech	To speech	To speech	3
	To pain	To pain	To pain	2
	None	None	None	1
Best verbal response	Oriented	Oriented, appropriate	Coos and babbles	5
	Confused	Confused	Irritable, cries	4
	Inappropriate words	Inappropriate words	Cries in response to pain	3
	Incomprehensible sounds	Incomprehensible words or nonspecific sounds	Moans in response to pain	2
	None	None	None	1
Best motor response‡	Obeys	Obeys commands	Moves spontaneously and purposely	6
	Localizes	Localizes painful stimulus	Withdraws in response to touch	5
	Withdraws	Withdraws in response to pain	Withdraws in response to pain	4
	Abnormal flexion	Flexion in response to pain	Decorticate posturing (abnormal flexion) in response to pain	3
	Extensor response	Extension in response to pain	Decerebrate posturing (abnormal extension) in response to pain	2
	None	None	None	1
Total score				**3-15**

*Teasdale G, Jennett B. Assessment of coma and impaired consciousness: a practical scale. *Lancet.* 1974;2(7872):81-84.

†Modified from Davis RJ, Dean JM, Goldberg AL, Carson BS, Rosenbaum AE, Rogers MC. Head and spinal cord injury. In: Rogers MC, ed. *Textbook of Pediatric Intensive Care.* Baltimore, MD: Williams & Wilkins; 1987:649-699, copyright Lippincott Williams & Wilkins; James HE, Trauner DA. The Glasgow Coma Scale. In: James HE, Anas NG, Perkin RM, eds. *Brain Insults in Infants and Children: Pathophysiology and Management.* Orlando, FL: Grune & Stratton; 1985:179-182; Jennett B, Teasdale G, Braakman R, Minderhoud J, Knill-Jones R. Predicting outcome in individual patients after severe head injury. *Lancet.* 1976;1:1031-1034; Morray JP, Tyler DC, Jones TK, Stuntz JT, Lemire RJ. Coma scale for use in brain-injured children. *Crit Care Med.* 1984;12:1018-1020; and Hazinski MF. Neurologic disorders. In: Hazinski MF. *Nursing Care of the Critically Ill Child.* 2nd ed. St Louis, MO: Mosby-Year Book; 1992:521-628, copyright Elsevier.

‡If the patient is intubated, unconscious, or preverbal, the most important part of this scale is motor response. Providers should carefully evaluate this component.

Pupil Response to Light

The response of pupils to light is a useful indicator of brainstem function. Normally pupils constrict in response to light and dilate in a dark environment. If the pupils fail to constrict in response to direct light (e.g., flashlight directed at the eyes), suspect that brainstem injury is present. The pupils are typically equal in size, although slight variations are normal. Irregularities in pupil size or response to light may occur as a result of ocular trauma or other conditions, such as increased intracranial pressure (ICP).

During the disability assessment, assess and record the following for each eye:

- Size of pupils (in millimeters)
- Equality of pupil size
- Constriction of pupils to light (i.e., the magnitude and rapidity of the response to light)

The acronym PERRL (Pupils Equal, Round, Reactive to Light) describes the normal pupil responses to light.

Exposure

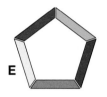

Exposure is the final component of the primary assessment. Undress the seriously ill or injured child as necessary to perform a focused physical examination. Remove clothing one area at a time to carefully observe the child's face and head, trunk (front and back), extremities, and skin. Maintain cervical spine precautions when turning any child with a suspected neck or spine injury. Keep the child comfortable and warm. If necessary, use blankets and, if available, heating lamps to prevent cold stress or hypothermia. Be sure to include an assessment of core temperature. Note any difference in warmth between trunk and extremities. Identify the presence of fever, which may indicate infection and early need for antibiotics (e.g., sepsis).

During this part of the examination, look for evidence of trauma, such as bleeding, burns, or unusual markings that suggest nonaccidental trauma. Signs include bruises in different stages of healing, injuries that don't correlate with the child's history, and delay from time of injury until the child receives medical attention.

Look for the presence and progression of petechiae and purpura (nonblanching purple discolourations in the skin caused by bleeding from capillaries and small vessels).

Petechiae appear as tiny red dots and suggest a low platelet count. Purpura appears as larger areas. Both petechiae and purpura may be signs of septic shock. Also look for other rashes that may be suggestive of shock (e.g., anaphylactic shock).

Look for signs of injury to the extremities, including deformities or bruising. Palpate the extremities and note the child's response. If there is tenderness, suspect injury; if necessary, immobilize the extremity.

Life-Threatening Problems

Signs of a life-threatening condition include the following:

Airway	Complete or severe airway obstruction
Breathing	Apnea, significant increased work of breathing, bradypnea
Circulation	Absence of palpable pulses, poor perfusion, hypotension, bradycardia
Disability	Unresponsiveness, decreased level of consciousness
Exposure	Significant hypothermia, significant bleeding, petechiae, or purpura consistent with septic shock

Interventions

Activate emergency response as indicated in your practice setting and begin lifesaving interventions in the following circumstances:

- If the child has a life-threatening condition
- If you are uncertain or "something feels wrong"

If the child does not have a life-threatening condition, begin the secondary assessment and diagnostic tests.

Secondary Assessment

After you complete the primary assessment and appropriate interventions to stabilize the child, perform the secondary assessment. Components of the secondary assessment are

- Focused history
- Focused physical examination

Focused History

Obtain a focused history to identify important aspects of the child's presenting complaint. Try to gain information that might help explain impaired respiratory or cardiovascular function. One memory aid for obtaining a focused history is "SAMPLE."

Signs and symptoms	Signs and symptoms at onset of illness, such as • Breathing difficulty (e.g., cough, rapid breathing, increased respiratory effort, breathlessness, abnormal breathing pattern, chest pain on deep inhalation) • Decreased level of consciousness • Agitation, anxiety • Fever • Decreased oral intake • Diarrhea, vomiting • Bleeding • Fatigue • Time course of symptoms
Allergies	• Medications, foods, latex, etc
Medications	• Medications • Last dose and time of recent medications
Past medical history	• Health history (e.g., premature birth) • Significant underlying medical problems (e.g., asthma, chronic lung disease, congenital heart disease, arrhythmia, congenital airway abnormality, seizures, head injury, brain tumor, diabetes, hydrocephalus, neuromuscular disease) • Past surgeries • Immunization status
Last meal	• Time and nature of last intake of liquid or food (including breast or bottle feeding in infants)
Events	• Events leading to current illness or injury (e.g., onset sudden or gradual, type of injury) • Hazards at scene • Treatment during interval from onset of disease or injury until evaluation • Estimated time of arrival (if out-of-hospital onset)

Focused Physical Examination

Next, perform a focused physical examination. The severity of the child's illness or injury should determine the extent of the physical examination. This should include careful assessment of the primary area of concern of the illness or injury (i.e., respiratory assessment with respiratory distress) as well as a brief head-to-toe evaluation.

Diagnostic Tests

Diagnostic tests help detect and identify the presence and severity of respiratory and circulatory problems. Some of these tests (such as rapid bedside glucose or point-of-care laboratory testing) may occur early in your evaluation. The timing of diagnostic tests is dictated by the clinical situation.

The following diagnostic tests help assess respiratory and circulatory problems:

- Arterial blood gas (ABG)
- Venous blood gas (VBG)
- Hemoglobin concentration
- Central venous O_2 saturation
- Arterial lactate
- Central venous pressure monitoring
- Invasive arterial pressure monitoring
- Chest x-ray
- ECG
- Echocardiogram
- Peak expiratory flow rate

Arterial Blood Gas

An ABG analysis measures the partial pressure of arterial O_2 (PaO_2) and CO_2 ($PaCO_2$) dissolved in the blood plasma (i.e., the liquid component of blood).

Measurement	Indicates
PaO_2	Adequacy of O_2 tension* in arterial blood (but not the O_2 content)
$PaCO_2$	Adequacy of ventilation

*An additional tool to assess the adequacy of arterial oxygenation is the pulse oximeter, a device that measures hemoglobin saturation with O_2.

Note that a normal PaO_2 does not confirm adequate O_2 content of the blood because it reflects only the O_2 dissolved in the blood plasma. If the child's hemoglobin is only 3 g/dL, the PaO_2 may be normal or high, but O_2 delivery to the tissues will be inadequate. Because most O_2 is carried by hemoglobin in the red blood cells rather than the plasma, a hemoglobin of 3 g/dL is inadequate to carry sufficient O_2. In this case the pulse oximeter may reflect 100% saturation despite inadequate O_2 content and delivery.

Identify respiratory failure on the basis of inadequate oxygenation (hypoxemia) or inadequate ventilation (hypercarbia). Use an ABG analysis to confirm your clinical impression and evaluate the child's response to therapy. An ABG analysis, however, is not required to initiate therapy. The following chart will help you interpret an ABG:

Diagnosis	ABG Result
Hypoxemia	Low PaO_2
Hypercarbia	High $PaCO_2$
Acidosis	pH <7.35
Alkalosis	pH >7.45

Don't wait for an ABG analysis to start treatment. Limitations of ABG analysis in pediatric critical care include the following:

- An ABG analysis may not be available (e.g., during transport); you should not delay initiation of therapy.
- A single ABG analysis provides only information at the time the sample was obtained. It does not provide information about trends in the child's condition. Monitoring clinical response to therapy is often more valuable than any single ABG analysis.
- Interpretation of ABG results requires consideration of the child's clinical appearance and condition.

For example, an infant with bronchopulmonary dysplasia (a form of chronic lung disease) is likely to have chronic hypoxemia and hypercarbia. Diagnosis of acute respiratory failure in this infant relies heavily on clinical examination and evaluation of arterial pH. The infant will compensate for chronic hypercarbia by renal retention of bicarbonate, and the arterial pH is likely to be normal or nearly normal at baseline. Deterioration will be apparent if the child's respiratory status (i.e., hypercarbia) is significantly worse than the baseline status and acidosis develops.

The arterial pH and bicarbonate (HCO_3^-) concentrations obtained with ABG analysis may be useful in the diagnosis of acid-base imbalances. ABG values do not reliably reflect O_2, CO_2, or acid-base status in the tissues. However, it is useful to monitor these values over time as an index of improving or worsening tissue oxygenation, as reflected by an increasing base deficit (accumulation of acid in the blood).

Venous Blood Gas

A venous blood pH, measured by VBG analysis, typically correlates well with the pH on ABG analysis. A VBG analysis is not as useful for monitoring blood gas status (PaO_2 and $PaCO_2$) in acutely ill children. If the child is well perfused, the venous PCO_2 is usually within 4 to 6 mm Hg of the arterial PCO_2. If the child is poorly perfused, however,

the gradient between arterial and venous PCO_2 increases. In general, venous PO_2 is not useful in the assessment of arterial oxygenation.

When interpreting a VBG, also consider the source of the venous specimen. A peripheral specimen that is free flowing may give results similar to the ABG, but if a tourniquet is used and the specimen is from a poorly perfused extremity, it often shows a much higher PCO_2 and lower pH than an arterial specimen. For this reason, a central venous specimen, if available, is preferred to a peripheral venous specimen. A VBG may be used if an arterial sample is unavailable. There is generally adequate correlation with ABG samples to make venous pH useful in the diagnosis of acid-base imbalance.

Hemoglobin Concentration

Hemoglobin concentration determines the O_2-carrying capacity of the blood. O_2 content is the total amount of O_2 bound to hemoglobin plus the unbound (dissolved) O_2 in arterial blood. O_2 content is determined chiefly by the hemoglobin concentration (in grams per deciliter) and its saturation with O_2 (SaO_2). At normal hemoglobin levels the amount of O_2 dissolved in the blood represents a very small part of total O_2 content. The amount of O_2 dissolved in the blood is determined by the partial pressure of arterial O_2 (PaO_2), also referred to as the *arterial oxygen tension*.

Central Venous Oxygen Saturation

Venous blood gases may provide a useful indicator of changes in the balance between O_2 delivery to the tissues and tissue O_2 consumption. Trends in venous O_2 saturation (SvO_2) may be used as a surrogate for monitoring trends in O_2 delivery (i.e., the product of cardiac output and arterial O_2 content). Such trending assumes that O_2 consumption remains stable (an assumption that is not always correct).

Normal SvO_2 is about 70% to 75%, assuming arterial O_2 saturation is 100%. If the arterial O_2 saturation is not normal, the SvO_2 should be about 25% to 30% below the arterial O_2 saturation. For example, if the child has cyanotic heart disease and the arterial O_2 saturation is 80%, the SvO_2 should be about 55%.

When O_2 delivery to the tissues is low, the tissues consume proportionately more O_2, so the difference between arterial O_2 saturation and SvO_2 is more substantial when shock

FYI **Measurement of Arterial O_2 Saturation**	The arterial O_2 saturation can be estimated by using a pulse oximeter, or it may be calculated from the PaO_2 and pH (by using an oxyhemoglobin dissociation curve). It may also be directly measured by using a co-oximeter. Obtain co-oximeter measurement if there is uncertainty about the calculated O_2 saturation and to rule out the presence of carbon monoxide intoxication or methemoglobinemia.

is present. For more information about SvO₂, see Part 7: "Management of Shock."

Arterial Lactate

The arterial concentration of lactate reflects the balance between lactate production and use. In a seriously ill or injured child, the arterial lactate can rise as a result of increased production of lactate (metabolic acidosis) associated with tissue hypoxia and anaerobic metabolism. Arterial lactate is easy to measure, is a good prognostic indicator, and may be followed sequentially to assess the child's response to therapy.

Lactate concentration also can be elevated in conditions associated with increased glucose production, such as stress hyperglycemia. An elevated lactate level does not always represent tissue ischemia, especially when there is no accompanying metabolic acidosis. In general, it is more helpful to monitor trends in lactate concentration over time than any single measurement. If treatment of shock is effective, the lactate concentration should decrease. Lack of response to therapy (i.e., the lactate concentration does not decrease) is more predictive of poor outcome than the initial elevated lactate concentration.

Central venous lactate concentration can be monitored if arterial blood samples are not readily available. Again, the trend in lactate concentration over time is more predictive than the initial concentration.

Central Venous Pressure Monitoring

Central venous pressure can be monitored through a central venous catheter. Measurement of central venous pressure may provide helpful information to guide fluid and vasoactive therapy.

The triad of low arterial blood pressure, high central venous pressure, and tachycardia is consistent with poor myocardial contractility or extrinsic cardiac compression (e.g., tension pneumothorax, cardiac tamponade, or excessive positive end-expiratory pressure [PEEP]). This triad is also consistent with obstruction of pulmonary arterial flow (severe pulmonary hypertension or massive pulmonary embolus).

Invasive Arterial Pressure Monitoring

Invasive arterial pressure monitoring enables continuous evaluation and display of the systolic and diastolic blood pressures. The arterial waveform pattern may provide information about SVR and visual indication of a compromised cardiac output (e.g., pulsus paradoxus, an exaggerated decrease in the systolic blood pressure during inspiration). Invasive arterial pressure monitoring requires an arterial catheter, a monitoring line, a transducer, and a monitoring system. Accurate measurement requires that the

transducer be appropriately zeroed, leveled, and calibrated. For more detailed information see the Hemodynamic Monitoring section in the Suggested Reading List.

Chest X-Ray

A chest x-ray is useful in respiratory illness to aid in the diagnosis of the following conditions:

- Airway obstruction (upper airway or lower airway)
- Lung tissue disease
- Barotrauma (complications related to mechanical ventilation)
- Pleural disease (pleural effusion/pneumothorax)

A chest x-ray will show the depth of ET tube placement, but an anterior-posterior (or posterior-anterior) x-ray will *not* help determine tracheal versus esophageal placement.

Use the chest x-ray in evaluation of circulatory abnormalities to assess heart size and presence or absence of congestive heart failure (pulmonary edema). A small heart implies that preload is reduced; a large heart suggests normal or increased preload or pericardial effusion.

Electrocardiogram

Obtain a 12-lead ECG to assess for cardiac arrhythmias. For more information, see Part 8: "Recognition and Management of Bradycardia" and Part 9: "Recognition and Management of Tachycardia."

Echocardiogram

Echocardiography is a valuable noninvasive tool for imaging

- Cardiac chamber size
- Ventricular wall thickness
- Ventricular wall motion (contractility)
- Valve configuration and motion
- Pericardial space
- Estimated ventricular pressures
- Interventricular septal position
- Congenital anomalies

It can be useful in the diagnosis and evaluation of cardiac disease. Technical expertise in performing and interpreting the echocardiogram is essential.

Peak Expiratory Flow Rate

The peak expiratory flow rate (PEFR) represents the maximum flow rate generated during forced expiration. Measurement of the PEFR requires cooperation, so it can only be evaluated in children who are alert, can follow directions, and can provide a maximum effort. The PEFR decreases in the presence of airway obstruction, such as asthma. Evaluate the child's PEFR by comparing measurements with the child's personal best and also with normal values predicted from the child's height and gender.

The PEFR measurement should improve in response to therapy. An asthmatic child in severe distress may not be able to cooperate with PEFR measurements. This suggests that the child has very significant respiratory distress.

Suggested Reading List

Dieckmann R, ed. *Pediatric Education for Prehospital Professionals*. 2nd ed. Sudbury, MA: Jones & Bartlett Publishers, American Academy of Pediatrics; 2006.

Dieckmann RA, Brownstein D, Gausche-Hill M. The pediatric assessment triangle: a novel approach for the rapid evaluation of children. *Pediatr Emerg Care.* 2010;26:312-315.

Downes JJ, Fulgencio T, Raphaely RC. Acute respiratory failure in infants and children. *Pediatr Clin North Am.* 1972;19:423-445.

Duncan H, Hutchison J, Parshuram CS. The Pediatric Early Warning System score: a severity of illness score to predict urgent medical need in hospitalized children. *J Crit Care.* 2006;21:271-278.

Hazinski MF. Children are different. In: Hazinski MF, ed. *Nursing Care of the Critically Ill Child*. 3rd ed. St Louis, MO: Mosby. In press.

Holmes JF, Palchak MJ, MacFarlane T, Kuppermann N. Performance of the pediatric Glasgow Coma Scale in children with blunt head trauma. *Acad Emerg Med.* 2005;12:814-819.

Nadkarni VM, Larkin GL, Peberdy MA, Carey SM, Kaye W, Mancini ME, Nichol G, Lane-Truitt T, Potts J, Ornato JP, Berg RA. First documented rhythm and clinical outcome from in-hospital cardiac arrest among children and adults. *JAMA.* 2006;295:50-57.

National High Blood Pressure Education Program Working Group on High Blood Pressure in Children and Adolescents. *The Fourth Report on the Diagnosis, Evaluation, and Treatment of High Blood Pressure in Children and Adolescents*. Bethesda, MD: National Heart, Lung, and Blood Institute; 2005. NIH publication 05-5267.

Ralston ME, Zaritsky AL. New opportunity to improve pediatric emergency preparedness: Pediatric Emergency Assessment, Recognition, and Stabilization course. *Pediatrics.* 2009;123:578-580.

Santamaria JP, Schafermeyer R. Stridor: a review. *Pediatr Emerg Care.* 1992;8:229-234.

Sarti A, Savron F, Ronfani L, Pelizzo G, Barbi E. Comparison of three sites to check the pulse and count heart rate in hypotensive infants. *Paediatr Anaesth.* 2006;16:394-398.

Schindler MB, Bohn D, Cox PN, McCrindle BW, Jarvis A, Edmonds J, Barker G. Outcome of out-of-hospital cardiac or respiratory arrest in children. *N Engl J Med.* 1996;335: 1473-1479.

Schultz AH, Localio AR, Clark BJ, Ravishankar C, Videon N, Kimmel SE. Epidemiologic features of the presentation of critical congenital heart disease: implications for screening. *Pediatrics.* 2008;121:751-757.

Singer JL, Losek JD. Grunting respirations: chest or abdominal pathology? *Pediatr Emerg Care.* 1992;8:354-358.

Thompson M. How well do vital signs identify children with serious infections in paediatric emergency care? *Arch Dis Child.* 2009;94:888-893.

Hemodynamic Monitoring

Dorr P. Pressure transducer systems. In: Verger JT, Lebet RM, eds. *AACN Procedure Manual for Pediatric Acute and Critical Care.* St Louis, MO: Saunders Elsevier; 2008:462-467.

Slota M. Bioinstrumentation. In: Hazinski MF, ed. *Nursing Care of the Critically Ill Child*. 3rd ed. St Louis, MO: Mosby. In press.

Part 3

Effective Resuscitation Team Dynamics

Overview

When a patient in cardiac arrest does not respond to CPR and shock delivery, a team of rescuers is needed. This team performs many tasks during resuscitation. Teamwork divides the tasks while multiplying the chances of a successful resuscitation.

Successful resuscitation teams not only have medical expertise and mastery of resuscitation skills, but they also demonstrate effective communication and team dynamics. This Part discusses the importance of team roles, behaviors of effective team leaders and team members, and elements of effective resuscitation team dynamics.

During the course you will have an opportunity to practice performing different roles as a member and leader of a simulated resuscitation team.

Learning Objectives

By the end of this Part you should:

- Understand the role of each resuscitation team member
- Understand how teamwork may increase resuscitation success

Preparation for the Course

During the course you will participate as both the team leader and a team member during case simulations. You will be expected to model the behaviors discussed in this Part.

Roles of the Team Leader and Team Members

Role of the Team Leader

The role of the team leader is multifaceted. The team leader:

- Organizes the group
- Monitors individual performance of team members
- Provides support for and is prepared to perform the skills of team members
- Models excellent team behavior
- Trains and coaches
- Facilitates understanding
- Focuses on comprehensive patient care

Every resuscitation team needs a leader to organize the efforts of the group. The team leader is responsible for making sure everything gets done at the right time in the right way by monitoring and integrating the individual performances of team members. The role of the team leader is similar to that of an orchestra conductor directing individual musicians. Like a conductor, the team leader does not play the instruments but instead knows how each member of the orchestra fits into the overall music.

The team leader must be proficient in all skills required during the resuscitation. This level of expertise is necessary because the team leader occasionally serves as a backup for a team member who may have trouble performing his or her role or assigned task.

Fundamental Fact **Understanding Team Roles**	Whether you are a team member or team leader during a resuscitation attempt, you should understand your role and the roles of other team members. This awareness will help you anticipate: • The actions that will be performed next • How to communicate and work as a member or leader of the team

The role of the team leader also includes modeling excellent team behavior and leadership skills for the team and other people who may be involved or interested in the resuscitation. The team leader should serve as a teacher or guide to help train future team leaders and improve team effectiveness. After resuscitation the team leader can provide analysis, critique, and practice in preparation for the next resuscitation attempt.

The team leader also helps team members understand why certain tasks are performed in a specific way. The team leader should be able to ensure that during CPR the rescuers push fast (at least 100 compressions per minute), push hard (at least one third of the AP diameter of the chest), allow complete chest recoil after each compression, minimize interruptions in chest compressions, and avoid excessive ventilation.

Whereas team members focus on their individual tasks, the team leader is attentive to comprehensive patient care.

Role of the Team Member

Team members must be proficient in performing the skills authorized by their scope of practice. It is essential to the success of the resuscitation attempt that team members are:

- Clear about role assignments
- Prepared to fulfill role responsibilities
- Well practiced in resuscitation skills
- Knowledgeable about the algorithms
- Committed to success

Students who do not have the real-world responsibility of performing as a resuscitation team leader may not master all the specific tasks of that role, such as selecting medications, interpreting rhythms, or making medical decisions. However, students should master their areas of responsibility and be committed to the success of the resuscitation attempt.

Elements of Effective Resuscitation Team Dynamics

Closed-Loop Communication

When communicating with resuscitation team members, the team leader should use closed-loop communication by taking these steps:

1. The team leader gives a message, order, or assignment to a team member.

2. By receiving a clear response and eye contact, the team leader confirms that the team member heard and understood the message.

3. The team leader listens for confirmation of task performance from the team member before assigning another task.

Correct Actions: Closed-Loop Communication	
Team leader	• Listen for verbal confirmation that requests are heard and understood. • Await confirmation that the previous task has been completed (e.g., "Vascular access in place") before assigning another task. • Confirm receipt of a completed assignment (e.g., "Good, now that the IV is in, give 1 mg of epinephrine").
Team members	• Confirm that the request is heard and understood (e.g., "I'll start the IV"). • Inform the team leader when a task begins or ends (e.g., "The IV is in"). • Verify orders for drugs or other treatments before administration (e.g., "Did you want the 5 mg/kg of IV amiodarone given now?")

Clear Messages

Clear messages consist of concise communication spoken with distinctive speech in a controlled tone of voice. All messages and orders should be delivered in a calm and direct manner without yelling or shouting. Communication that is unclear can lead to unnecessary delays in treatment or to medication errors. For example, "Did the patient get IV propofol so I can proceed with the cardioversion?" "No, I thought you said to give him *propranolol*."

Yelling or shouting can impair effective team interaction. Only 1 person should be talking at any time.

Correct Actions: Clear Messages	
Team leader	• Provide clear messages and orders. • Encourage team members to speak clearly and distinctly. • Request clarification of any ambiguous messages. • Speak in a calm and normal tone of voice.
Team members	• Repeat the prescription medication order. • Question an order if it is ambiguous or not understood.

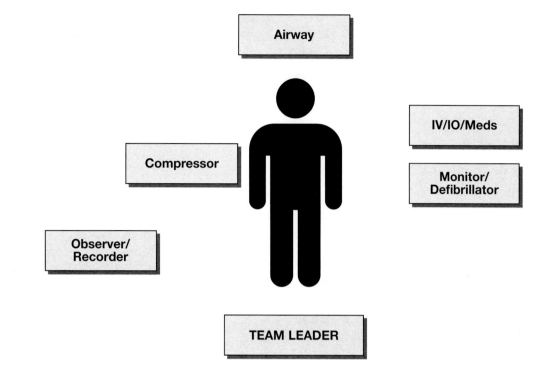

Figure 1. Potential locations for the team leader and team members during the case simulations.

Clear Roles and Responsibilities

Every member of the team should know his or her role and responsibilities. Just as different-shaped pieces make up a jigsaw puzzle, each team member's role is unique and critical to the effective performance of the team. Figure 1 identifies 6 team roles for resuscitation. When fewer than 6 team members are available, all tasks must be divided among the rescuers present.

When roles are unclear, team performance suffers. Signs of unclear roles include:

- Performing the same task more than once
- Missing essential tasks
- Performing unnecessary tasks or tasks that are not in correct sequence

To avoid inefficiencies, the team leader should clearly delegate tasks. Team members should question ambiguous or incorrect requests. In addition, team members should communicate when and if they can handle additional responsibilities. The team leader should encourage team members to provide input and feedback to the team leader as needed.

Correct Actions: Clear Roles and Responsibilities	
Team leader	• Clearly define all roles of team members in the clinical setting. • Assign roles and responsibilities according to competence of each team member. • Distribute assignments evenly so resources (skills) of team members are used as efficiently and effectively as possible.
Team members	• Seek out and perform tasks that are clearly defined and appropriate to level of competence. • Inform the team leader if the role or requested task is too difficult based on experience or competence. • Be prepared to assist with tasks as needed.

Knowing Limitations

Each member of the team must know his or her own limitations and capabilities. In addition, the team leader must be aware of the skills and limitations of each team member. This knowledge allows the team leader to evaluate team resources and call for additional assistance when needed. Team members should anticipate situations in which they might require assistance and inform the team leader.

During the stress of an attempted resuscitation, do not practice or explore a new skill. If you need extra help, request it early. It is not a sign of weakness or incompetence to call for help; it is better to have more help than needed than to have inadequate help. Inadequate resources can compromise the quality and success of the resuscitation.

Correct Actions: Knowing Limitations	
Team leader and team members	• Call for assistance early rather than waiting until the patient deteriorates and it is too late to get the help needed. • Ask other team members to help if one team member is having difficulty completing tasks. • Seek advice from more experienced personnel when the patient's condition worsens despite initial treatment.

Knowledge Sharing

Sharing information is a critical component of effective team performance. Team leaders may become focused on a specific treatment or diagnostic approach and neglect to consider others. Three common types of narrow-focus errors (also called *fixation errors*) are:

- "Everything is okay"
- "This and only this is the correct path"
- "Anything but this"

When resuscitative efforts are ineffective, the team leader must review the basics and talk with the team. "Let's consider the reversible causes of arrest, the H's and T's.... Have we missed something?" Team members should discuss any changes in the patient's condition with the team leader to ensure that decisions are made with all available information.

Correct Actions: Knowledge Sharing	
Team leader	• Encourage an environment of information sharing and ask for suggestions if uncertain of the next best interventions. • Ask the opinions and suggestions of team members regarding reversible causes of arrest and factors that may be limiting effectiveness of the resuscitation effort. • Ask if anything has been overlooked (e.g., IV access should have been obtained or drugs should have been administered). • Consider all clinical signs that are relevant to treatment.
Team members	• Share information with other team members. • Try to identify factors that may be limiting effectiveness of resuscitation effort.

Constructive Intervention

During a resuscitation attempt the team leader or a team member may need to intervene if an action that is about to occur may be inappropriate. Although constructive intervention is necessary, it should be tactful. Team leaders should avoid confrontation with team members. Instead, conduct a debriefing after the resuscitation if constructive criticism is needed.

Correct Actions: Constructive Intervention	
Team leader	• Intervene if a team member is preparing to perform an incorrect action. • Take corrective action to ensure that team members are performing the correct tasks in the appropriate sequence. • Reassign a team member if that team member is not able to perform assigned tasks.
Team members	• Ask the team leader or a team member to verify action if you think that a team member is about to make a mistake. • Suggest an alternative drug, drug dose, or therapy if you observe an error in the drug, drug dose, or therapy ordered or prepared for administration.

Reevaluation and Summarizing

An essential role of the team leader is monitoring and reevaluating:

- The patient's status
- Interventions that have been performed
- Assessment findings

It is helpful for the team leader to summarize patient information periodically to the team during the resuscitation attempt. Review the status of the resuscitation attempt and announce the plan for the next few steps. Remember that the patient's condition can change. Remain flexible to changing treatment plans and revisiting the initial differential diagnosis. Ask for information and summaries from the code recorder and suggestions from the team members.

Correct Actions: Reevaluation and Summarizing	
Team leader	• Ask for suggestions from team members regarding differential diagnoses and factors that may be contributing to unsuccessful resuscitation efforts. • Frequently review drugs and treatments administered and the patient's response with the team. • Change the treatment strategy when new information or patient response (or failure to respond) suggests the need for such a change. • Inform arriving personnel of the patient's current status and plans for further action.
Team leader and team members	• Clearly draw attention to significant changes in the patient's clinical condition and increase monitoring (e.g., frequency of respirations and blood pressure) when the patient's condition deteriorates.

Mutual Respect

The best teams are composed of members who share mutual respect and work together in a collegial, supportive manner. To have a high-performing resuscitation team, members of the team must respect one another, regardless of differences in training or experience.

Correct Actions: Mutual Respect	
Team leader and team members	• Speak in a friendly, controlled tone of voice. • Provide positive feedback to team members. • Intervene if team members begin to raise voices or speak disrespectfully. • Remember that all team members are trying to perform well despite the stress present during the attempted resuscitation.
Team members	• Speak in friendly, controlled tone of voice. • Remember that the team leader and all team members are trying to perform well in a stressful situation.

Suggested Reading List

Brilli RJ, Gibson R, Luria JW, Wheeler TA, Shaw J, Linam M, Kheir J, McLain P, Lingsch T, Hall-Haering A, McBride M. Implementation of a medical emergency team in a large pediatric teaching hospital prevents respiratory and cardiopulmonary arrests outside the intensive care unit. *Pediatr Crit Care Med.* 2007;8:236-246.

Henderson SO, Ballesteros D. Evaluation of a hospital-wide resuscitation team: does it increase survival for in-hospital cardiopulmonary arrest? *Resuscitation.* 2001;48:111-116.

Hunt EA, Vera K, Diener-West M, Haggerty JA, Nelson KL, Shaffner DH, Pronovost PJ. Delays and errors in cardiopulmonary resuscitation and defibrillation by pediatric residents during simulated cardiopulmonary arrests. *Resuscitation.* 2009;80:819-825.

Sharek PJ, Parast LM, Leong K, Coombs J, Earnest K, Sullivan J, Frankel LR, Roth SJ. Effect of a rapid response team on hospital-wide mortality and code rates outside the ICU in a children's hospital. *JAMA.* 2007;298:2267-2274.

Tibballs J, Kinney S. Reduction of hospital mortality and of preventable cardiac arrest and death on introduction of a pediatric medical emergency team. *Pediatr Crit Care Med.* 2009;10:306-312.

Tibballs J, Kinney S, Duke T, Oakley E, Hennessy M. Reduction of paediatric in-patient cardiac arrest and death with a medical emergency team: preliminary results. *Arch Dis Child.* 2005;90:1148-1152.

Part 4

Recognition of Respiratory Distress and Failure

Overview

Respiratory distress is a condition of abnormal respiratory rate or effort. It encompasses a spectrum of signs from tachypnea with retractions to agonal gasps. Respiratory distress includes increased work of breathing, inadequate respiratory effort (e.g., hypoventilation or bradypnea), and irregular breathing. Any of these breathing patterns can be a sign that a child's condition is deteriorating toward respiratory failure.

PALS providers must identify respiratory conditions that are treatable with simple measures, such as clearing of airway secretions or administration of O_2. Yet it may be even more important to identify those respiratory conditions that are subtly but rapidly progressing toward respiratory failure. These conditions require timely interventions with more advanced airway techniques (e.g., assisted bag-mask ventilation).

In infants and children respiratory distress can quickly progress to respiratory failure and finally to cardiac arrest. Good outcome (i.e., neurologically intact survival to hospital discharge) is more likely following respiratory arrest than following cardiac arrest. Once the child is in cardiac arrest, outcome is often poor. You can greatly improve outcome by early identification and management of respiratory distress and respiratory failure before the child deteriorates to cardiac arrest.

Learning Objectives

After completing this section you should be able to:

- Recognize signs and symptoms of inadequate oxygenation and ventilation
- Describe respiratory distress and respiratory failure
- Identify the respiratory problem by type and severity

Preparation for the Course

You need to understand the concepts in this Part to be able to quickly identify signs of respiratory distress and respiratory failure. You also must be able to recognize respiratory problems by type so that you can choose appropriate interventions.

Fundamental Issues Associated With Respiratory Problems

Children with respiratory problems have impairment of oxygenation, ventilation, or both. This section discusses

- Impairment of oxygenation and ventilation in respiratory problems
- Physiology of respiratory disease

Impairment of Oxygenation and Ventilation in Respiratory Problems

Physiology of the Respiratory System

The main function of the respiratory system is gas exchange. Air is taken into the lungs with inspiration. O_2 diffuses from the alveolus into the blood, where some

Identify and Intervene	The earlier you detect respiratory distress or respiratory failure and start appropriate therapy, the better the chance for a good outcome.
Respiratory Distress and Failure	

O_2 dissolves in plasma. Most O_2 that enters the blood is attached to hemoglobin. The percentage of hemoglobin that becomes bound to O_2 is called *oxygen saturation*. When blood passes through the lungs, CO_2 diffuses from the blood into the alveoli; it is exhaled. Acute respiratory problems can result from alterations in any part of this system, from the alveoli (lung parenchyma) to the airway. Central nervous system disease, such as seizures or head trauma, can impair control of respiration, leading to decreased respiratory rate. Muscle weakness, either primary (e.g., muscular dystrophy) or secondary (e.g., fatigue), may also impair oxygenation or ventilation.

Children have a high metabolic rate, so O_2 demand per kilogram of body weight is high. O_2 consumption in infants is 6 to 8 mL/kg per minute, compared with 3 to 4 mL/kg per minute in adults. Therefore, hypoxemia and tissue hypoxia can develop more rapidly in a child than in an adult if apnea or inadequate alveolar ventilation occurs.

Respiratory problems can result in:

- Hypoxemia
- Hypercarbia
- A combination of both hypoxemia and hypercarbia

Hypoxemia

Hypoxemia is a low arterial O_2 tension (PaO_2) that is associated with a low O_2 saturation assessed by pulse oximetry (SpO_2). Hypoxemia indicates inadequate oxygenation. An $SpO_2 \leq 94\%$ in a child who is breathing room air indicates hypoxemia.

It is important to distinguish between *hypoxemia* and *tissue hypoxia*. Hypoxemia is low arterial O_2 saturation ($SpO_2 \leq 94\%$). In tissue hypoxia, O_2 delivery is not adequate to meet tissue O_2 demand. Hypoxemia does not always lead to tissue hypoxia. Compensatory mechanisms can increase O_2-carrying capacity (e.g., increased hemoglobin concentration) or blood flow (e.g., increased cardiac output) to maintain tissue oxygenation despite hypoxemia. For example, a child with cyanotic congenital heart disease has decreased arterial O_2 saturation but does not have tissue hypoxia as long as cardiac output remains adequate and hemoglobin concentration is slightly elevated. Conversely, O_2 delivery to the tissues can be inadequate (e.g., shock or severe anemia) despite adequate arterial O_2 saturation.

In response to tissue hypoxia the child may initially compensate by increasing respiratory rate and depth. This is known as *hyperventilation*. Tachycardia may also develop in response to hypoxemia as a means of increasing cardiac output. As tissue hypoxia worsens, these signs of cardiopulmonary distress become more severe.

Signs of tissue hypoxia include:

- Tachycardia (early sign)
- Tachypnea
- Nasal flaring, retractions
- Agitation, anxiety, irritability
- Pallor
- Cyanosis (late sign)
- Decreased level of consciousness (late sign)
- Bradypnea, apnea (late sign)
- Bradycardia (late sign)

FYI **Arterial O_2 Content**	Arterial O_2 content is the total amount of O_2 carried in the blood (in milliliters O_2 per deciliter of blood). It is the sum of the quantity of O_2 bound to hemoglobin plus the O_2 dissolved in arterial blood. O_2 content is determined largely by the hemoglobin (Hgb) concentration (grams per deciliter) and its saturation with O_2 (SaO_2). Use the following equation to calculate arterial O_2 content: **Arterial O_2 Content = [1.36 × Hgb concentration × SaO_2] + (0.003 × PaO_2)** Under normal conditions dissolved O_2 (0.003 × PaO_2) is an inconsequential portion of the total arterial O_2 content. But an increase in dissolved O_2 can produce a relatively significant increase in arterial O_2 content for a child with severe anemia.

Hypoxemia can be caused by a number of different mechanisms leading to respiratory distress and failure (Table 1).

Table 1. Mechanisms of Hypoxemia

Factor	Causes	Mechanism	Treatment
Low atmospheric P_{O_2}	High altitude (decreased barometric pressure)	Decreased Pa_{O_2}	Supplementary O_2
Alveolar hypoventilation	• CNS infection • Traumatic brain injury • Drug overdose • Neuromuscular weakness • Apnea	Increased arterial CO_2 tension (hypercarbia) displaces alveolar O_2, resulting in decreased alveolar and arterial O_2 tension (low Pa_{O_2} or hypoxemia).	Restore normal ventilation; supplementary O_2
Diffusion defect	• Pulmonary edema • Interstitial pneumonia • Alveolar proteinosis	Impaired movement of O_2 and CO_2 between the alveolus and blood results in decreased Pa_{O_2} (hypoxia) and, if severe, an increased Pa_{CO_2} (hypercarbia).	Supplementary O_2 with CPAP or ventilation with an advanced airway and PEEP
Ventilation/perfusion (V/Q) imbalance	• Pneumonia • Atelectasis • ARDS • Asthma • Bronchiolitis • Foreign body	Mismatch of ventilation and perfusion: blood flow through areas of the lung that are inadequately ventilated results in incomplete oxygenation of the blood returning to the left side of the heart. The result is a decreased arterial O_2 saturation and Pa_{O_2} and, to a lesser extent, increased Pa_{CO_2}.	PEEP to increase mean airway pressure*; supplementary O_2; ventilatory support
Right-to-left shunt	• Cyanotic congenital heart disease • Extracardiac (anatomical) vascular shunt Same causes listed for V/Q imbalance†	Shunting of unoxygenated blood from the right side of the heart to the left (or from the pulmonary artery into the aorta) results in a low Pa_{O_2}. Effects are similar to right-to-left shunt in the lungs.	Correction of defect (supplementary O_2 alone is insufficient)

Abbreviations: ARDS, acute respiratory distress syndrome; CNS, central nervous system; CPAP, continuous positive airway pressure; PEEP, positive end-expiratory pressure.

*PEEP should be used carefully in children with asthma; expert consultation is advised.

†With pneumonia, ARDS, and other lung tissue diseases, the pathophysiology is often characterized by a mix of mechanisms of hypoxemia. The most extreme form of V/Q mismatch would be a segment of lung with blood flow (Q) but no ventilation (V). In such a situation the blood does

Fundamental Fact **Detection of Hypercarbia**	Hypercarbia is more difficult to detect than hypoxemia because it produces no obvious clinical sign, such as cyanosis. Precise measurement of Pco_2 requires a blood sample (arterial, capillary or venous). Exhaled CO_2 detectors are now available for use in children with or without advanced airways. The end-tidal CO_2 measured by capnography may not be identical to the arterial CO_2. However, if the airway is patent, there is no increased dead space from air trapping (e.g., asthma), and cardiac output is adequate, the end-tidal CO_2 will increase in the presence of hypercarbia.

not become oxygenated. When it returns to the left side of the heart, it mixes with the oxygenated blood. The result is a lower O_2 saturation. The degree of desaturation depends on the size of the unventilated lung segment.

Hypercarbia

Hypercarbia is an increased CO_2 tension in the arterial blood ($Paco_2$). When hypercarbia is present, ventilation is inadequate.

CO_2 is a by-product of tissue metabolism. Normally it is eliminated by the lungs to maintain acid-base homeostasis. When ventilation is inadequate, CO_2 elimination is inadequate. The resulting increase in $Paco_2$ causes the blood to become acidic (respiratory acidosis). Inadequate ventilation may be due to airway or lung tissue disease. It may also result from decreased respiratory effort (central hypoventilation).

Most children with hypercarbia present with respiratory distress and tachypnea. Children may become tachypneic in an attempt to eliminate excess CO_2. However, hypercarbia may also present with poor respiratory effort, including decreased respiratory rate. In this case hypercarbia results from inadequate ventilation secondary to impaired respiratory drive. This inadequate ventilation may result from drugs, such as a narcotic overdose. It may also result from a central nervous system disorder with respiratory muscle weakness preventing the development of compensatory tachypnea. Detection of an inadequate respiratory drive requires careful observation and assessment. Consequences of inadequate ventilation become more severe as the arterial Pco_2 increases and respiratory acidosis worsens.

Decreased level of consciousness is a critical symptom of both inadequate ventilation and hypoxia. If a child's clinical condition deteriorates from agitation and anxiety to decreased responsiveness despite administration of supplementary O_2, this may indicate that the Pco_2 is rising. Note that even if the pulse oximeter indicates adequate O_2 saturation, ventilation may be impaired. If a child with respiratory distress has a decreased level of consciousness despite adequate oxygenation, suspect that ventilation is inadequate and that hypercarbia and respiratory acidosis may be present.

Signs of inadequate ventilation are nonspecific and include one or more of the following:

- Tachypnea or inadequate respiratory rate for age and clinical condition
- Nasal flaring, retractions
- Agitation, anxiety
- Decreased level of consciousness

Physiology of Respiratory Disease

Normal spontaneous breathing is accomplished with minimal work. Breathing is quiet with unlabored, smooth inspiration and passive expiration. In children with respiratory disease, "work of breathing" becomes more apparent. Important factors associated with increased work of breathing include:

- Increased airway resistance (upper and lower)
- Decreased lung compliance
- Use of accessory muscles of respiration
- Disordered central nervous system control of breathing

Airway Resistance

Airway resistance is the impedance to airflow within the airways. Resistance is primarily increased by a reduction in the size of the conducting airways (either by airway constriction or inflammation). Turbulent airflow also causes increased airway resistance. Airflow may become turbulent when the flow rate is increased, even if the size of the airway is unchanged. When airway resistance increases, work of breathing increases in an attempt to maintain airflow despite the increase in airway resistance.

Larger airways provide lower resistance to airflow than smaller airways. Airway resistance decreases as lung volume increases (inflation) because airway dilation accompanies lung inflation. Edema, bronchoconstriction, secretions, mucus, or a mediastinal mass impinging on large or small airways can decrease airway size, thereby increasing airway resistance. Resistance in the upper airway, particularly in the nasal or nasopharyngeal

---

FYI

Airway Resistance

Airway Resistance in Laminar Airflow

During normal breathing, airflow is laminar and airway resistance is relatively low. That is, only a small driving pressure (difference in pressure between the pleural space and the atmosphere) is needed to produce adequate airflow. When airflow is laminar (quiet), resistance to airflow is inversely proportional to the *fourth* power of the airway radius, so even a small reduction in airway diameter results in an exponential increase in airway resistance and work of breathing (Figure 1).

Airway Resistance in Turbulent Airflow

When airflow is turbulent, resistance is inversely proportional to the *fifth* power of the radius of the airway lumen, a 10-fold increase over normal laminar flow. In this state a larger driving pressure is required to produce the same rate of airflow. Therefore, patient agitation (causing rapid, turbulent airflow) results in a much greater increase in airway resistance and work of breathing than with quiet, laminar flow. To prevent generation of turbulent airflow (e.g., during crying), try to keep a child with airway obstruction as calm as possible.

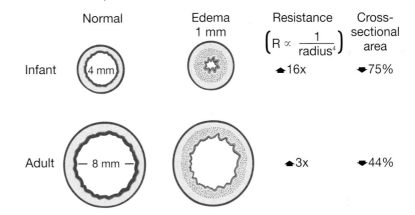

Figure 1. Effects of edema on airway resistance in the infant versus the adult. Normal airways are shown on the left; edematous airways (with 1 mm of circumferential edema) are on the right. Resistance to flow is inversely proportional to the fourth power of the radius of the airway lumen for laminar flow and to the fifth power for turbulent flow. The net result is a 75% decrease in cross-sectional area and a 16-fold increase in airway resistance in the infant versus a 44% decrease in cross-sectional area and a 3-fold increase in airway resistance in the adult during quiet breathing. Turbulent flow in the infant (e.g., crying) increases airway resistance and thus the work of breathing from 16- to 32-fold. Modified from Coté CJ, Todres ID. The pediatric airway. In: Coté CJ, Ryan JF, Todres ID, Goudsouzian NG, eds. *A Practice of Anesthesia for Infants and Children.* 2nd ed. Philadelphia, PA: WB Saunders Co; 1993: 55-83, copyright Elsevier.

---

passages, can represent a significant portion of total airway resistance, especially in infants.

Lung Compliance

Compliance refers to the distensibility of the lung, chest wall, or both. *Lung compliance* is defined as the change in lung volume produced by a change in driving pressure across the lung. When lung compliance is high, the lungs are easily distended (there is a large change in volume produced by a slight change in driving pressure). In a child with low lung compliance, the lungs are stiffer; more effort is needed to inflate the alveoli. The increased pressure required to inflate stiff lungs results in increased work of breathing. This increased inspiratory effort reduces the

intrathoracic pressure to a level significantly less than atmospheric pressure to create sufficient airflow into the lung. During mechanical ventilation, increased positive airway pressure is needed to achieve adequate ventilation when lung compliance is decreased.

Compliance varies within the lung according to the degree of lung inflation. Extrapulmonary conditions that cause decreased compliance are pneumothorax and pleural effusion. Pneumonia and inflammatory lung tissue disease (e.g., ARDS, fibrosis, pulmonary edema) cause decreased compliance. These conditions are associated with an increase in the water content in the interstitial space and alveoli. The impact of this increase in water content on lung

The chest wall in infants and young children is compliant. Therefore, relatively small pressure changes can move the chest wall. During normal breathing, diaphragm contraction in infants pulls the lower ribs slightly inward but does not result in chest retraction. Conversely, forceful contraction of the diaphragm results in a large drop in pressure within the chest, pulling the chest inward during inspiration. When lung compliance is reduced, maximum inspiratory effort may not produce adequate tidal volume because marked retractions of the chest wall limit lung expansion during inspiration.

Children with neuromuscular disorders have a weak chest wall and weak respiratory muscles that can make breathing and coughing ineffective. Muscle weakness can result in characteristic seesaw breathing (simultaneous retraction of the chest wall and expansion of the abdomen).

The normal diaphragm is dome-shaped and contracts most forcefully in this shape. When the diaphragm is flattened, as occurs with lung hyperinflation (e.g., acute asthma), contraction is less forceful and ventilation is less efficient. Respiration is compromised if movement of the diaphragm is impeded by abdominal distention and high intra-abdominal pressure (e.g., gastric inflation) or by air trapping caused by airway obstruction. During infancy and early childhood the intercostal muscles cannot effectively lift the chest wall to increase intrathoracic volume and compensate for loss of diaphragm motion.

compliance is similar to the expansion that occurs when a sponge becomes saturated with water. A normal sponge re-expands quickly when it is compressed. A wet sponge is harder to compress and re-expands more slowly because its normal elasticity is opposed by the extra weight of the fluid.

Inspiratory and Expiratory Flow

The inspiratory muscles of respiration include the diaphragm, intercostals, and accessory muscles (primarily of the abdomen and neck). During spontaneous breathing, inspiratory muscles (chiefly the diaphragm) increase intrathoracic volume, resulting in a decrease in intrathoracic pressure. When intrathoracic pressure is less than atmospheric pressure, air flows into the lungs (*inspiration*). The intercostal muscles normally stiffen the chest wall as the diaphragm contracts. Accessory muscles of respiration are not typically needed during normal ventilation. In respiratory disorders that increase airway resistance or reduce lung compliance, accessory muscles help create a decrease in intrathoracic pressure and maintain adequate chest wall stiffness needed to produce inspiratory flow.

Expiratory flow results from relaxation of the inspiratory muscles and elastic recoil of the lung and chest wall. These changes increase intrathoracic pressure to a level that is higher than the atmospheric pressure. During spontaneous breathing, expiratory flow is primarily a passive process. Expiration may become an active process in the presence of increased lower airway resistance and may require involvement of muscles of the abdominal wall and the intercostals.

Central Nervous System Control of Breathing

Breathing is controlled by complex mechanisms involving:

- Brainstem respiratory centres
- Central and peripheral chemoreceptors
- Voluntary control

Spontaneous breathing is controlled by a group of respiratory centres located in the brainstem. Breathing also can be overridden by voluntary control from the cerebral cortex. Examples of voluntary control include breath holding, panting, and sighing. Conditions such as infection of the central nervous system, traumatic brain injury, and

Central chemoreceptors respond to changes in the hydrogen ion concentration of cerebrospinal fluid, which is largely determined by the arterial CO_2 tension ($PaCO_2$). Peripheral chemoreceptors (carotid body) respond primarily to a decrease in arterial O_2 (PaO_2); some receptors also respond to an increase in $PaCO_2$.

drug overdose can impair respiratory drive, resulting in hypoventilation or even apnea.

Identification of Respiratory Problems by Severity

Identifying the severity of a respiratory problem will help you decide the most appropriate interventions. Be alert for signs of:

- Respiratory distress
- Respiratory failure

Respiratory Distress

Respiratory distress is a clinical state characterized by abnormal respiratory rate (e.g., tachypnea) or effort. The respiratory effort may be increased (e.g., nasal flaring, retractions, and use of accessory muscles) or inadequate (e.g., hypoventilation or bradypnea). Assess for respiratory distress by looking for changes in airway sounds and associated changes in skin colour and mental status.

Respiratory distress can range from mild to severe. For example, a child with mild tachypnea and a mild increase in respiratory effort with changes in airway sounds is in *mild* respiratory distress. A child with marked tachypnea, significantly increased respiratory effort and changes in airway sounds, deterioration in skin colour, and changes in mental status is in *severe* respiratory distress. Severe respiratory distress can be an indication of respiratory failure.

Clinical signs of respiratory distress typically include some or all of the following:

- Tachypnea
- Increased respiratory effort (e.g., nasal flaring, retractions)
- Inadequate respiratory effort (e.g., hypoventilation or bradypnea)
- Abnormal airway sounds (e.g., stridor, wheezing, grunting)
- Tachycardia
- Pale, cool skin
- Changes in level of consciousness

These indicators may vary in severity.

Respiratory distress is apparent when a child tries to maintain adequate gas exchange despite airway obstruction, reduced lung compliance, or lung tissue

disease. As the child tires or as respiratory function or effort or both deteriorate, adequate gas exchange cannot be maintained. When this happens, clinical signs of respiratory failure develop.

Respiratory Failure

Respiratory failure is a clinical state of inadequate oxygenation, ventilation, or both. Respiratory failure is often the end stage of respiratory distress. If there is abnormal central nervous system control of breathing or muscle weakness, the child may show little or no respiratory effort despite the development of respiratory failure. In these situations you may need to identify respiratory failure based on clinical findings. Confirm the diagnosis with objective measurements, such as pulse oximetry or blood gas analysis.

Suspect *probable respiratory failure* if some of the following signs are present:

- Marked tachypnea (early)
- Bradypnea, apnea (late)
- Increased, decreased, or no respiratory effort
- Poor to absent distal air movement
- Tachycardia (early)
- Bradycardia (late)
- Cyanosis
- Stupor, coma (late)

Respiratory failure can result from upper or lower airway obstruction, lung tissue disease, and disordered control of breathing (e.g., apnea or shallow, slow respirations). *When respiratory effort is inadequate, respiratory failure can occur without typical signs of respiratory distress.* Respiratory failure is a clinical state that *requires intervention* to prevent deterioration to cardiac arrest.

Identification of Respiratory Problems by Type

Respiratory distress or failure can be classified into one or more of the following types:

- Upper airway obstruction
- Lower airway obstruction
- Lung tissue disease
- Disordered control of breathing

Respiratory problems do not always occur in isolation. A child may have more than a single cause of respiratory

FYI	It is difficult to define strict criteria for respiratory failure because the baseline respiratory function of an infant or child may be abnormal. For example, an infant with cyanotic congenital heart disease and a baseline arterial O_2 saturation (SaO_2) of 75% is not in respiratory failure on the basis of O_2 saturation. But the same degree of hypoxemia would be one sign of respiratory failure in a child with normal baseline cardiopulmonary physiology.
Respiratory Failure and Baseline Physiology	

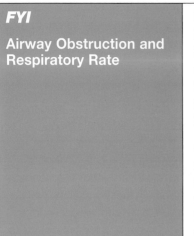

In children with acute lower airway obstruction (e.g., status asthmaticus), the increase in intrapleural pressure produced by forced expiration compresses airways proximal to the alveoli. This airway compression leads to further expiratory obstruction with no increase in expiratory flow. If this small airway collapse is severe, it leads to air trapping and lung hyperinflation. In acute severe asthma the respiratory rate may slow and the child may attempt to increase tidal volume. These responses minimize frictional forces and the work of breathing.

An infant with lower airway obstruction, by comparison, typically has a rapid respiratory rate. The infant has a compliant chest wall. If the infant attempts to breathe more deeply, the resulting decrease in intrapleural pressure may result in greater chest wall collapse. When there is significant lower airway obstruction, it is more efficient for the infant to breathe at a fast rate with small tidal volumes to maintain minute ventilation, keeping a relatively larger volume of gas in the lungs.

distress or failure. For example, a child may have disordered control of breathing due to a head injury and then develop pneumonia (lung tissue disease).

Upper Airway Obstruction

Obstruction of the upper airways (i.e., the airways outside the thorax) can occur in the nose, pharynx, or larynx. Obstruction can range from mild to severe. Common causes of upper airway obstruction are foreign-body aspiration (e.g., food or a small object) and swelling of the airway (e.g., anaphylaxis, tonsillar hypertrophy, croup, or epiglottis). Other causes of upper airway obstruction are a mass that compromises the airway lumen (e.g., pharyngeal or peritonsillar abscess, retropharyngeal abscess, or tumor), thick secretions obstructing the nasal passages, or any congenital airway abnormality resulting in narrowing (e.g., congenital subglottic stenosis). Upper airway obstruction also may be iatrogenic. For example, subglottic stenosis may develop secondary to trauma induced by endotracheal intubation.

Signs of upper airway obstruction occur most often during *inspiration* and may include:

- Tachypnea
- Increased inspiratory respiratory effort (e.g., inspiratory retractions, nasal flaring)
- Change in voice (e.g., hoarseness), cry, or presence of a barking cough
- Stridor (usually inspiratory but may be biphasic)

- Poor chest rise
- Poor air entry on auscultation

Other signs are cyanosis, drooling, cough, or seesaw breathing. The respiratory rate is often only mildly elevated because rapid rates create turbulent flow and further increase resistance to airflow.

Lower Airway Obstruction

Obstruction of the lower airways (i.e., the airways within the thorax) can occur in the lower trachea, the bronchi, or the bronchioles. Asthma and bronchiolitis are common causes of lower airway obstruction.

Typical signs of lower airway obstruction occur during *expiration* and include:

- Tachypnea
- Wheezing (most commonly expiratory but may be inspiratory or biphasic)
- Increased respiratory effort (retractions, nasal flaring, and prolonged expiration)
- Prolonged expiratory phase associated with increased expiratory effort (i.e., expiration is an active rather than a passive process)
- Cough

Lung Tissue Disease

Lung tissue disease is a term given to a heterogeneous group of clinical conditions that generally affects the lung

Children with lung tissue disease can often maintain ventilation (i.e., CO_2 elimination) with a relatively small number of functional alveoli, but they cannot maintain oxygenation as effectively. Compromised ventilation, indicated by hypercarbia, is typically a late manifestation of the disease process.

Grunting produces early glottic closure during expiration. Grunting is a compensatory mechanism to maintain positive airway pressure and prevent collapse of the alveoli and small airways.

at the level of the point where gas exchange occurs. It is often characterized by alveolar and small airway collapse or fluid-filled alveoli. As a result abnormalities in oxygenation and, with severe disease, ventilation are typical. Lung compliance is commonly reduced, and pulmonary infiltrates are present on chest x-ray.

Lung tissue disease has many causes. Pneumonia from any cause (e.g., bacterial, viral, chemical), pulmonary edema (from congestive heart failure and ARDS) can cause lung tissue disease. Other potential causes are pulmonary contusion (trauma), allergic reaction, toxins, vasculitis, and infiltrative disease.

Signs of lung tissue disease are:

- Tachypnea (often marked)
- Increased respiratory effort
- Grunting
- Crackles (rales)
- Diminished breath sounds
- Tachycardia
- Hypoxemia (may be refractory to administration of supplementary O_2)

Disordered Control of Breathing

Disordered control of breathing is an abnormal breathing pattern that produces signs of inadequate respiratory rate, effort, or both. Often the parents will say the child is "breathing funny." Common causes are neurologic disorders (e.g., seizures, central nervous system infections, head injury, brain tumor, hydrocephalus, neuromuscular disease). Because disordered control of breathing is typically associated with conditions that impair neurologic function, these children often have a decreased level of consciousness.

Signs of disordered control of breathing include:

- Variable or irregular respiratory rate (tachypnea alternating with bradypnea)
- Variable respiratory effort
- Shallow breathing (frequently resulting in hypoxemia and hypercarbia)
- Central apnea (i.e., apnea without any respiratory effort)

Summary: Recognition of Respiratory Problems Flowcharts

Figure 2 summarizes recognition and identification of respiratory problems. Note that this chart does not include all respiratory emergencies; it provides key characteristics for a limited number of diseases.

Pediatric Advanced Life Support
Signs of Respiratory Problems

	Clinical Signs	Upper Airway Obstruction	Lower Airway Obstruction	Lung Tissue Disease	Disordered Control of Breathing
A	Patency	Airway open and maintainable/not maintainable			
B	Respiratory Rate/Effort	Increased			Variable
	Breath Sounds	Stridor (typically inspiratory) Barking cough Hoarseness	Wheezing (typically expiratory) Prolonged expiratory phase	Grunting Crackles Decreased breath sounds	Normal
	Air Movement	Decreased			Variable
C	Heart Rate	Tachycardia (early) Bradycardia (late)			
	Skin	Pallor, cool skin (early) Cyanosis (late)			
D	Level of Consciousness	Anxiety, agitation (early) Lethargy, unresponsiveness (late)			
E	Temperature	Variable			

Pediatric Advanced Life Support
Identification of Respiratory Problems by Severity

Respiratory Distress ➡ Respiratory Failure

A	Open and maintainable ⟹ Not maintainable
B	Tachypnea ⟹ Bradypnea to apnea
	Work of breathing (nasal flaring/retractions) Increased effort ⟹ Decreased effort ⟹ Apnea
	Good air movement ⟹ Poor to absent air movement
C	Tachycardia ⟹ Bradycardia
	Pallor ⟹ Cyanosis
D	Anxiety, agitation ⟹ Lethargy to unresponsiveness
E	Variable temperature

Figure 2. Signs of respiratory problems and identification of respiratory problems by severity.

Suggested Reading List

Arnold DH, Jenkins CA, Hartert TV. Noninvasive assessment of asthma severity using pulse oximeter plethysmograph estimate of pulsus paradoxus physiology. *BMC Pulm Med*. 2010;10:17.

Coté CJ, Ryan J, Todres ID, Goudsouzian NG. *A Practice of Anesthesia for Infants and Children.* Philadelphia, PA: WB Saunders; 1993.

Downes JJ, Fulgencio T, Raphaely RC. Acute respiratory failure in infants and children. *Pediatr Clin North Am*. 1972;19:423-445.

Nitu ME, Eigen H. Respiratory failure. *Pediatr Rev.* 2009;30:470-477.

Madden K, Khemani RG, Newth CJL. Paediatric applied respiratory physiology: the essentials. *Paediatr Child Health*. 2009;19:249-256.

Santamaria JP, Schafermeyer R. Stridor: a review. *Pediatr Emerg Care*. 1992;8:229-234.

Singer JL, Losek JD. Grunting respirations: chest or abdominal pathology? *Pediatr Emerg Care*. 1992;8:354-358.

Thompson, M. How well do vital signs identify children with serious infections in paediatric emergency care? *Arch Dis Child*. 2009;94:888-893.

Management of Respiratory Distress and Failure

Overview

Respiratory problems are a major cause of cardiac arrest in children. In fact, many infants and children who require CPR (both in and out of hospital) have respiratory problems that progress to cardiopulmonary failure. It may not be possible to differentiate between respiratory distress and respiratory failure on the basis of clinical examination alone. Respiratory failure can develop even without significant signs of distress. In children, clinical deterioration in respiratory function may progress rapidly, so there is little time to waste. Prompt recognition and effective management of respiratory problems are fundamental to pediatric advanced life support.

Learning Objectives

After completing this Part you should be able to:

- Describe initial interventions to manage respiratory distress and respiratory failure
- Discuss specific interventions for management of upper airway obstruction, lower airway obstruction, lung tissue disease, and disordered control of breathing

Preparation for the Course

During the course you will participate in the Management of Respiratory Emergencies Skills Station. You will have an opportunity to practice and demonstrate your proficiency in performing basic airway management skills, such as insertion of airway adjuncts, effective bag-mask ventilation, and suctioning. See the Appendix for a checklist of required competencies. See the section "Resources for Management of Respiratory Emergencies" that follows this Part for details on bag-mask ventilation. You will also need to have an understanding of respiratory function monitoring devices (e.g., monitoring of O_2 saturation by pulse oximetry, monitoring of exhaled CO_2) and O_2 delivery systems.

Initial Management of Respiratory Distress and Failure

The first priority in the management of a seriously ill or injured child who is not in cardiac arrest is evaluation of airway and breathing. If there are signs of respiratory distress or failure, initial interventions must support or restore adequate oxygenation and ventilation.

Respiratory conditions are a major cause of cardiac arrest in infants and children. As a result, when respiratory distress or failure is detected, it is important to begin appropriate interventions quickly.

Initial interventions are a rapid, focused evaluation of respiratory function to identify the type and severity, rather than the precise etiology, of the respiratory problem. Once oxygenation and ventilation are stabilized, identify the cause of the problem to facilitate targeted interventions. Use the evaluate-identify-intervene sequence to monitor progression of symptoms or response to therapy and to prioritize further interventions.

Initial stabilization and management of a child in respiratory distress or respiratory failure may include the interventions listed in Table 1.

Critical Concept **Intervene Quickly to Restore Respiratory Function**	PALS providers must intervene quickly to restore adequate respiratory function. You can greatly improve outcome by early identification and prompt management of respiratory distress and failure. Once respiratory failure progresses to cardiac arrest, outcome is often poor.

Table 1. Initial Management of Respiratory Distress or Failure

Evaluate	Interventions (as Indicated)
Airway	• Support an open airway (allow child to assume position of comfort) or, if necessary, open the airway with: – Head tilt–chin lift – Jaw thrust without head tilt if cervical spine injury is suspected. If this maneuver does not open the airway, use the head tilt–chin lift or jaw thrust with gentle head extension. • Clear the airway if indicated (e.g., suction nose and mouth, remove visualized foreign body). • Consider an oropharyngeal airway (OPA) or nasopharyngeal airway (NPA) to improve airway patency.
Breathing	• Monitor O_2 saturation by pulse oximetry. • Provide O_2 (humidified if available). Use a high-concentration delivery device such as a nonrebreathing mask for treatment of severe respiratory distress or possible respiratory failure. • Administer inhaled medication (e.g., salbutamol, epinephrine) as needed. • Assist ventilation with bag-mask device and supplementary O_2 if needed. • Prepare for endotracheal intubation if indicated.
Circulation	• Monitor heart rate, heart rhythm, and blood pressure. • Establish vascular access (for fluid therapy and medications) as indicated.

Principles of Targeted Management

Once oxygenation and ventilation are stabilized, identify the type of the respiratory problem to help prioritize the next interventions. This Part reviews principles of targeted management for the following 4 types of respiratory problems:

- Upper airway obstruction
- Lower airway obstruction
- Lung tissue disease
- Disordered control of breathing

Management of Upper Airway Obstruction

Upper airway obstruction is an obstruction of the large airways outside the thorax; the obstruction can range from mild to severe. Causes of upper airway obstruction are airway swelling, infection, or an aspirated foreign body. Other causes of obstruction are an increase in the soft tissue of the upper airway (large tonsils or adenoids) or poor control of the upper airway due to a decreased level of consciousness.

Infants and small children are especially prone to upper airway obstruction. An infant's tongue is large in proportion to the oropharyngeal cavity. If the infant has a decreased level of consciousness, the muscles may relax, allowing the tongue to fall back and obstruct the oropharynx. Infants also have a prominent occiput. If the infant with a decreased level of consciousness is supine, resting on the large occiput can cause flexion of the neck, resulting in upper airway obstruction. In young infants, nasal obstruction can impair ventilation. Secretions, blood, and debris in the nose, pharynx, and larynx from infection,

inflammation, or trauma also can obstruct the airway. It is important to remember that the smaller the airway is, the more easily it can become obstructed.

General Management of Upper Airway Obstruction

General management of upper airway obstruction includes initial interventions listed in Table 1. Additional measures focus on relieving the obstruction. These measures may include opening the airway by:

- Allowing the child to assume a position of comfort
- Performing manual airway maneuvers, such as a jaw thrust or head tilt–chin lift
- Removing a foreign body
- Suctioning the nose or mouth
- Reducing airway swelling with medications
- Minimizing agitation (agitation often worsens upper airway obstruction)
- Deciding whether an airway adjunct or advanced airway is needed
- Deciding early if a surgical airway (tracheostomy or needle cricothyroidotomy) is needed

Suctioning is helpful in removing secretions, blood, or debris; *however, if the upper airway obstruction is caused by edema from infection (e.g., croup) or allergic reaction, carefully weigh advantages versus disadvantages of suctioning.* Suctioning may increase the child's agitation and may increase respiratory distress. Instead, consider allowing the child to assume a position of comfort. Give nebulized epinephrine, particularly if the swelling is beyond the tongue. Corticosteroids (inhaled, IV, oral, or intramuscular [IM]) also may be helpful in this situation.

When upper airway obstruction is severe, *call early* for advanced help. The provider with the greatest skill and experience in airway management is the most likely to safely establish an airway. Failure to aggressively treat an acute partial upper airway obstruction may lead to complete airway obstruction and, ultimately, to cardiac arrest.

In less severe cases of upper airway obstruction, infants and children may benefit from specific airway adjuncts. For example, in a child with a decreased level of consciousness, an OPA or NPA may be helpful in relieving obstruction caused by the tongue. Use an OPA only if the child is deeply unconscious with no gag reflex. A child with a gag reflex may tolerate an NPA. Insert an NPA carefully to avoid nasopharyngeal trauma and bleeding. Avoid using an NPA in children with increased bleeding risk.

An infant or child with upper airway obstruction from redundant tissues or tissue edema may benefit from the application of CPAP.

Specific Management of Upper Airway Obstruction by Etiology

Specific causes of upper airway obstruction require specific interventions. This section reviews management of upper airway obstruction due to:

- Croup
- Anaphylaxis
- FBAO

Management of Croup Based on Severity

Croup is managed according to your assessment of clinical severity. The following characteristics of croup are listed by degree of severity:

- **Mild croup:** Occasional barking cough, little or no stridor at rest, absent or mild retractions
- **Moderate croup:** Frequent barking cough, easily audible stridor at rest, retractions at rest, little or no agitation, good air entry by auscultation of the peripheral lung fields
- **Severe croup:** Frequent barking cough, prominent inspiratory and occasional expiratory stridor, marked retractions, significant agitation, decreased air entry by auscultation of the lungs
- **Impending respiratory failure:** Barking cough (may not be prominent if the child's respiratory effort is growing weaker because of severe hypoxemia and hypercarbia), audible stridor at rest (can be difficult to hear with failing respiratory effort), retractions (may not be severe if respiratory effort is failing), lethargy or decreased level of consciousness, and, sometimes, pallor or cyanosis despite administration of supplementary O_2, poor air movement on auscultation

O_2 saturation may be slightly low in mild and moderate croup and is commonly well below normal in severe croup.

General management for upper airway obstruction includes the initial interventions listed in Table 1. *Specific interventions for management of croup* may include the following:

Severity of Croup	Intervention
Mild	• Consider dexamethasone.
Moderate to severe	• Administer humidified O_2. • Give nothing by mouth. • Administer nebulized epinephrine. • Observe for at least 2 hours after giving nebulized epinephrine to ensure continued improvement (no recurrence of stridor). • Administer dexamethasone. • Consider use of heliox (helium-oxygen mixture) for severe disease.
Impending respiratory failure	• Administer a high concentration of O_2; use a nonrebreathing mask if available. • Assist ventilation (i.e., bag-mask ventilation) if necessary (e.g., persistent, severe hypoxemia [<90% O_2 saturation] despite O_2 administration, inadequate ventilation, or changes in level of consciousness). • Administer dexamethasone IV/IM. • Perform endotracheal intubation if indicated; to avoid injury to the subglottic area, use a smaller ET tube size (a half size smaller than predicted for the child's age). • Prepare for surgical airway if needed. *Endotracheal intubation of the child with upper airway obstruction is a high-risk procedure and should be performed by a team with significant airway expertise. Use neuromuscular blockade only if you are confident the child can be supported with manual ventilation.*

Management of Anaphylaxis

In addition to the initial interventions listed in Table 1, specific interventions for *management of anaphylaxis* may include the following:

Intervention
Administer IM epinephrine by autoinjector or regular syringe every 10 to 15 minutes as needed. Repeated doses may be needed.
• Treat bronchospasm (wheezing) with salbutamol administered by metered-dose inhaler (MDI) or nebulizer solution. • Give continuous nebulization if indicated (i.e., severe bronchospasm).
For severe respiratory distress, anticipate further airway swelling and prepare for endotracheal intubation.
To treat hypotension: • Place the child in the Trendelenburg position as tolerated. • Administer isotonic crystalloid (e.g., normal saline [NS] or lactated Ringer's [LR]) 20 mL/kg bolus IV (repeat as needed). • For hypotension unresponsive to fluids and IM epinephrine, administer an epinephrine infusion titrated to achieve adequate blood pressure for age.
• Administer diphenhydramine and H₂ blocker (e.g., ranitidine) IV.
• Administer methylprednisolone or equivalent corticosteroid IV.

Management of Foreign-Body Airway Obstruction

If you suspect an FBAO that is not complete (the child is able to make sounds and cough), do not intervene. Call for help and allow the child to try to clear the obstruction by coughing. If you suspect complete airway obstruction (no sound, unable to cough, unable to breathe adequately) by a foreign body, perform the following maneuvers:

Intervention

• For a conscious infant or child, use manual techniques appropriate for age. Repeat the following as needed:
  – <1 year: Give 5 back slaps followed by 5 chest thrusts
  – ≥1 year: Give abdominal thrusts
• If the infant or child becomes unresponsive, start CPR, beginning with chest compressions (even if a pulse is palpable), until additional expertise is available. The chest compressions may help to dislodge the foreign body. Before you deliver breaths, look into the mouth. If you see a foreign body that can be easily removed, remove it.
• *Note:* Do not perform a *blind finger sweep* in an effort to dislodge a foreign body. This may push the foreign body further into the airway. It also may cause trauma and bleeding.

Management of Lower Airway Obstruction

Lower airway obstruction involves the smaller bronchi and bronchioles inside the thorax. Common causes are bronchiolitis and asthma.

General Management of Lower Airway Obstruction

General management of lower airway obstruction includes the initial interventions listed in Table 1.

In a child with respiratory failure or severe respiratory distress, your first priority is to restore adequate oxygenation; correction of hypercarbia to normal levels is not required because most children can tolerate hypercarbia without adverse effects. If assisted ventilation is required for lower airway obstruction, perform bag-mask ventilation at a relatively slow respiratory rate.

Specific Management of Lower Airway Obstruction by Etiology

Specific causes of lower airway obstruction require specific interventions. This section reviews management of lower airway obstruction due to the following:

- Bronchiolitis
- Acute asthma

Fundamental Fact **Ventilate at a Slow Rate When Lower Airway Obstruction Is Present**	Ventilating at a slow rate allows more time for expiration and reduces the risk of air trapping. With a slow rate you can also lengthen the inspiratory time to prevent creation of high airway pressure and its complications. High airway pressure results in gastric distention (air preferentially enters the stomach). Gastric distention may interfere with normal movement of the diaphragm, thus limiting effective ventilation. It also increases the risk of regurgitation and aspiration. High airway pressure also increases the risk of pneumothorax and may compromise venous return to the heart and decrease cardiac output.

Note: Distinguishing between bronchiolitis and asthma in a wheezing infant can be difficult. A history of previous wheezing episodes suggests that the infant has reversible bronchospasm (i.e., asthma). Consider a trial of bronchodilators if the diagnosis is unclear.

Management of Bronchiolitis

In addition to initial management in Table 1, specific measures for the *management of bronchiolitis* may include the following:

Intervention
Perform oral or nasal suctioning as needed.
Consider laboratory and other tests, which may include viral studies, chest x-ray, and ABG.

Randomized controlled trials of bronchodilator or corticosteroid therapy for bronchiolitis have shown mixed results. Some infants improve when treated with nebulized epinephrine or salbutamol. In some infants, however, respiratory symptoms are aggravated by nebulizer therapy. Consider a trial of nebulized epinephrine or salbutamol treatment. Discontinue it if there is no improvement. Administer supplementary O_2 if O_2 saturation is <94%.

Management of Acute Asthma

Manage asthma according to your assessment of clinical severity (Table 2). In addition to initial interventions listed in Table 1, specific interventions for the *management of acute asthma* may include the following:

Asthma Severity	Intervention
Mild to moderate	• Administer humidified O_2 in high concentration via nasal cannula or O_2 mask; titrate according to pulse oximetry. Keep O_2 saturation ≥94%. • Administer salbutamol by MDI or nebulizer solution. • Administer oral corticosteroids.

(continued)

(continued)

Asthma Severity	Intervention
Moderate to severe	• Administer humidified O_2 in high concentrations to keep O_2 saturation ≥94%; use a nonrebreathing mask if needed. • Administer salbutamol by MDI (with spacer) or nebulizer solution. If wheezing and aeration are not alleviated, continuous salbutamol administration may be required. • Administer ipratropium bromide by nebulizer solution. Salbutamol and ipratropium may be mixed for nebulization. Consider establishing vascular access for administration of fluids and medications. • Administer corticosteroids PO/IV. • Consider administering magnesium sulfate by slow (15 to 30 minutes) IV bolus infusion while monitoring heart rate and blood pressure. • Perform diagnostic tests (e.g., ABG, chest x-ray) as indicated.
Impending respiratory failure	All of the above therapies are indicated in addition to the following: • Administer O_2 in high concentrations; use a nonrebreathing mask if available. • Administer salbutamol by continuous nebulizer. • Administer corticosteroid IV if not already given. • Consider giving terbutaline subcutaneously or by continuous IV; titrate to response while monitoring for toxicity. You may administer subcutaneous or IM epinephrine as an alternative. • Consider bilevel positive airway pressure (noninvasive positive-pressure ventilation), especially in alert, cooperative children. • Consider endotracheal intubation for children with refractory hypoxemia (low O_2 saturation), worsening clinical condition (e.g., decreasing level of consciousness, irregular breathing), or both despite the aggressive medical management described above. Intubation in an asthmatic child carries significant risk for respiratory and circulatory complications. Consider using a cuffed ET tube.

Table 2. Severity Score: Classification of Mild, Moderate, and Severe Asthma

Parameter*	Mild	Moderate	Severe	Respiratory Arrest Imminent
Breathless	Walking Can lie down	Talking (Infant will have softer, shorter cry; difficulty feeding) Prefers sitting	At rest (Infant will stop feeding) Hunched forward	
Talks in	Sentences	Phrases	Words	
Alertness	May be agitated	Usually agitated	Usually agitated	Drowsy or confused
Respiratory rate	Increased	Increased	Often >30/min	
	Age <2 months 2-12 months 1-5 years 6-8 years	**Normal rate** <60/min <50/min <40/min <30/min		
Accessory muscles and suprasternal retractions	Usually not	Usually	Usually	Paradoxical thoraco-abdominal movement
Wheeze	Moderate, often only end-expiration	Loud	Usually loud	Absence of wheeze
Pulse/min	<100	100-120	>120	Bradycardia
	Guide to limits of normal pulse rate in children: **Age** Infants (2-12 months) Toddler (1-2 years) Preschool/school age (2-8 years)	**Normal rate** <160/min <120/min <110/min		
Pulsus paradoxus	Absent <10 mm Hg	May be present 10-25 mm Hg	Often present >25 mm Hg (adult) 25-40 mm Hg (child)	Absence suggests respiratory muscle fatigue
PEF after initial bronchodilator % predicted or % personal best	>80%	Approximately 60%-80%	<60% predicted or personal best (<100 L/min adults) or response lasts <2 hours	
Pao₂ (on air) and/or Paco₂	Normal, test usually not necessary <45 mm Hg†	>60 mm Hg <45 mm Hg†	<60 mm Hg Possible cyanosis >45 mm Hg; possible respiratory failure	
Sao₂ %	>95%	91%-95%	<90%	

*The presence of several parameters, but not necessarily all, indicates the general classification of the attack.

†Hypercapnia (hypoventilation) develops more readily in young children than in adults and adolescents.

Reproduced from National Heart, Lung, and Blood Institute and World Health Organization. *Global Strategy for Asthma Management and Prevention NHLBI/WHO Workshop Report.* Bethesda, MD: US Department of Health and Human Services; 1997. Publication 97-4051.

Management of Lung Tissue Disease

Lung tissue disease (also called *parenchymal lung disease*) refers to a heterogeneous group of clinical conditions. Common causes of lung tissue disease are pneumonia (e.g., infectious, chemical, aspiration) and cardiogenic pulmonary edema. ARDS and traumatic pulmonary contusion are other causes. Lung tissue disease can also result from allergic, vascular, infiltrative, environmental, and other factors.

General Management of Lung Tissue Disease

General management of lung tissue disease includes the initial interventions listed in Table 1. In children with hypoxemia refractory to high inspired O_2 concentrations, positive expiratory pressure (CPAP, noninvasive ventilation, or mechanical ventilation with PEEP) is usually helpful in the management of lung tissue disease.

Specific Management of Lung Tissue Disease by Etiology

Specific causes of lung tissue disease require specific interventions. This section reviews the management of lung tissue disease from the following causes:

- Infectious pneumonia
- Chemical pneumonitis
- Aspiration pneumonitis
- Cardiogenic pulmonary edema
- Noncardiogenic pulmonary edema (ARDS)

Management of Infectious Pneumonia

Infectious pneumonia results from viral, bacterial, or fungal inflammation of the alveoli. The common causes of acute community-acquired pneumonia in children include viruses, bacteria (*Streptococcus pneumoniae*), and atypical bacteria (*Mycoplasma pneumoniae* and *Chlamydia pneumoniae*). Methicillin-resistant *Staphylococcus aureus* is increasingly common and may cause empyema.

In addition to initial interventions listed in Table 1, specific interventions for the *management of acute infectious pneumonia* may include the following:

Intervention
Perform diagnostic tests (e.g., ABG, chest x-ray, viral studies, complete blood count, blood culture, sputum gram stain and culture) as indicated.
Administer antibiotic therapy.

(continued)

(continued)

Intervention
Treat wheezing with salbutamol by MDI or nebulizer solution.
Consider using CPAP or noninvasive ventilation. In severe cases endotracheal intubation and mechanical ventilation may be required.
Reduce metabolic demand by normalizing temperature and reducing the work of breathing.

Management of Chemical Pneumonitis

Chemical pneumonitis is an inflammation of the lung tissue caused by inhalation or aspiration of toxic liquids, gases, or particulate matter such as dust or fumes. Aspiration of hydrocarbons or inhalation of irritant gases (e.g., chlorine) can result in noncardiogenic pulmonary edema with increased capillary permeability.

In addition to initial interventions listed in Table 1, specific interventions for the *management of chemical pneumonitis* may include the following:

Intervention
Treat wheezing with nebulized bronchodilator.
Consider using CPAP or noninvasive ventilation. Intubation and mechanical ventilation may be required.
In a child with rapidly progressive symptoms, obtain early consultation. Refer to a specialized centre because advanced technologies (e.g., high-frequency oscillation or pediatric extracorporeal membrane oxygenation [ECMO]) may be required.

Management of Aspiration Pneumonitis

Aspiration pneumonitis is a form of chemical pneumonitis that results from the toxic effects of oral secretions or stomach acid and enzymes and the subsequent inflammatory response.

General management of lung tissue disease includes the initial interventions listed in Table 1. Specific interventions for the *management of aspiration pneumonitis* may include the following:

Intervention
Consider using CPAP or noninvasive ventilation. Intubation and mechanical ventilation may be required in severe cases.
Consider administration of antibiotics if the child has an elevated temperature and an infiltrate is present on chest x-ray. Prophylactic antimicrobial therapy is not indicated.

Management of Cardiogenic Pulmonary Edema

In cardiogenic pulmonary edema, high pressure in the pulmonary vessels causes fluid to leak into the lung interstitium and alveoli. The most common cause of acute cardiogenic pulmonary edema in children is left ventricular myocardial dysfunction. This can be caused by congenital heart disease, myocarditis, inflammatory processes, hypoxia, and cardiac-depressant drugs (e.g., β-adrenergic blockers, tricyclic antidepressants, calcium channel blockers).

In addition to initial interventions listed in Table 1, specific interventions for the *management of cardiogenic pulmonary edema* may include the following:

Intervention
Provide ventilatory support (i.e., noninvasive ventilation or mechanical ventilation with PEEP) as needed.
Consider diuretics to reduce left atrial pressure, inotropic infusions and afterload-reducing agents to improve myocardial function. Obtain expert consultation.
Reduce metabolic demand by normalizing temperature and reducing the work of breathing.

Indications for ventilatory support (noninvasive ventilation or endotracheal intubation with mechanical ventilation) in children with cardiogenic pulmonary edema include:

- Persistent hypoxemia despite noninvasive ventilation
- Impending respiratory failure
- Hemodynamic compromise (e.g., hypotension, severe tachycardia, signs of shock)

PEEP is added during mechanical ventilation to help reduce the need for high O_2 concentrations. It is usually started at 6 to 10 cm H_2O and adjusted upward until O_2 saturation improves. Too much PEEP may create pulmonary hyperinflation that impedes pulmonary venous return and thus cardiac output and O_2 delivery.

Management of Noncardiogenic Pulmonary Edema

ARDS usually follows a pulmonary (e.g., pneumonia or aspiration) or systemic (e.g., sepsis, pancreatitis, trauma) disease process that injures the interface between alveoli and pulmonary vessels and triggers release of inflammatory mediators. Early recognition and treatment of bacteremia,

shock, and respiratory failure may help prevent the progression to ARDS.

The following are characteristics of ARDS:

- Acute onset
- PaO_2/FIO_2 <200 (regardless of PEEP)
- Bilateral infiltrates on chest x-ray
- No evidence for a cardiogenic cause of pulmonary edema

In addition to initial interventions listed in Table 1, specific interventions for the *management of ARDS* may include the following:

Intervention
Monitor heart rate and rhythm, blood pressure, respiratory rate, pulse oximetry, and end-tidal CO_2.
Obtain laboratory studies, including ABG, central venous blood gas, and complete blood count.
Provide ventilatory support (i.e., noninvasive ventilation or mechanical ventilation with PEEP) as needed.

Indications for ventilatory support (noninvasive ventilation or endotracheal intubation with mechanical ventilation) in children with ARDS are:

- Worsening clinical and radiographic lung disease
- Hypoxemia refractory to high concentrations of inspired O_2

Correction of hypoxemia is the most important intervention. This is accomplished by increasing PEEP until O_2 saturation is adequate. "Permissive" hypercarbia is a treatment approach that recognizes that correction of increased $PaCO_2$ is less important than correction of hypoxemia. Maintaining low tidal volumes (5 to 7 mL/kg) and keeping peak inspiratory pressure <30 to 35 cm H_2O is more important than correcting the $PaCO_2$.

Management of Disordered Control of Breathing

Disordered control of breathing results in an abnormal respiratory pattern that produces inadequate minute ventilation. Common causes of disordered control of breathing are increased intracranial pressure (ICP) and neuromuscular disease (weakness). Conditions that depress the level of consciousness (e.g., central nervous system infection, seizures, metabolic disorders such as

---

FYI **Endotracheal Intubation in Children with Lung Tissue Disease**	When endotracheal intubation is anticipated in children with lung tissue disease, providers should anticipate the need to use PEEP and higher airway pressures. To ensure that both can be provided effectively, a cuffed ET tube is helpful to prevent glottic air leak. When using a cuffed tube, carefully monitor cuff inflation pressure and maintain it according to manufacturer's recommendations (typically <20 to 25 cm H_2O).

hyperammonemia, poisoning or drug overdose) also cause disordered control of breathing.

General Management of Disordered Control of Breathing

General management for treatment of disordered control of breathing includes the initial interventions listed in Table 1.

Specific Management of Disordered Control of Breathing by Etiology

Specific causes of *disordered control of breathing* require specific interventions. This section reviews the management of disordered control of breathing caused by the following:

- Increased ICP
- Poisoning or drug overdose
- Neuromuscular disease

Management of Respiratory Distress/Failure With Increased ICP

Increased ICP can be a complication of meningitis, encephalitis, intracranial abscess, subarachnoid hemorrhage, subdural or epidural hematoma, traumatic brain injury, hypoxic/ischemic insult, hydrocephalus, and central nervous system tumor. An irregular respiratory pattern is one sign of increased ICP. A combination of irregular breathing or apnea, an increase in mean arterial pressure, and bradycardia is called *Cushing's triad*. This triad suggests a marked increase in ICP and impending brain herniation. However, children with increased ICP also can present with irregular breathing, hypertension, and tachycardia rather than with bradycardia.

If increased ICP is suspected, obtain neurosurgical consult. In addition to initial interventions listed in Table 1, specific interventions for *disordered control of breathing due to increased ICP* may include the following:

Intervention
If trauma is suspected and you need to open the airway, manually stabilize the cervical spine, and use a jaw-thrust maneuver.
Verify patent airway, adequate oxygenation, and adequate ventilation. A brief period of hyperventilation may be used as temporizing rescue therapy in response to signs of impending brain herniation (e.g., irregular respirations or apnea, bradycardia, hypertension, unequal or dilated pupil[s] not responsive to light, decerebrate or decorticate posturing).
If the child has poor perfusion or other evidence of poor end-organ function, administer 20 mL/kg IV isotonic crystalloid (NS or LR).

(continued)

(continued)

Intervention
Administer pharmacologic therapy for management of increased ICP (e.g., hypertonic saline, osmotic agents).
Treat agitation and pain aggressively once the airway is established and ventilation is adequate.
Avoid hyperthermia.

Management of Respiratory Distress/Failure in Poisoning or Drug Overdose

One of the most common causes of respiratory distress or failure after a poisoning or drug overdose is depression of central respiratory drive; a less common cause is weakness or paralysis of respiratory muscles.

Complications of disordered breathing in this setting include upper airway obstruction, poor respiratory effort and rate, hypoxemia, aspiration, and respiratory failure. Complications from a decreased level of consciousness (e.g., aspiration pneumonitis and noncardiogenic pulmonary edema) may also result in respiratory failure. If you suspect poisoning, contact your local poison control centre. For more information on toxicology, see Part 12.7 of the *2010 Guidelines for CPR and ECC*.

Support of airway and ventilation is the main therapeutic intervention. In addition, interventions for *disordered control of breathing due to poisoning or drug overdose* may include the following:

Intervention
Contact your local poison control centre.
Be prepared to suction the airway in case of vomiting.
Administer antidote as indicated.
Perform diagnostic tests as indicated (e.g., ABG, ECG, chest x-ray, electrolytes, glucose, serum osmolality, and drug screen).

Respiratory Management in Neuromuscular Disease

Chronic progressive neuromuscular diseases can affect the muscles of respiration. Affected children can develop an ineffective cough and difficulty managing secretions. Complications include atelectasis, restrictive lung disease, pneumonia, chronic respiratory insufficiency, and respiratory failure. Consider the initial interventions listed in Table 1 for disordered control of breathing due to neuromuscular disease. For children with advanced restrictive lung disease, long-term noninvasive ventilation may be used.

Summary: Management of Respiratory Emergencies Flowchart

The Management of Respiratory Emergencies Flowchart summarizes general management of respiratory emergencies and specific management by etiology. Note that this chart does not include all respiratory emergencies; it provides key management strategies for a limited number of diseases.

Management of Respiratory Emergencies Flowchart

- Airway positioning
- Suction as needed
- Oxygen
- Pulse oximetry
- ECG monitor (as indicated)
- BLS as indicated

Upper Airway Obstruction
Specific Management for Selected Conditions

Croup	Anaphylaxis	Aspiration Foreign Body
• Nebulized epinephrine • Corticosteroids	• IM epinephrine (or autoinjector) • Salbutamol • Antihistamines • Corticosteroids	• Allow position of comfort • Specialty consultation

Lower Airway Obstruction
Specific Management for Selected Conditions

Bronchiolitis	Asthma
• Nasal suctioning • Bronchodilator trial	• Salbutamol ± ipratropium • Corticosteroids • Subcutaneous epinephrine • Magnesium sulfate • Terbutaline

Lung Tissue Disease
Specific Management for Selected Conditions

Pneumonia/Pneumonitis Infectious Chemical Aspiration	Pulmonary Edema Cardiogenic or Noncardiogenic (ARDS)
• Salbutamol • Antibiotics (as indicated)	• Consider noninvasive or invasive ventilatory support with PEEP • Consider vasoactive support • Consider diuretic

Disordered Control of Breathing
Specific Management for Selected Conditions

Increased ICP	Poisoning/Overdose	Neuromuscular Disease
• Avoid hypoxemia • Avoid hypercarbia • Avoid hyperthermia	• Antidote (if available) • Contact poison control	• Consider noninvasive or invasive ventilatory support

Figure 1. Management of Respiratory Emergencies Flowchart.

Suggested Reading List

Frazier M, Cheifetz I. The role of heliox in paediatric respiratory disease. *Paediatr Respir Rev.* 2010;11:46-53.

Kairys SW, Olmstead EM, O'Connor GT. Steroid treatment of laryngotracheitis: a meta-analysis of the evidence from randomized trials. *Pediatrics.* 1989;83:683-693.

Munoz-Bonet JI, Flor-Macian EM, Rosello PM, Llopis MC, Lizondo A, Lopez-Prats JL, Brines J. Noninvasive ventilation in pediatric acute respiratory failure by means of a conventional volumetric ventilator. *World J Pediatr.* 2010;6:323-330.

Yanez LJ, Yunge M, Emilfork M, Lapadula M, Alcantara A, Fernandez C, Lozano J, Contreras M, Conto L, Arevalo C, Gayan A, Hernandez F, Pedraza M, Feddersen M, Bejares M, Morales M, Mallea F, Glasinovic M, Cavada G. A prospective, randomized, controlled trial of noninvasive ventilation in pediatric acute respiratory failure. *Pediatr Crit Care Med.* 2008;9:484-489.

Anaphylaxis

Ben-Shoshan M, Clarke AE. Anaphylaxis: past, present and future. *Allergy.* 2011;66:1-14.

ARDS

Randolph AG. Management of acute lung injury and acute respiratory distress syndrome in children. *Crit Care Med.* 2009;37:2448-2454.

Bronchiolitis

American Academy of Pediatrics Subcommittee on Diagnosis and Management of Bronchiolitis. Diagnosis and management of bronchiolitis. *Pediatrics.* 2006;118: 1774-1793.

Fernandes RM, Bialy LM, Vandermeer B, Tjosvold L, Plint AC, Patel H, Johnson DW, Klassen TP, Hartling L. Glucocorticoids for acute viral bronchiolitis in infants and young children. *Cochrane Database Syst Rev.* 2010;(10):CD004878.

Langley JM, Smith MB, LeBlanc JC, Joudrey H, Ojah CR, Pianosi P. Racemic epinephrine compared to salbutamol in hospitalized young children with bronchiolitis: a randomized controlled clinical trial [ISRCTN46561076]. *BMC Pediatr.* 2005;5:7.

Ralston S, Hartenberger C, Anaya T, Qualls C, Kelly HW. Randomized, placebo-controlled trial of albuterol and epinephrine at equipotent beta-2 agonist doses in acute bronchiolitis. *Pediatr Pulmonol.* 2005;40:292-299.

Zorc JJ, Hall CB. Bronchiolitis: recent evidence on diagnosis and management. *Pediatrics.* 2010;125:342-349.

Croup

Bjornson CL, Johnson DW. Croup. *Lancet.* 2008;371: 329-339.

Bjornson CL, Klassen TP, Williamson J, Brant R, Mitton C, Plint A, Bulloch B, Evered L, Johnson DW. A randomized trial of a single dose of oral dexamethasone for mild croup. *N Engl J Med.* 2004;351:1306-1313.

Cetinkaya F, Tufekci BS, Kutluk G. A comparison of nebulized budesonide, and intramuscular, and oral dexamethasone for treatment of croup. *Int J Pediatr Otorhinolaryngol.* 2004;68:453-456.

Cherry JD. Clinical practice. Croup. *N Engl J Med.* 2008; 358:384-391.

Geelhoed GC, Turner J, Macdonald WB. Efficacy of a small single dose of oral dexamethasone for outpatient croup: a double blind placebo controlled clinical trial. *BMJ.* 1996;313:140-142.

Kristjansson S, Berg-Kelly K, Winso E. Inhalation of racemic adrenaline in the treatment of mild and moderately severe croup: clinical symptom score and oxygen saturation measurements for evaluation of treatment effects. *Acta Paediatr.* 1994;83:1156-1160.

Luria JW, Gonzalez-del-Rey JA, DiGiulio GA, McAneney CM, Olson JJ, Ruddy RM. Effectiveness of oral or nebulized dexamethasone for children with mild croup. *Arch Pediatr Adolesc Med.* 2001;155:1340-1345.

Vorwerk C, Coats T. Heliox for croup in children. *Cochrane Database Syst Rev.* 2010;(2):CD006822.

Vorwerk C, Coats TJ. Use of helium-oxygen mixtures in the treatment of croup: a systematic review. *Emerg Med J.* 2008; 25:547-550.

Status Asthmaticus

Andrews T, McGintee E, Mittal MK, Tyler L, Chew A, Zhang X, Pawlowski N, Zorc JJ. High-dose continuous nebulized levalbuterol for pediatric status asthmaticus: a randomized trial. *J Pediatr.* 2009;155:205-210.

Bigham MT, Jacobs BR, Monaco MA, Brilli RJ, Wells D, Conway EM, Pettinichi S, Wheeler DS. Helium/oxygen-driven albuterol nebulization in the management of children with status asthmaticus: a randomized, placebo-controlled trial. *Pediatr Crit Care Med.* 2010;11:356-361.

Browne L, Gorelick M. Asthma and pneumonia. *Pediatr Clin North Am.* 2010;57:1347-1356.

Ciarallo L, Brousseau D, Reinert S. Higher-dose intravenous magnesium therapy for children with moderate to severe acute asthma. *Arch Pediatr Adolesc Med*. 2000;154: 979-983.

Expert Panel Report 3 (EPR-3): Guidelines for the Diagnosis and Management of Asthma—Summary Report 2007. *J Allergy Clin Immunol*. 2007;120(suppl):S94-S138.

Plotnick LH, Ducharme FM. Acute asthma in children and adolescents: should inhaled anticholinergics be added to β_2-agonists? *Am J Respir Med*. 2003;2:109-115.

Plotnick LH, Ducharme FM. Combined inhaled anticholinergic agents and β_2-agonists for initial treatment of acute asthma in children. *Cochrane Database Syst Rev*. 2000;(2):CD000060.

Szefler S. Advances in pediatric asthma in 2010: addressing the major issues. *J Allergy Clin Immunol.* 2011;127:102-115.

Resources for Management of Respiratory Emergencies

Bag-Mask Ventilation
Overview

Bag-mask ventilation can provide adequate oxygenation and ventilation for a child with no breathing or inadequate breathing despite a patent airway. Signs of inadequate breathing are apnea, abnormal respiratory rate, inadequate breath sounds, and hypoxemia despite supplementary O_2. When properly performed, bag-mask ventilation is as effective as ventilation through an ET tube for short periods and may be safer. In the out-of-hospital setting, bag-mask ventilation is especially useful if the transport time is short or providers are inexperienced in insertion of advanced airways or have insufficient opportunities to maintain competence in this skill.

Preparation for the Course

All healthcare providers who care for infants and children should be able to provide ventilation effectively with a bag and mask. In the PALS Provider Course you will be required to demonstrate effective bag-mask ventilation during BLS testing, in the respiratory management skills station, and in some case simulations.

How to Select and Prepare the Equipment

For ventilation to be effective with a bag-mask device, you must know how to select the face mask, prepare the ventilation bag, and provide supplementary O_2 if needed.

Face Mask

Select a face mask that extends from the bridge of the child's nose to the cleft of the chin, covering the nose and mouth but not compressing the eyes (Figure 1). The mask should have a soft rim (e.g., flexible cuff) that molds easily to create a tight seal against the face. If the face-mask seal

is not tight, O_2 intended for ventilation will escape under the mask, and ventilation will not be effective.

Select a transparent mask if available. A transparent mask allows you to see the colour of the child's lips and condensation on the mask (which indicates exhalation). You will also be able to observe for regurgitation.

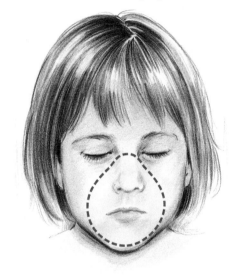

Figure 1. Proper area of the face for face-mask application. Note that no pressure is applied to the eyes.

Ventilation Bag

There are 2 basic types of ventilation bags:

- Self-inflating bag
- Flow-inflating bag

Self-Inflating Bag

A self-inflating bag is typically used for initial resuscitation. A self-inflating bag consists of a bag with an intake valve and a nonrebreathing outlet valve. The intake valve allows

---

Critical Concept

Use O_2 During Resuscitation

Attach an O_2 reservoir to the self-inflating bag as soon as possible during resuscitation. Frequently verify that O_2 is attached and flowing to the bag. Remember to:

- Listen for O_2 flow
- Check O_2 tank pressure or verify connection to a wall O_2 source

Once circulation is adequate and when appropriate equipment is available, titrate O_2 administration to maintain an O_2 saturation of 94% to 99%.

the bag to fill with either room air (Figures 2C and D) or O_2 (Figures 2A and B). When you compress the bag, the intake valve closes and the nonrebreathing outlet valve opens, allowing either room air or an air-O_2 gas mixture to flow to the child. When the child exhales, the nonrebreathing outlet valve closes and exhaled gases are vented. The nonrebreathing outlet valve is designed to prevent the child from rebreathing CO_2.

Even when supplementary O_2 is attached, the concentration of delivered O_2 varies from 30% to 80%. The amount of delivered O_2 is affected by tidal volume and peak inspiratory flow rate. To deliver a high O_2 concentration (60% to 95%), attach an O_2 reservoir to the intake valve (Figures 2A and

B). Maintain an O_2 flow of 10 to 15 L/min into a reservoir attached to a pediatric bag and a flow of at least 15 L/min into an adult bag.

Check to see if the bag has a pop-off valve. Many self-inflating bags have a pressure-limited pop-off valve set at 35 to 45 cm H_2O to prevent development of excessive airway pressures. If the child's lung compliance is poor or airway resistance is high or CPR is needed, an automatic pop-off valve may prevent delivery of sufficient tidal volume, resulting in inadequate ventilation and chest expansion. Ventilation bags used during CPR should have *no pop-off valve* or the valve should be twisted into the closed position.

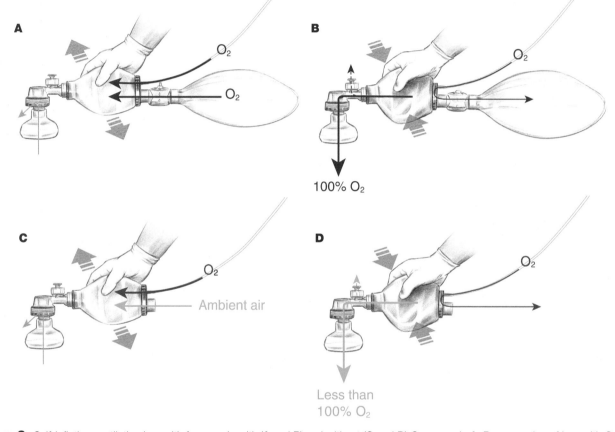

Figure 2. Self-inflating ventilation bag with face mask, with (**A** and **B**) and without (**C** and **D**) O_2 reservoir. **A,** Re-expansion of bag with O_2 reservoir. When the provider's hand releases the bag, O_2 flows into the bag from the O_2 source and from the reservoir, so the concentration of O_2 in the bag remains 100%. **B,** Compression of bag with O_2 reservoir delivers 100% O_2 to the patient (purple arrow). O_2 continuously flows into the reservoir. **C,** Re-expansion of the bag without an O_2 reservoir. When the provider's hand releases the bag, O_2 flows into the bag from the O_2 source, but ambient air is also entrained into the bag, so the bag becomes filled with a mixture of O_2 and ambient air. **D,** Compression of the bag without O_2 reservoir delivers O_2 mixed with room air (aqua arrow). Note that with both setups exhaled patient air flows into the atmosphere near the connection of the mask and bag (see gray arrows from mask in **A** and **C**).

Critical Concept	Self-inflating bag-mask devices with a fish-mouth or leaf-flap–operated nonrebreathing outlet valve do not provide a continuous flow of O_2 to the mask. Such valves open *only* if the bag is squeezed *or* the mask is sealed tightly to the face and the child generates significant inspiratory force to open the valve. Many infants cannot generate the inspiratory pressure required to open the outlet valve. *Do not use this type of bag to provide supplementary O_2 to a spontaneously breathing infant or child.*
Caution: Continuous O_2 Flow Not Possible With Some Self-Inflating Bags	

FYI **Providing PEEP During Bag-Mask Ventilation**	Use of PEEP may improve oxygenation in children with lung tissue disease or low lung volumes. Provide PEEP during ventilation with a bag by adding a compatible spring-loaded ball or disk or a magnetic-disc PEEP valve to the bag-mask or bag-tube system. Do *not* use self-inflating bag-mask devices equipped with PEEP valves to provide CPAP *during spontaneous breathing* because the outlet valve in the bag will not open (and provide gas flow) unless the child generates very high negative inspiratory pressure.

Flow-Inflating Bag

A flow-inflating bag (Figure 3), also called an *anesthesia bag*, may be used in the intensive care unit, delivery room, and operating room. It requires O_2 flow to operate. Safe and effective ventilation with a flow-inflating bag requires more experience than is needed to use a self-inflating bag. To provide effective ventilation with a flow-inflating bag, the provider must be able to adjust the flow of O_2, adjust the outlet control valve, ensure a proper seal with the face mask, and deliver the appropriate tidal volume at the correct rate. For these reasons, flow-inflating bags should be used only by trained and experienced providers.

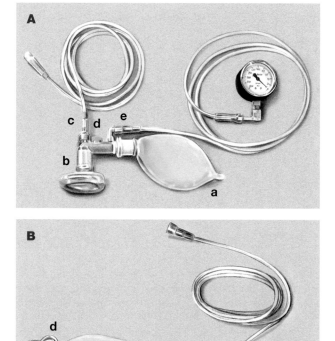

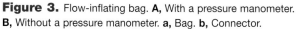

Figure 3. Flow-inflating bag. **A,** With a pressure manometer. **B,** Without a pressure manometer. **a,** Bag. **b,** Connector. **c,** Oxygen inflow port. **d,** Outlet port with adjustable valve. **e,** Pressure monitoring port.

Bag Size

Use a self-inflating bag with a volume of at least 450 to 500 mL for infants and young children. Smaller bags may not deliver an effective tidal volume over the longer inspiratory times required by full-term neonates and infants. In older children or adolescents, you may need to use an adult self-inflating bag (1000 mL) to achieve chest rise.

How to Test the Device

Check all components of the self-inflating bag and mask before use to ensure proper function. To test the device:

- Check the bag for leaks by occluding the patient outlet valve with your hand and squeezing the bag.
- Check the gas flow control valves to verify proper function.
- Check the pop-off valve (if present) to ensure that it can be closed.
- Check that the O_2 tubing is securely connected to the device and the O_2 source.
- Listen for the sound of O_2 flowing into the bag.
- Ensure that the cuff of the mask (if present) is adequately inflated.

How to Position the Child

Properly position the child to maintain an open airway. During bag-mask ventilation it may be necessary to move the child's head and neck gently through a range of positions to optimize ventilation. A "sniffing" position without hyperextension of the neck is usually best for infants and toddlers.

To achieve a "sniffing" position, place the child supine. Flex the child's neck forward at the level of the shoulders while extending the head. Position the opening of the external ear canal at the level of or in front of the anterior aspect of the shoulder while the head is extended (Figure 4). Avoid hyperextending the neck because this may obstruct the airway.

Children >2 years of age may require padding under the occiput. Younger children and infants may need padding under the shoulders or upper torso to prevent excessive flexion of the neck that can occur when the prominent occiput rests on a flat surface.

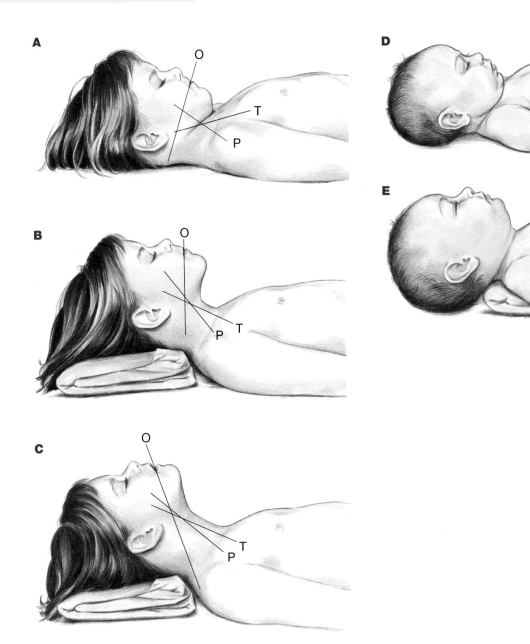

Figure 4. Correct positioning of the child >2 years of age for ventilation and endotracheal intubation. **A,** With the child on a flat surface (e.g., bed or table), the oral (O), pharyngeal (P), and tracheal (T) axes pass through 3 divergent planes. **B,** A folded sheet or towel placed under the occiput aligns the pharyngeal and tracheal axes. **C,** Extension of the atlanto-occipital joint results in the alignment of the oral, pharyngeal, and tracheal axes. Note that proper positioning places the external ear canal anterior to the shoulder. **D,** Incorrect position with neck flexion. **E,** Correct position for infant. Note that the external ear canal is anterior to the shoulder. Reproduced from Coté CJ, Todres ID. The pediatric airway. In: Coté CJ, Ryan JF, Todres ID, Goudsouzian NG, eds. *A Practice of Anesthesia for Infants and Children.* 2nd ed. Philadelphia, PA: WB Saunders Co; 1993:55-83, copyright Elsevier.

How to Perform Bag-Mask Ventilation

Bag-mask ventilation can be performed by 1 or 2 providers. Because effective bag-mask ventilation requires complex steps, bag-mask ventilation is not recommended for a lone rescuer during CPR. During CPR the lone rescuer should use the mouth-to–barrier device technique for ventilation. Bag-mask ventilation can be provided effectively during 2-rescuer CPR.

1-Person Bag-Mask Ventilation Technique

If 1 healthcare provider is performing bag-mask ventilation, the provider must open the airway and keep the mask sealed to the child's face with one hand (Figure 5) and squeeze the bag with the other hand. Effective bag-mask ventilation requires a tight seal between the mask and the child's face. Use the E-C clamp technique described below to open the airway and achieve a tight seal.

Step	Action
1	To open the airway and make a seal between the mask and the face *in the absence of suspected cervical spine injury*, tilt the head back. Use the E-C clamp technique to lift the jaw against the mask, pressing and sealing the mask on the face. This technique moves the tongue away from the posterior pharynx, moves the jaw forward, and opens the mouth. Lifting the jaw toward the mask helps seal the mask against the face. If possible, the mouth should be open under the mask, as a result of either lifting the jaw or insertion of an oropharyngeal airway.
2	With the other hand, squeeze the ventilation bag until the chest rises. Deliver each breath over 1 second. Avoid excessive ventilation (see "How to Deliver Effective Ventilation" in this section).

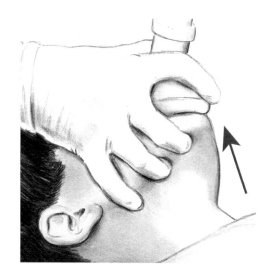

Figure 5. One-handed E-C clamp face-mask application technique. Three fingers of one hand lift the jaw (they form the "E") while the thumb and index finger hold the mask to the face (making a "C").

2-Person Bag-Mask Ventilation Technique

If 2 healthcare providers are available to perform bag-mask ventilation, one provider uses both hands to open the airway and keep the mask sealed to the child's face and the other provider squeezes the bag (Figure 6). Both providers should observe the child's chest to ensure that chest rise is visible. Be careful to avoid delivering too high a tidal volume, which may result in excessive ventilation.

Critical Concept **E-C Clamp Technique**	The technique of opening the airway and making a seal between the mask and the face is called the *E-C clamp technique*. The third, fourth, and fifth fingers of one hand (forming an "E") are positioned along the jaw to lift it forward; then the thumb and index finger of the same hand (forming a "C") make a seal to hold the mask to the face. Avoid pressure on the soft tissues underneath the chin (the submental area) because this can push the tongue into the posterior pharynx, resulting in airway compression and obstruction.
Critical Concept **Effective Ventilation With a Bag-Mask**	Give each breath slowly over about 1 second. Watch for chest rise. If the chest does not rise, reopen the airway. Verify that there is a tight seal between the mask and the face. Reattempt ventilation.
FYI **Feeling for Changes in Lung Compliance**	When performing bag-mask ventilation, be aware of the child's lung compliance. A poorly compliant lung is "stiff" or difficult to inflate. A sudden increase in lung stiffness during ventilation with a bag may indicate airway obstruction, decreased lung compliance, or pneumothorax. Lung overdistention from excessive inflating pressures, PEEP, or rapid assisted respiratory rates with short exhalation time may also cause the feel of "stiff lungs" during ventilation.

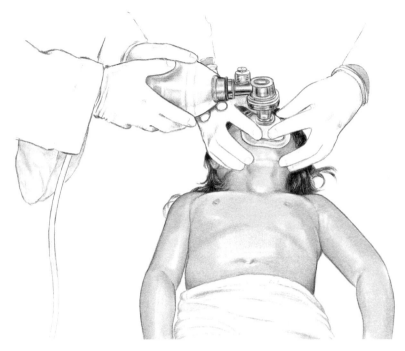

Figure 6. Two-person bag-mask ventilation technique may provide more effective ventilation than 1-person ventilation when there is significant airway obstruction or poor lung compliance. One provider uses both hands to open the airway and maintain a tight mask-to-face seal while the other provider squeezes the ventilation bag.

The 2-person technique may provide more effective bag-mask ventilation than a 1-person technique. Also, 2-person bag-mask ventilation may be necessary when:

- There is difficulty making a seal between the face and the mask
- The provider's hands are too small to reach from the front of the mask to behind the jaw or to open the airway and create a seal between the face and mask
- There is significant airway resistance (i.e., asthma) or poor lung compliance (i.e., pneumonia or pulmonary edema)
- Cervical spine immobilization is necessary

How to Deliver Effective Ventilation

Avoid excessive ventilation; use only the force and tidal volume necessary to just make the chest rise.

Precaution

Healthcare providers often deliver excessive ventilation during CPR. Excessive ventilation is harmful because it:

- Increases intrathoracic pressure and impedes venous return, which decreases cardiac output, coronary perfusion, and cerebral blood flow
- Causes air trapping and barotrauma in children with small airway obstruction
- Increases the risk of regurgitation and aspiration in children without an advanced airway

Parameters of Oxygenation and Ventilation

Frequently monitor the following parameters to assess the effectiveness of oxygenation and ventilation:

- Visible chest rise with each breath
- O_2 saturation
- Exhaled CO_2
- Heart rate
- Blood pressure
- Distal air entry
- Signs of improvement or deterioration (e.g., appearance, colour, agitation)

If effective ventilation is not achieved (i.e., the chest does not rise), do the following:

- Reposition/reopen the airway: attempt to further lift the jaw and ensure that the child is placed in a sniffing position.
- Verify mask size and ensure a tight face-mask seal.
- Suction the airway if needed.
- Check the O_2 source.
- Check the ventilation bag and mask.
- Treat gastric inflation.

Gastric Inflation and Cricoid Pressure

Gastric inflation may interfere with effective ventilation and cause regurgitation. To minimize gastric inflation:

- Avoid creation of excessive peak inspiratory pressures by delivering each breath over about 1 second

- Consider application of cricoid pressure, but only in an unresponsive victim if another healthcare provider is present
- Avoid excessive cricoid pressure so as not to obstruct the trachea and interfere with delivering positive pressure breaths

There is insufficient evidence to recommend routine cricoid pressure application to prevent aspiration during endotracheal intubation in children.

Endotracheal Intubation

Potential Indications

Consider endotracheal intubation if the child is unable to maintain effective airway, oxygenation, or ventilation despite initial intervention.

Preparation for Endotracheal Intubation

In the Management of Respiratory Emergencies Skills Station you will need to know the equipment needed for endotracheal intubation (Table 1).

Table 1. Pre-event Equipment Checklist for Endotracheal Intubation

❏	Universal precautions (gloves, mask, eye protection)
❏	Cardiac monitor, pulse oximeter, and blood pressure monitoring device
❏	End-tidal CO_2 detector or exhaled CO_2 capnography (or esophageal detector device, if appropriate)
❏	Intravenous and intraosseous infusion equipment
❏	Oxygen supply, bag mask (appropriate size)
❏	Oral/tracheal suction equipment (appropriate size); confirm that it is working
❏	Oral and nasopharyngeal airways (appropriate size)
❏	Endotracheal tubes with stylets (all sizes, with and without cuffs) and sizes 0.5 mm (i.d.) above and below anticipated size for patient
❏	Laryngoscope (curved and straight blades) and/or video laryngoscope; backup laryngoscope available
❏	Cuff pressure monitor (if using cuffed tubes)
❏	3-, 5-, and 10-mL syringes to test inflate endotracheal tube balloon
❏	Adhesive/cloth tape or commercial endotracheal tube holder to secure tube
❏	Towel or pad to align airway by placing under head or torso
❏	Specialty equipment as needed for difficult airway management or anticipated complications (supraglottic, transtracheal, and/or cricothyrotomy)

Part 6

Recognition of Shock

Overview

When shock is present, rapid identification and prompt intervention are critical to improving outcome. If left untreated, shock can quickly progress to cardiopulmonary failure followed by cardiac arrest. Once an infant or child develops cardiac arrest, the outcome is poor.

This Part discusses the following:

- Pathophysiology of shock
- Effect of different types of shock on blood pressure
- Systolic blood pressure as a method of categorizing the severity of shock (i.e., compensated or hypotensive)
- Etiology and signs of the 4 most common types of shock
- Systematic approach to evaluation of the cardiovascular system

Your evaluation will help you identify the child's shock based on type and severity. These clinical findings will direct your interventions, as discussed in Part 7: "Management of Shock."

Learning Objectives

After completing this Part you should be able to

- Explain the pathophysiology of shock
- Evaluate clinical signs of systemic perfusion
- Differentiate between compensated shock and hypotensive shock
- Describe 4 types of shock (hypovolemic, distributive, cardiogenic, and obstructive) and the signs and symptoms of each

Preparation for the Course

During the PALS Course you will need to identify different types and severities of shock. Your evaluation will help determine effective interventions.

Definition of Shock

Shock is a critical condition that results from inadequate tissue delivery of O_2 and nutrients to meet tissue metabolic demand. Shock is often, but not always, characterized by inadequate peripheral and end-organ perfusion. The definition of shock does not depend on blood pressure measurement; shock can occur with a normal, increased, or decreased systolic blood pressure. In children most shock is characterized by low cardiac output; however, in some types of shock (e.g., caused by sepsis or anaphylaxis), cardiac output may be high. All types of shock can result in impaired function of vital organs, such as the brain (decreased level of consciousness) and kidneys (low urine output, ineffective filtering).

Shock can result from:

- Inadequate blood volume or oxygen-carrying capacity (hypovolemic shock, including hemorrhagic shock)
- Inappropriate distribution of blood volume and flow (distributive shock)
- Impaired cardiac contractility (cardiogenic shock)
- Obstructed blood flow (obstructive shock)

Conditions such as fever, infection, injury, respiratory distress, and pain may contribute to shock by increasing tissue demand for O_2 and nutrients. Whether due to inadequate

Identify and Intervene **Shock**	The earlier you recognize shock, establish priorities, and start therapy, the better the child's chance for a good outcome.

supply, increased demand, or a combination of both, *O_2 and nutrient delivery to the tissues is inadequate relative to metabolic needs*. Inadequate tissue perfusion can lead to tissue hypoxia, anaerobic metabolism, accumulation of lactic acid and CO_2, irreversible cell damage, and, ultimately, organ damage. Death may then result rapidly from cardiovascular collapse or more slowly from multiorgan failure.

Pathophysiology of Shock

The major function of the cardiopulmonary system is to deliver O_2 to body tissues and remove metabolic by-products of cellular metabolism (primarily CO_2). When O_2 delivery is inadequate to meet tissue demand, cells use anaerobic metabolism to produce energy, but this generates lactic acid as a by-product. Anaerobic metabolism can only maintain limited cell function. Unless O_2 delivery is restored, organ dysfunction or failure will result.

Components of Tissue Oxygen Delivery

Adequate tissue O_2 delivery (Figure 1) depends on:

- Sufficient O_2 content in the blood
- Adequate blood flow to the tissues (cardiac output)
- Appropriate distribution of blood flow to the tissues

O_2 content of the blood is determined primarily by the hemoglobin concentration and percent of the hemoglobin that is saturated with O_2 (SaO_2).

Adequate blood flow to the tissues is dependent on cardiac output and vascular resistance. Cardiac output (the volume of blood pumped by the heart per minute) is the product of stroke volume (the volume of blood pumped with each beat) and heart rate (number of beats per minute):

Cardiac Output = Stroke Volume × Heart Rate

According to this formula, if the heart rate decreases, stroke volume must increase to maintain the cardiac output. It also shows that cardiac output can increase either by an increase in heart rate, stroke volume, or both. Increasing the cardiac output by increasing heart rate does, however, have its limit. If the heart rate is too fast, as can happen with certain ingestions or a tachyarrhythmia (e.g., supraventricular tachycardia), stroke volume decreases because there is inadequate time to fill the heart (i.e., the diastolic phase is too short).

Infants have a very small stroke volume that cannot increase very much. Infants are therefore dependent on an

| **FYI**
Central Venous O_2 Saturation and Cardiac Output | In healthy children with normal metabolic demand, the arterial blood contains more O_2 than the tissues need. If demand increases and/or O_2 delivery decreases, the tissues will extract a greater percent of the O_2 delivered. This results in reduced O_2 saturation in the venous blood returning to the heart. The central venous O_2 saturation therefore can be used to assess the balance between O_2 delivery and demand. If metabolic demand and O_2 content are unchanged, a decreased central venous O_2 saturation indicates a fall in cardiac output and, therefore, a fall in O_2 delivered to the tissues. In addition, greater extraction of O_2 has occurred as the result of reduced delivery. |

FYI **Compensatory Mechanisms for Hypoxemia**	Tissue hypoxia is present when a region of the body or an organ is deprived of adequate O_2 supply. Low blood O_2 saturation (hypoxemia) alone does not necessarily result in tissue hypoxia. Tissue oxygenation and O_2 delivery are determined by the volume of blood pumped per minute (cardiac output) and the blood's arterial O_2 content (determined chiefly by the hemoglobin concentration and its saturation with O_2). O_2 delivery may be normal despite hypoxemia if cardiac output increases commensurate with the decrease in O_2 content.
	When hypoxemia is chronic (e.g., unrepaired cyanotic heart disease), hemoglobin concentration increases (polycythemia). The increased hemoglobin concentration will increase the O_2-carrying capacity of the blood and help maintain arterial O_2 content at near-normal levels, despite the fact that hemoglobin saturation is low.
	If cardiac output decreases or hypoxemia worsens, these compensatory mechanisms may not be sufficient to maintain tissue O_2 delivery, and tissue hypoxia will likely develop.

adequate heart rate to maintain or increase cardiac output. With growth, children develop the ability to increase stroke volume, and cardiac output becomes less dependent on the heart rate.

Appropriate distribution of blood flow is determined by the size of the blood vessels supplying a specific organ. This property is known as *vascular resistance*. If the vessel is large, vascular resistance is low; if the vessel is small, vascular resistance is high. Vascular resistance is adjusted by tissues to locally regulate blood flow to meet metabolic demands. Abnormally increased resistance (vasoconstriction) or decreased resistance (vasodilation) can interfere with blood flow distribution, even if cardiac output is adequate.

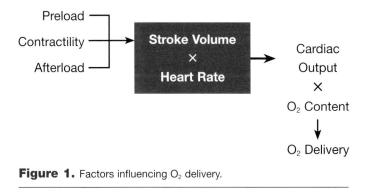

Figure 1. Factors influencing O_2 delivery.

Stroke Volume

Stroke volume is the amount of blood ejected by the heart with each beat. Stroke volume is determined by 3 factors:

Factor	Clinical Definition
Preload	Volume of blood present in the ventricle before contraction
Contractility	Strength of contraction
Afterload	Resistance against which the ventricle is ejecting

Inadequate *preload* is the most common cause of low stroke volume and, therefore, low cardiac output. A number of conditions (e.g., hemorrhage, severe dehydration, or vasodilation) can cause inadequate preload. Inadequate preload results in hypovolemic shock.

Poor contractility (also referred to as *myocardial dysfunction*) impairs stroke volume and cardiac output. It can lead to cardiogenic shock. Poor contractility can be due to an intrinsic problem with pump function or an acquired abnormality, such as an inflamed heart muscle (i.e., myocarditis). Poor contractility also can occur from metabolic problems, such as hypoglycemia, or from toxic ingestions (e.g., calcium channel blockers).

Increased afterload is an uncommon primary cause of low stroke volume and impaired cardiac output in children. Certain conditions, such as severe pulmonary hypertension or congenital abnormalities of the aorta, can increase afterload so significantly that cardiogenic shock results.

FYI Preload	Preload is often estimated by the central venous pressure, but the relationship between central venous pressure and volume of blood in the ventricles is complex. Preload to the ventricles is the volume of blood in the ventricles before a contraction (end-diastolic volume). In general, for the right ventricle, this corresponds with the central venous pressure, measured in the superior vena cava or right atrium. In most cases an increase in the central venous pressure reflects an increase in right ventricular end-diastolic volume and preload. However, if there is increased pressure around the right atrium from a tension pneumothorax or pericardial tamponade, end-diastolic volume may be decreased despite increased central venous pressure. This is because venous return to the heart is obstructed. If congenital heart disease or pulmonary hypertension is present, preload to the right ventricle may differ from preload to the left ventricle.
	Preload is not the same as total blood volume. At steady state most of the blood (about 70%) is in the veins. If the veins are dilated, the total blood volume may be normal or increased, but an inadequate amount of blood may be returning to the heart. This is part of the problem with sepsis: there is inappropriate vasodilation and maldistribution of blood flow and blood volume, so preload to the heart may be inadequate.

FYI

Negative Effects of High Afterload in Cardiogenic Shock

High afterload in children with poor myocardial function can further impair stroke volume and cardiac output. When cardiac output is reduced, the body responds with vasoconstriction in an attempt to maintain blood pressure and blood flow to vital organs. Paradoxically, vasoconstriction increases impedance to ventricular ejection and further decreases stroke volume and cardiac output. An essential component of the advanced treatment of cardiogenic shock is afterload reduction.

Compensatory Mechanisms

As shock develops, compensatory mechanisms attempt to maintain O_2 delivery to vital organs. These include

- Tachycardia
- Increase in systemic vascular resistance (SVR) (vasoconstriction)
- Increase in strength of cardiac contraction (contractility)
- Increase in venous smooth muscle tone

The body's first action to maintain cardiac output is to increase heart rate (tachycardia). *Tachycardia* can increase cardiac output to a limited degree. The more rapid the heart rate, the shorter the ventricular filling time until ventricular filling time becomes so short that stroke volume and cardiac output decrease. A decrease in cardiac output will produce a decrease in O_2 delivery to the tissues.

When O_2 delivery to the tissues is compromised, blood flow is redirected or shunted from nonvital organs and tissues (e.g., skin, skeletal muscles, gut, kidneys) to vital organs (e.g., brain, heart). This redirection occurs by a selective *increase in SVR (vasoconstriction).* Clinically this results in reduced peripheral perfusion (i.e., delayed capillary refill, cool extremities, less easily palpable peripheral pulses), and reduced perfusion to the gut and kidneys (decreased urine volume).

Another compensatory mechanism to maintain stroke volume and cardiac output is an *increase in strength of cardiac contractions (contractility)* with more complete emptying of the ventricles. Stroke volume may also be supported by an *increase in venous smooth muscle tone,* improving venous return to the heart and preload.

Effect on Blood Pressure

Blood pressure is the product of cardiac output and SVR. As cardiac output decreases, blood pressure is maintained as long as SVR increases. In children with shock, this compensatory mechanism can be so effective that systolic blood pressure may initially remain normal or even slightly elevated. Pulse pressure, the difference between the systolic and diastolic blood pressure, is often narrowed because an increase in SVR raises the diastolic pressure. In contrast, if SVR is low (as in sepsis), diastolic blood pressure decreases and pulse pressure widens.

If cardiac output is inadequate, tissue perfusion is compromised, even if blood pressure is normal. Signs of poor tissue perfusion, including lactic acidosis and end-organ dysfunction, will be present even if blood pressure is normal.

When SVR cannot increase further, blood pressure begins to decline. At that point, delivery of O_2 to vital organs is severely compromised. Clinical signs include metabolic acidosis and evidence of end-organ dysfunction (e.g., impaired mental status and decreased urine output). Ultimately O_2 delivery to the myocardium becomes inadequate, causing myocardial dysfunction, decreased stroke volume, and hypotension. These may rapidly lead to cardiovascular collapse, cardiac arrest, and irreversible end-organ injury.

Identification of Shock by Severity (Effect on Blood Pressure)

The severity of shock is frequently characterized by its effect on systolic blood pressure. Shock is described as *compensated* if compensatory mechanisms are able to maintain a systolic blood pressure within a normal range (i.e., at least the 5th percentile systolic blood pressure for age). When compensatory mechanisms fail and systolic blood pressure declines, shock is classified as *hypotensive* (previously referred to as *decompensated*).

You can easily identify hypotensive shock by measuring blood pressure; compensated shock is more difficult to diagnose. Shock can range from mild to severe. Its manifestations are affected by the type of shock and the child's compensatory responses. Blood pressure is used to determine severity of shock; however, children with both compensated and hypotensive shock are at high risk for deterioration. The child with low cardiac output (i.e., hypovolemic shock) but normal blood pressure due to vasoconstriction may have more end-organ compromise than the child with normal or increased cardiac output (i.e., septic shock) and low systolic blood pressure.

Because blood pressure is one method of categorizing the severity of shock, it is important to recognize that automated blood pressure devices are accurate only when there is adequate distal perfusion. If you cannot palpate distal pulses and the extremities are cool and poorly perfused, automated blood pressure readings may not be reliable. Treat the child based on your entire clinical evaluation. If measurement of blood pressure is not feasible, use clinical evaluation of tissue perfusion to guide treatment.

Critical Concept Systolic Blood Pressure in Identification of Shock	Note that the term *compensated shock* refers to the child with signs of poor perfusion but a normal systolic blood pressure (i.e., with blood pressure compensation). Systolic blood pressure is used by convention and consensus to determine the presence or absence of hypotension with shock. Infants and children with compensated shock may be critically ill despite an adequate systolic blood pressure.

Compensated Shock

If systolic blood pressure is within the normal range but there are signs of inadequate tissue perfusion, the child is in *compensated* shock. In this stage of shock the body is able to maintain blood pressure despite impaired delivery of O_2 and nutrients to the vital organs.

When O_2 delivery is limited, compensatory mechanisms try to maintain normal blood flow to the brain and heart. These compensatory mechanisms are clues to the presence of shock and vary according to the type of shock. Table 1 lists common compensatory mechanisms in shock and the cardiovascular signs associated with these mechanisms.

Table 1. Common Signs of Shock Resulting From Cardiovascular Compensatory Mechanisms

Compensatory Mechanism	Area	Sign
Increased heart rate	Heart	Tachycardia
Increased SVR	Skin	Cold, pale, mottled, diaphoretic
	Peripheral circulation	Delayed capillary refill
	Pulses	Weak peripheral pulses; narrow pulse pressure (increased diastolic blood pressure)
Increased renal and splanchnic vascular resistance (redistribution of blood flow away from these areas)	Kidney	Oliguria (decreased urine output)
	Intestine	Vomiting, ileus

Signs specific to shock type are discussed in "Identification of Shock by Type" later in this Part.

Hypotensive Shock

Hypotension develops when physiologic attempts to maintain systolic blood pressure and perfusion are no longer effective. A key clinical sign of deterioration is a change in level of consciousness as brain perfusion declines. Hypotension is a late finding in most types of shock and may signal impending cardiac arrest. Hypotension can occur early in septic shock because mediators of sepsis produce vasodilation and reduce SVR. In this setting the child may initially appear to have warm extremities, brisk capillary refill, and full peripheral pulses despite hypotension.

Hypotension Formula

In children 1 to 10 years of age, hypotension is present if the systolic blood pressure reading is less than

70 mm Hg + [child's age in years × 2] mm Hg

For more information, see Part 2, Table 4: Definition of Hypotension by Systolic Blood Pressure and Age.

Physiologic Continuum

Be alert to the progression of clinical signs that may signal a worsening of the child's condition. These signs will develop along a continuum from compensated shock to hypotensive shock and ultimately to cardiac arrest. Decreased peripheral pulses and prolonged capillary refill time occur early in shock progression. Progressive tachypnea and tachycardia are indicators of worsening status. Later warning signs include loss of peripheral pulses and decreasing level of consciousness. Bradycardia and weak central pulses in a child with signs of shock are ominous signs of impending cardiac arrest.

Accelerating Process

Shock progression is unpredictable. It may take hours for compensated shock to progress to hypotensive shock but only minutes for hypotensive shock to progress to cardiopulmonary failure and cardiac arrest. This progression is typically an *accelerating process.*

Critical Concept Hypotension in Septic Shock	SVR may be increased or decreased in septic shock. When SVR is decreased, hypotension will be an early rather than a late sign of shock.

Critical Concept	Early recognition and rapid intervention are critical to halting the progression from compensated shock to hypotensive shock to cardiopulmonary failure and cardiac arrest.
Halting the Progression	

Compensated Shock

⬇ Possibly hours

Hypotensive Shock

⬇ Potentially minutes

Cardiac Arrest

These and other clinical manifestations are discussed in greater detail later in this Part.

Identification of Shock by Type

Shock can be categorized into 4 basic types (see Figure 2 near the end of this Part):

- Hypovolemic
- Distributive
- Cardiogenic
- Obstructive

Hypovolemic Shock

Hypovolemia is the most common cause of shock in children worldwide. Fluid loss from diarrhea is the leading cause of hypovolemic shock and a major worldwide cause of infant mortality. Volume loss that can lead to hypovolemic shock can result from

- Diarrhea
- Vomiting
- Hemorrhage (internal and external)
- Inadequate fluid intake
- Osmotic diuresis (e.g., DKA)
- Third-space losses (fluid leak into tissues)
- Large burns

Hypovolemic shock is the result of an absolute deficiency of intravascular blood volume, but in fact it typically represents depletion of both intravascular and extravascular fluid volume. As a result, adequate fluid resuscitation often requires administration of fluid boluses that exceed the volume of the estimated intravascular deficit.

Tachypnea, a respiratory compensation to maintain acid-base balance, is often present in hypovolemic shock. The respiratory alkalosis that results from hyperventilation partially compensates for the metabolic acidosis (lactic acidosis) that accompanies shock.

Physiology of Hypovolemic Shock

Hypovolemic shock is characterized by decreased preload leading to reduced stroke volume and low cardiac output.

Tachycardia, increased SVR, and increased cardiac contractility are the main compensatory mechanisms.

Hypovolemic Shock		
Preload	**Contractility**	**Afterload**
Decreased	Normal or increased	Increased

Signs of Hypovolemic Shock

Table 2 outlines typical signs of hypovolemic shock found during the initial impression and primary assessment.

Although septic, anaphylactic, neurogenic, and other distributive forms of shock are not classified as hypovolemic, they are characterized by *relative* hypovolemia. The relative hypovolemia results from arterial and venous vasodilation, increased capillary permeability, and plasma loss into the interstitium ("third spacing" or capillary leak).

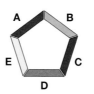

Table 2. Findings Consistent With Hypovolemic Shock

Primary Assessment	Finding
A	Typically patent unless level of consciousness is significantly impaired
B	Tachypnea without increased effort (quiet tachypnea)
C	• Tachycardia • Adequate systolic blood pressure, narrow pulse pressure, or systolic hypotension with a narrow pulse pressure • Weak or absent peripheral pulses • Normal or weak central pulses • Delayed capillary refill • Cool to cold, pale, mottled, diaphoretic skin • Dusky/pale distal extremities • Changes in level of consciousness • Oliguria
D	Changes in level of consciousness
E	Extremities often cooler than trunk

Distributive Shock

Distributive shock is characterized by inappropriate distribution of blood volume with inadequate organ and tissue perfusion (especially the splanchnic vascular bed).

The most common forms of distributive shock are

- Septic shock
- Anaphylactic shock
- Neurogenic shock (e.g., head injury, spinal injury)

Distributive shock caused by sepsis is characterized by reduced or increased SVR resulting in maldistribution of blood flow. The vasodilation and venodilation cause pooling of blood in the venous system and a relative hypovolemia. Septic shock also causes increased capillary permeability, so there is loss of plasma from the vascular space. This increases the severity of the hypovolemia. Myocardial contractility may also be depressed in septic shock.

In anaphylactic shock, venodilation, arterial vasodilation, and increased capillary permeability combined with pulmonary vasoconstriction reduce cardiac output. The low cardiac output is caused by relative hypovolemia and increased right ventricular afterload.

Neurogenic shock is characterized by generalized loss of vascular tone, most often following a high cervical spine injury. The loss of vascular tone leads to severe vasodilation and hypotension. Normally, the sympathetic nervous system increases heart rate in response to hypotension. Children with neurogenic shock may be unable to generate a faster heart rate in response to hypotension. As a result cardiac output and blood flow to tissues decrease dramatically.

Pathophysiology of Distributive Shock

In distributive shock cardiac output may be increased, normal, or decreased. Although myocardial dysfunction may be present, stroke volume can be adequate, particularly if there is aggressive volume resuscitation. Tachycardia and an increase in ventricular end-diastolic volume help maintain cardiac output. Tissue perfusion is compromised by maldistribution of blood flow. Some tissue beds (e.g., splanchnic circulation) may be inadequately perfused; in other tissues (e.g., some skeletal muscle and skin) perfusion may exceed metabolic needs. Hypoxic tissues generate lactic acid, leading to metabolic acidosis. Early in the clinical course a child with distributive shock may present with decreased SVR and increased blood flow to the skin. This produces warm extremities and bounding peripheral pulses ("warm shock").

The high cardiac output and low SVR often observed in distributive shock differ from the low cardiac output and high SVR seen in hypovolemic, cardiogenic, and obstructive shock. As distributive shock progresses, concomitant hypovolemia and/or myocardial dysfunction produce a decrease in cardiac output. SVR can then increase, resulting in inadequate blood flow to the skin, cold extremities, and weak pulses ("cold shock"). The late phase of distributive shock therefore can be similar to the clinical picture of hypovolemic and cardiogenic shock.

Distributive Shock		
Preload	**Contractility**	**Afterload**
Normal or decreased	Normal or decreased	Variable

Distributive shock is most often characterized by many changes in cardiovascular function, including

- Low SVR, which causes the wide pulse pressure characteristic of distributive shock and contributes to early hypotension. Late in the clinical course, SVR may increase.
- Increased blood flow to some peripheral tissue beds
- Inadequate perfusion of the splanchnic (gut and kidney) vascular bed
- Release of inflammatory and other mediators and vaso-active substances

FYI **Central Venous O$_2$ Saturation in Septic Shock**	In contrast to hypovolemic and cardiogenic shock, central venous O$_2$ saturation may be normal or increased in septic shock. There are 2 mechanisms to explain this observation: • Children with low SVR and increased cardiac output will extract less O$_2$ from the blood because some tissues are receiving more blood flow than they need. Other tissues don't receive enough blood flow so they don't have the opportunity to extract the O$_2$. • Children with sepsis may be unable to utilize O$_2$ at the cellular level. Toxins and inflammatory mediators circulating in sepsis can prevent aerobic metabolism even in the setting of adequate O$_2$ delivery. As a result, lactic acidosis and end-organ dysfunction can occur even in the setting of normal or increased central venous O$_2$ saturation.

Critical Concept **Relative Hypovolemia**	Although most types of distributive shock are not typically classified as hypovolemic shock, all are characterized by relative hypovolemia unless adequate fluid resuscitation is provided.

- Volume depletion caused by capillary leak
- Accumulation of lactic acid in poorly perfused tissue beds

Signs of Distributive Shock

Table 3 outlines typical signs of distributive shock seen during the initial impression and primary assessment. The **bold** text denotes type-specific signs that distinguish distributive shock from other forms of shock.

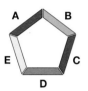

Table 3. Findings Consistent With Distributive Shock

Primary Assessment	Finding
A	Usually patent unless level of consciousness is significantly impaired
B	Tachypnea, usually without increased work of breathing ("quiet tachypnea") unless the child has pneumonia or is developing ARDS or cardiogenic pulmonary edema
C	• Tachycardia • **Bounding peripheral pulses** • **Brisk or delayed capillary refill** • **Warm, flushed skin peripherally (warm shock)** *or* **Pale, mottled skin with vasoconstriction (cold shock)** • **Hypotension with a wide pulse pressure (warm shock)** *or* **Hypotension with a narrow pulse pressure (cold shock)** *or* • Normotension • Changes in level of consciousness • Oliguria
D	Changes in level of consciousness

(continued)

(continued)

Primary Assessment	Finding
E	• Fever or hypothermia • Extremities warm or cool • Petechial or purpuric rash (septic shock)

Septic Shock

Septic shock is the most common form of distributive shock. It is caused by infectious organisms or their by-products (e.g., endotoxin) that stimulate the immune system and trigger release or activation of inflammatory mediators.

Pathophysiology of Septic Shock

Septic shock in children typically evolves along a continuum from a systemic inflammatory response in the early stages to septic shock in the late stages. This continuum may evolve over days or just a few hours; there is wide variability in clinical presentation and progression.

Septic Shock		
Preload	**Contractility**	**Afterload**
Decreased	Normal to decreased	Variable

For more information about the definition and characteristics of pediatric sepsis, see the Suggested Reading List at the end of this Part.

Signs of Septic Shock

In the early stages, signs of septic shock are often subtle and may be difficult to recognize because peripheral perfusion may appear to be good. Because septic shock is triggered by an infection or its by-products, the child may have fever or hypothermia, and the white blood cell (WBC) count may be decreased, normal, or increased.

In addition to the findings listed in Table 3, the child with septic shock may have other abnormalities identified by diagnostic tests. Examples include metabolic acidosis, respiratory alkalosis, leukocytosis (high WBC count), leukopenia (low WBC count), or left shift (increased percent of bands or immature white blood cells).

| FYI

Inflammatory Cascade Response to Sepsis | The pathophysiology of the septic cascade includes the following, often referred to as the *systemic inflammatory response:*

- The infectious organism or its by-products (e.g., endotoxin) activates the immune system, including neutrophils, monocytes, and macrophages.
- These cells, or their interaction with the infecting organism, stimulate release or activation of inflammatory mediators (cytokines).
- Cytokines produce vasodilation and damage to the lining of the blood vessels (endothelium), causing increased capillary permeability.
- Cytokines activate the coagulation cascade, and may result in microvascular thrombosis and disseminated intravascular coagulation (DIC).
- Specific inflammatory mediators can impair cardiac contractility and cause myocardial dysfunction. |

| FYI

The Difficulty of Treating Septic Shock | In septic shock the combination of inadequate perfusion and possible microvascular thrombosis leads to ischemia, which is diffuse and patchy so that individual organs have varying levels of hypoxia and ischemia within and between them. The variability of perfusion throughout the body is what makes treatment of sepsis so difficult. |

| FYI

Adrenal Insufficiency in Septic Shock | The adrenal glands are especially prone to microvascular thrombosis and hemorrhage in septic shock. Because adrenal glands produce cortisol, an important hormone in the body's stress response, children with sepsis may develop absolute or relative adrenal insufficiency. Adrenal insufficiency contributes to low SVR and myocardial dysfunction in septic shock. |

| *Identify and Intervene*

Septic Shock | *Early recognition and treatment of septic shock are critically important determinants of outcome.* You should evaluate systemic perfusion and clinical signs of end-organ function to identify sepsis before hypotensive shock develops. If you suspect sepsis, and especially if shock develops, provide aggressive volume resuscitation and hemodynamic support (see Part 7: "Management of Shock" for details). Search for and treat the underlying cause. |

Anaphylactic Shock

Anaphylactic shock is an acute multisystem allergic response caused by a severe reaction to a drug, vaccine, food, toxin, plant, venom, or other antigen. The reaction is characterized by venodilation, arterial vasodilation, increased capillary permeability, and pulmonary vasoconstriction. It can occur within seconds to minutes after a sensitized child is exposed to the offending allergen.

Physiology of Anaphylactic Shock

Pulmonary vasoconstriction acutely increases right heart afterload. It may reduce pulmonary blood flow, pulmonary venous return, and preload to the left ventricle, thus decreasing cardiac output. Death may occur immediately or the child may develop acute-phase symptoms, which typically begin 5 to 10 minutes after exposure.

Anaphylactic Shock		
Preload	**Contractility**	**Afterload**
Decreased	Variable	Left ventricle: Decreased

Right ventricle: Increased |

Signs of Anaphylactic Shock

Signs and symptoms may include

- Anxiety or agitation
- Nausea and vomiting
- Urticaria (hives)
- Angioedema (swelling of the face, lips, and tongue)
- Respiratory distress with stridor or wheezing
- Hypotension
- Tachycardia

Angioedema may cause partial or complete upper airway obstruction. Hypotension results from vasodilation, hypovolemia, and diminished cardiac output. Relative hypovolemia is caused by the vasodilation, and absolute volume loss is caused by capillary leak.

Neurogenic Shock

Neurogenic shock, also known as *spinal shock*, results from a cervical (neck) or upper thoracic (above T6) injury that disrupts the sympathetic nervous system innervation of blood vessels and the heart.

Physiology of Neurogenic Shock

The sudden loss of sympathetic nervous system signals to the smooth muscle in the vessel walls results in uncontrolled vasodilation. The same disruption prevents development of tachycardia as a compensatory mechanism.

Neurogenic Shock		
Preload	**Contractility**	**Afterload**
Decreased	Normal	Decreased

Signs of Neurogenic Shock

Primary signs of neurogenic shock are

- Hypotension with a wide pulse pressure
- Normal heart rate or bradycardia

Other signs may include increased respiratory rate, diaphragmatic breathing (use of muscles in the diaphragm rather than the chest wall), and other evidence of a high thoracic or cervical spine injury (i.e., motor or sensory deficits).

Neurogenic shock must be differentiated from hypovolemic shock. Hypovolemic shock is typically associated with hypotension, a narrow pulse pressure from compensatory vasoconstriction, and compensatory tachycardia. In neurogenic shock, these compensatory mechanisms cannot take place because sympathetic innervation of the heart and blood vessels is interrupted.

Cardiogenic Shock

Cardiogenic shock results from inadequate tissue perfusion secondary to myocardial dysfunction. Common causes of cardiogenic shock include

- Congenital heart disease
- Myocarditis (inflammation of the heart muscle)
- Cardiomyopathy (an inherited or acquired abnormality of pumping function)
- Arrhythmias
- Sepsis
- Poisoning or drug toxicity
- Myocardial injury (e.g., trauma)

Physiology of Cardiogenic Shock

Cardiogenic shock is characterized by marked tachycardia, high SVR, and decreased cardiac output. End-diastolic volume within the left and right ventricles is increased, resulting in congestion within the pulmonary and systemic venous systems. Pulmonary venous congestion leads to pulmonary edema and increased work of breathing. Typically, intravascular volume is normal or increased unless a concurrent illness causes hypovolemia (e.g., in a child who has viral myocarditis with recent vomiting and fever).

Cardiogenic Shock		
Preload	**Contractility**	**Afterload**
Variable	Decreased	Increased

Cardiogenic shock is often characterized by sequential compensatory and pathologic mechanisms, including

- Increase in heart rate and left ventricular afterload, which increases left ventricular work and myocardial O_2 consumption
- Compensatory increase in SVR to redirect blood from peripheral and splanchnic tissues to the heart and brain
- Decrease in stroke volume due to decreased myocardial contractility and increased afterload
- Increased venous tone, which increases central venous (right atrial) and pulmonary capillary (left atrial) pressures
- Diminished renal blood flow resulting in fluid retention
- Pulmonary edema resulting from myocardial failure and high left ventricular end-diastolic, left atrial, and pulmonary venous pressure, and from increased venous tone and fluid retention

The same compensatory mechanisms that maintain perfusion to the brain and heart in hypovolemic shock are often detrimental during cardiogenic shock. For example, compensatory peripheral vasoconstriction can maintain blood pressure in hypovolemic shock. However, because it increases left ventricular afterload (increased resistance to left ventricular ejection), compensatory vasoconstriction has detrimental effects in cardiogenic shock.

Because the heart muscle also needs O_2, almost all children with severe or sustained shock may eventually have inadequate myocardial O_2 delivery relative to myocardial O_2 demand. Therefore, severe or sustained shock of any type eventually causes impaired myocardial function (i.e., these children develop cardiogenic shock in addition to the primary cause of shock). Once myocardial function declines, the child's clinical status usually deteriorates rapidly.

Signs of Cardiogenic Shock

Table 4 outlines signs of cardiogenic shock typically found during the initial impression and primary assessment of the child. The **bold** text denotes type-specific signs that distinguish cardiogenic shock from other forms of shock.

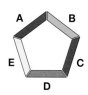

Table 4. Findings Consistent With Cardiogenic Shock

Primary Assessment	Finding
A	Usually patent unless level of consciousness is significantly impaired
B	• Tachypnea • **Increased respiratory effort (retractions, nasal flaring, grunting) resulting from pulmonary edema**
C	• Tachycardia • Normal or low blood pressure with a narrow pulse pressure • Weak or absent peripheral pulses • Normal and then weak central pulses • Delayed capillary refill with cool extremities • **Signs of congestive heart failure (e.g., pulmonary edema, hepatomegaly, jugular venous distention)** • **Cyanosis (caused by cyanotic congenital heart disease or pulmonary edema)** • Cold, pale, mottled, diaphoretic skin • Changes in level of consciousness • Oliguria
D	Changes in level of consciousness
E	Extremities often cooler than trunk

Rapid volume resuscitation of *cardiogenic* shock in the setting of poor myocardial function can aggravate pulmonary edema and further impair myocardial function. This can further compromise oxygenation, ventilation, and cardiac output. Volume resuscitation for cardiogenic shock should be gradual. Give smaller (5 to 10 mL/kg) boluses of isotonic crystalloid and deliver over a longer period of time (i.e., over 10 to 20 minutes). Carefully monitor hemodynamic parameters during fluid infusion and repeat infusion as needed.

Infants and children with cardiogenic shock often require medications to increase and redistribute cardiac output, improve myocardial function, and reduce SVR. Direct treatment to reduce metabolic demand, such as decreasing work of breathing and controlling fever. This will allow a limited cardiac output to better meet tissue metabolic demands. For more details, see Part 7: "Management of Shock."

Obstructive Shock

In obstructive shock, cardiac output is impaired by a physical obstruction of blood flow. Causes of obstructive shock include

- Cardiac tamponade
- Tension pneumothorax
- Ductal-dependent congenital heart lesions
- Massive pulmonary embolism

The physical obstruction to blood flow results in low cardiac output, inadequate tissue perfusion, and a compensatory increase in SVR. The early clinical presentation of obstructive shock can be indistinguishable from hypovolemic shock. Careful clinical examination, however, may reveal signs of systemic or pulmonary venous congestion that are not consistent with hypovolemia. As the condition progresses, increased respiratory effort, cyanosis, and signs of vascular congestion become more apparent.

Obstructive Shock		
Preload	**Contractility**	**Afterload**
Variable	Normal	Increased

Critical Concept

Distinguishing Signs of Cardiogenic Shock

Increased respiratory effort often distinguishes cardiogenic shock from hypovolemic shock. Hypovolemic shock is characterized by "quiet tachypnea," while children with cardiogenic shock may demonstrate retractions, grunting, and use of accessory muscles.

In cardiogenic shock there may be decreased arterial O_2 saturation secondary to pulmonary edema.

Pathophysiology and Clinical Signs of Obstructive Shock

Pathophysiology and clinical signs vary according to the cause of the obstructive shock.

Cardiac Tamponade

Cardiac tamponade is caused by an accumulation of fluid, blood, or air in the pericardial space. Increased intrapericardial pressure and compression of the heart impede systemic venous and pulmonary venous return. This reduces ventricular filling and causes a decrease in stroke volume and cardiac output. If untreated, cardiac tamponade results in cardiac arrest with pulseless electrical activity (PEA).

In children, cardiac tamponade most often occurs after penetrating trauma or cardiac surgery. It also may develop as a result of pericardial effusion complicating an inflammatory disorder, a tumor or extremely high white blood cell count, or an infection of the pericardium. Table 5 outlines signs of cardiac tamponade typically found during the initial impression and primary assessment. The signs unique to pericardial tamponade are in **bold** type.

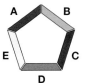

Table 5. Findings Consistent With Cardiac Tamponade

Primary Assessment	Finding
A	Usually patent unless level of consciousness is significantly impaired
B	Respiratory distress with increased respiratory rate and effort
C	• Tachycardia • Poor peripheral perfusion (weak distal pulses, cool extremities, delayed capillary refill) • **Muffled or diminished heart sounds** • Narrowed pulse pressure • **Pulsus paradoxus** (decrease in systolic blood pressure by >10 mm Hg during inspiration) • Distended neck veins (may be difficult to see in infants, especially with severe hypotension)
D	Changes in level of consciousness
E	Extremities often cooler than trunk

FYI	
Pulsus Paradoxus	*Pulsus paradoxus* is an exaggerated manifestation of a normal variation in stroke volume that occurs during the phases of respiration. Stroke volume decreases slightly during inspiration and increases slightly during expiration. In pulsus paradoxus the blood pressure declines by >10 mm Hg on inspiration, compared with expiration. True assessment for pulsus paradoxus requires measurement of blood pressure with a manual pressure cuff. Inflate the cuff until no sounds are heard (as usual). Slowly decrease the cuff pressure and note the point at which the first Korotkoff sounds are initially heard, which will be when the child is exhaling. Continue to slowly deflate the cuff and note the point at which the Korotkoff sounds are heard consistently throughout the respiratory cycle. If the difference between these 2 points is >10 mm Hg, the child has a clinically significant pulsus paradoxus. You may be able to detect a significant pulsus paradoxus by palpation of the pulse, noting a distinct variation in pulse amplitude as the child inhales and exhales. Pulsus paradoxus may also be apparent on arterial and pulse oximetry waveforms but is not as easily quantified unless the waveform can be saved on the monitor screen or printed for review.

Note that after cardiovascular surgery in children, signs of tamponade may be indistinguishable from those of cardiogenic shock. Favorable outcome depends on urgent diagnosis and immediate treatment. In children with a large pericardial effusion, the ECG typically shows small QRS complexes (low voltage), but echocardiography provides a definitive diagnosis.

Tension Pneumothorax

Tension pneumothorax is caused by the entry of air into the pleural space and accumulation under pressure. This air can enter from lung tissue injured by an internal tear or a penetrating chest injury. An air leak that enters the pleural space but then stops spontaneously is called a *simple pneumothorax*. An ongoing leak can result from positive-pressure ventilation or chest trauma that forces air out of the injured lung and into the pleural space. If air continues to leak into the pleural space, it accumulates under pressure, creating a tension pneumothorax. As this pressure increases, it compresses the underlying lung and pushes the mediastinum to the opposite side of the chest. Compression of the lung rapidly causes respiratory failure. The high intrathoracic pressure and direct pressure on mediastinal structures (heart and great vessels) impede venous return, resulting in a rapid decline in cardiac output and hypotension. Untreated tension pneumothorax leads to cardiac arrest characterized by PEA.

Suspect tension pneumothorax in a victim of chest trauma or in any intubated child who deteriorates suddenly while receiving positive-pressure ventilation (including bag-mask or noninvasive ventilation). Table 6 outlines signs of tension pneumothorax typically found during the initial impression and primary assessment. Signs unique to tension pneumothorax are in **bold** type.

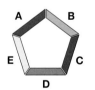

Table 6. Findings Consistent With Tension Pneumothorax

Primary Assessment	Finding
A	• Variable depending on situation and primary cause of respiratory distress • Advanced airway may already be in place • **Tracheal deviation toward contralateral side (may be difficult to appreciate in infants)**

(continued)

(continued)

Primary Assessment	Finding
B	• Respiratory distress with increased respiratory rate and effort • **Hyperresonance of affected side; hyperexpansion of affected side** • **Diminished breath sounds on affected side**
C	• Distended neck veins (may be difficult to appreciate in infants or in children with severe hypotension) • Pulsus paradoxus (decrease in systolic blood pressure by >10 mm Hg during inspiration) • Rapid deterioration in perfusion; commonly, rapid evolution from tachycardia to bradycardia and hypotension as cardiac output decreases
D	Changes in level of consciousness
E	Extremities often cooler than trunk

Favorable outcome depends on immediate diagnosis and treatment.

Ductal-Dependent Lesions

Ductal-dependent congenital cardiac abnormalities are usually present in the first days to weeks of life. Ductal-dependent lesions include

- Cyanotic congenital heart lesions (ductal dependent for pulmonary blood flow)
- Left ventricular outflow obstructive lesions (ductal dependent for systemic blood flow)

The ductal-dependent pulmonary blood flow lesions present with cyanosis rather than signs of shock. The left ventricular outflow obstructive lesions often present with signs of obstructive shock in the first few days or weeks of life when the ductus arteriosus closes. These left-sided lesions include coarctation of the aorta, interrupted aortic arch, critical aortic valve stenosis, and hypoplastic left heart syndrome. Restoring and maintaining patency of the ductus arteriosus is critical for survival, because the ductus serves as a conduit for systemic blood flow that bypasses the left-sided obstruction.

Table 7 outlines findings consistent with left ventricular outflow obstructive lesions that may be found during evaluation of the child. Those unique to left ventricular outflow obstructive lesions are in **bold** type.

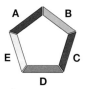

Table 7. Findings Consistent With Left Ventricular Outflow Obstructive Lesions

Primary Assessment	Finding
A	Usually patent unless level of consciousness is significantly impaired
B	Respiratory failure with signs of pulmonary edema or inadequate respiratory effort
C	• Rapid progressive deterioration in systemic perfusion • Congestive heart failure (cardiomegaly, hepatomegaly) • **Higher preductal versus postductal blood pressure (coarctation or interrupted aortic arch)** • **Higher (greater than 3% to 4%) preductal versus postductal arterial O$_2$ saturation (coarctation or interrupted aortic arch)** • Absence of femoral pulses (coarctation or interrupted aortic arch) • Metabolic acidosis (elevated lactate)
D	Rapid deterioration in level of consciousness
E	Cool skin

Massive Pulmonary Embolism

Pulmonary embolism is a total or partial obstruction of the pulmonary artery or its branches by a blood clot, fat, air, amniotic fluid, catheter fragment, or injected matter. Most commonly, a pulmonary embolus is a thrombus that migrates to the pulmonary circulation. Pulmonary embolism is rare in children but may develop when an underlying condition predisposes the child to intravascular thrombosis. Examples include central venous catheters, sickle cell

disease, malignancy, connective tissue disorders, and inherited disorders of coagulation (e.g., antithrombin III, protein S, and protein C deficiencies).

Pulmonary embolism results in ventilation/perfusion mismatch, hypoxemia, increased pulmonary vascular resistance leading to right heart failure, decreased left ventricular filling, and decreased cardiac output. Pulmonary embolism may be difficult to diagnose because signs may be subtle and nonspecific (cyanosis, tachycardia, and hypotension). Providers may not suspect pulmonary embolus, especially in children. Signs of congestion and right heart failure, however, do help distinguish it from hypovolemic shock. Some children with pulmonary embolism will complain of chest pain, reflecting lack of oxygenated blood flow to the lung tissue itself.

Table 8 outlines findings consistent with pulmonary embolism that may be found during evaluation of the child.

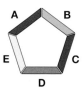

Table 8. Findings Consistent With Pulmonary Embolism

Primary Assessment	Finding
A	Usually patent unless level of consciousness is significantly impaired
B	Respiratory distress with increased respiratory rate and effort
C Assessment of Cardiovascular Function	• Tachycardia • Cyanosis • Hypotension • Systemic venous congestion and right heart failure • Chest pain
D	Changes in level of consciousness
E	Extremities may be cooler than trunk

Identify and Intervene **Ductal-Dependent Lesions**	If the infant is to survive, you must quickly recognize ductal-dependent lesions and promptly provide treatment to open and maintain a patent ductus arteriosus.

Identify and Intervene **Obstructive Shock**	Without early recognition and immediate treatment, children with obstructive shock often progress rapidly to cardiopulmonary failure and cardiac arrest.

Treatment of obstructive shock is cause specific; immediate recognition and correction of the underlying cause of the obstruction can be lifesaving. The most critical tasks for PALS providers are prompt recognition, diagnosis, and treatment of obstructive shock.

Recognition of Shock Flowchart

	Clinical Signs	Hypovolemic Shock	Distributive Shock	Cardiogenic Shock	Obstructive Shock
A	Patency	Airway open and maintainable/not maintainable			
B	Respiratory rate	Increased			
	Respiratory effort	Normal to increased		Labored	
	Breath sounds	Normal	Normal (± crackles)	Crackles, grunting	
C	Systolic blood pressure	Compensated Shock ➞ Hypotensive Shock			
	Pulse pressure	Narrow	Variable	Narrow	
	Heart rate	Increased			
	Peripheral pulse quality	Weak	Bounding or weak	Weak	
	Skin	Pale, cool	Warm or cool	Pale, cool	
	Capillary refill	Delayed	Variable	Delayed	
	Urine output	Decreased			
D	Level of consciousness	Irritable early Lethargic late			
E	Temperature	Variable			

Figure 2. Recognition of Shock Flowchart.

Suggested Reading List

Brierley J, Carcillo JA, Choong K, Cornell T, Decaen A, Deymann A, Doctor A, Davis A, Duff J, Dugas MA, Duncan A, Evans B, Feldman J, Felmet K, Fisher G, Frankel L, Jeffries H, Greenwald B, Gutierrez J, Hall M, Han YY, Hanson J, Hazelzet J, Hernan L, Kiff J, Kissoon N, Kon A, Irazuzta J, Lin J, Lorts A, Mariscalco M, Mehta R, Nadel S, Nguyen T, Nicholson C, Peters M, Okhuysen-Cawley R, Poulton T, Relves M, Rodriguez A, Rozenfeld R, Schnitzler E, Shanley T, Kache S, Skippen P, Torres A, von Dessauer B, Weingarten J, Yeh T, Zaritsky A, Stojadinovic B, Zimmerman J, Zuckerberg A. Clinical practice parameters for hemodynamic support of pediatric and neonatal septic shock: 2007 update from the American College of Critical Care Medicine. *Crit Care Med*. 2009;37:666-688.

Carcillo JA. Pediatric septic shock and multiple organ failure. *Crit Care Clin*. 2003;19:413-440, viii.

Finfer S, Bellomo R, Boyce N, French J, Myburgh J, Norton R. A comparison of albumin and saline for fluid resuscitation in the intensive care unit. *N Engl J Med*. 2004;350:2247-2256.

Part 7

Management of Shock

Overview

Once you identify shock in a critically ill or injured child, early intervention can reduce morbidity and mortality. This Part discusses goals and priorities of shock management, fundamentals of treatment, general and advanced management, and specific management according to etiology.

Learning Objectives

After completing this Part you should be able to

- Describe the general goals of shock management, including initial treatment priorities, monitoring, and ongoing management
- Describe effective fluid resuscitation
- Manage shock based on type and severity
- Summarize the principles of acute management of hypovolemic, distributive, cardiogenic, and obstructive shock

Preparation for the Course

During the course you will be asked to manage a child in shock. To do this you will need to know general and specific treatment based on the different types of shock.

Goals of Shock Management

The goals in treatment of shock are to improve O_2 delivery, balance tissue perfusion and metabolic demand, reverse perfusion abnormalities, restore organ function, and prevent progression to cardiac arrest. Speed of intervention is crucial: having the knowledge to identify shock and the skill to respond quickly may be lifesaving. The longer the interval

is between the precipitating event and the restoration of adequate O_2 delivery and organ perfusion, the poorer the outcome is. Once a child is in cardiac arrest, prognosis is very poor.

Warning Signs

Be alert to signs that compensatory mechanisms are failing in a seriously ill or injured child. Once you recognize that the child's condition is deteriorating, act decisively with the resuscitation team to provide effective resuscitative therapy. Warning signs that indicate progression from compensated to hypotensive shock include

- Increasing tachycardia
- Diminishing or absent peripheral pulses
- Weakening central pulses
- Narrowing pulse pressure
- Cold distal extremities with prolonged capillary refill
- Decreasing level of consciousness
- Hypotension (late finding)

Once the child is hypotensive, organ perfusion is typically severely compromised, and organ dysfunction may develop even if the child does not progress to cardiac arrest.

Fundamentals of Shock Management

The acute treatment of shock focuses on restoring O_2 delivery to the tissues and improving the balance between tissue perfusion and metabolic demand. The acute treatment of shock consists of

Identify and Intervene **Compensated Shock**	Early identification of compensated shock is critical to effective treatment and good outcome.

85

- Optimizing O_2 content of the blood
- Improving volume and distribution of cardiac output
- Reducing O_2 demand
- Correcting metabolic derangements

Try to identify and reverse the underlying cause of shock while providing prompt interventions.

Optimizing Oxygen Content of the Blood

O_2 content of the blood is determined by the oxygenation of hemoglobin and the hemoglobin concentration. To optimize O_2 content

- Administer a high concentration of O_2 (use nonrebreathing mask to deliver 100% O_2)
- Use invasive or noninvasive mechanical ventilation to improve oxygenation by correcting a ventilation/blood flow (V/Q) mismatch or other respiratory disorders
- If hemoglobin concentration is low, consider packed red blood cell (PBRC) transfusion

Improving Volume and Distribution of Cardiac Output

Measures to improve the volume and distribution of cardiac output are based on the type of shock:

- Hypovolemic
- Distributive
- Cardiogenic
- Obstructive

Hypovolemic Shock

Rapid administration of isotonic crystalloid fluids is indicated for most children who present with signs and symptoms of hypovolemic shock. Use vital signs and physical examination to assess the child's response to each fluid bolus. Look for ongoing evidence of hypovolemia or fluid loss to determine the need for additional fluids.

Distributive Shock

Suspect distributive shock when there is evidence of low systemic vascular resistance (SVR, wide pulse pressure) and maldistribution of blood flow (e.g., vasodilation and warm skin). Although the end result is inadequate O_2 delivery to organs, the primary abnormality is low SVR caused by the host response to invading organisms (e.g., sepsis) or loss of vasomotor tone (e.g., anaphylaxis or spinal cord injury) and increased capillary permeability.

Management of distributive shock is aimed at rapidly restoring intravascular volume to better fill the vasodilated vascular space. If hypotension persists despite administration of fluids, consider vasopressors to combat the primary problem of low SVR. Although cardiac output is typically increased early in distributive shock if there are

signs of myocardial dysfunction, use inotropic agents to improve cardiac contractility.

Cardiogenic Shock

Suspect cardiogenic shock when there are signs of poor perfusion and pulmonary or systemic venous congestion (e.g., increased work of breathing, grunting respirations, distended neck veins, or hepatomegaly). In addition, consider cardiogenic shock when there is clinical deterioration in perfusion and respiratory function in response to fluid resuscitation.

If signs are consistent with cardiogenic shock, focus treatment on improving cardiac output while reducing metabolic demand when possible. Specific treatments may include noninvasive or invasive positive-pressure ventilation to reduce the work of breathing and improve oxygenation. Consider a cautious, slow infusion of IV fluid using 5 to 10 mL/kg over 10 to 20 minutes with careful observation for any signs of deterioration. Selection of inotropic and vasodilator therapy is determined by the need to maintain adequate blood pressure, restore tissue perfusion, and/or minimize the adverse effects of inotropes on myocardial O_2 demand. See the section "Medication Therapy" later in this Part.

Expert consultation is recommended early in the management of children with cardiogenic shock. Selection of the best vasoactive drug may be guided by information from echocardiography or other studies. Children may benefit from vasodilator, inodilator, and/or inotropic therapy to reduce afterload, improve contractility, and increase blood flow to vital organs.

Obstructive Shock

Suspect obstructive shock when the child demonstrates signs of elevated central venous pressure, venous congestion with poor peripheral perfusion, and rapid development of hypotension. Support cardiovascular function (e.g., with bolus fluid administration and possible vasoactive agents) while you perform further assessment and diagnostic studies and obtain expert consultation. The key to management of obstructive shock is to quickly identify and treat the cause.

Reducing Oxygen Demand

For all forms of shock, try to improve the balance between O_2 delivery and supply by using measures to reduce O_2 demand. The most common factors that contribute to increased O_2 demand are

- Increased work of breathing
- Pain and anxiety
- Fever

Support breathing with noninvasive ventilation or endotracheal intubation and assisted ventilation. To facilitate intubation and mechanical ventilation, you may need to administer sedatives or analgesics and neuromuscular blockade. Control pain and anxiety with analgesics and sedatives. Use sedative and analgesic agents cautiously; they may suppress the child's endogenous stress response and impair compensatory mechanisms, such as tachycardia. Control fever by administering antipyretics and other cooling measures.

Correcting Metabolic Derangements

Many conditions that lead to shock may result in or be complicated by metabolic derangements, including

- Hypoglycemia
- Hypocalcemia
- Hyperkalemia
- Metabolic acidosis

All of these conditions can adversely affect cardiac contractility. Metabolic acidosis is characteristic of all forms of shock.

Hypoglycemia is low serum glucose. Glucose is vital for proper cardiac and brain function. Glucose stores may be low in infants and chronically ill children. Untreated hypoglycemia can cause seizures and brain injury.

Hypocalcemia is a low serum ionized plasma calcium concentration. Calcium is essential for effective cardiac function and vasomotor tone.

Hyperkalemia is a high serum potassium concentration, which may result from renal dysfunction, cell death, iatrogenic excess administration, or acidosis. Acidosis causes a shift of potassium from the intracellular to the extracellular, including the intravascular space. As a result, acidosis may cause a rise in serum potassium.

Metabolic acidosis develops from production of acids, such as lactic acid, when tissue perfusion is inadequate. Renal or gastrointestinal dysfunction can cause metabolic acidosis. Renal dysfunction can cause retention of organic acids or loss of bicarbonate ions. Gastrointestinal dysfunction, such as diarrhea, can result in loss of bicarbonate ions.

Severe metabolic acidosis may depress myocardial contractility and reduce the effect of vasopressors. Unless metabolic acidosis is due solely to bicarbonate losses, it does not respond well to buffer therapy. Treat the acidosis by attempting to restore tissue perfusion with fluid resuscitation and vasoactive agents. If treatment is effective, the metabolic acidosis will resolve.

On occasion, buffers (e.g., sodium bicarbonate) may be needed to acutely correct profound metabolic acidosis that is impairing vital organ function. Sodium bicarbonate works by combining with hydrogen ions (acids) to produce carbon dioxide and water; carbon dioxide is then eliminated through increased alveolar ventilation. Support of ventilation is always important in the critically ill child, but is especially important if metabolic acidosis is treated with sodium bicarbonate.

Correction of metabolic derangements may be essential to optimizing organ function. Measure ionized calcium concentration (active form of calcium in the body) and glucose concentration. Replenish them as indicated. Consider administration of sodium bicarbonate to treat metabolic acidosis refractory to attempts at increasing cardiac output or redistributing blood flow to vital organs.

Therapeutic End Points

No single resuscitation end point has been identified as a consistent marker of adequate tissue perfusion and cellular homeostasis. Signs that indicate clinical improvement toward a normal hemodynamic state are

- Normal heart rate and blood pressure for age
- Normal pulses
- Capillary refill time <2 seconds
- Warm extremities
- Normal mental status
- Urine output >1 mL/kg per hour
- Decreased serum lactate
- Reduced base deficit
- Central venous oxygen saturation ($ScvO_2$) >70%

Monitor these therapeutic end points in addition to addressing the underlying cause of the child's shock.

General Management of Shock

Fundamental Fact Accurate Assessment of Tissue Perfusion	Although blood pressure is easily measured, it is important to assess other clinical parameters to evaluate tissue perfusion. Remember that blood pressure may be normal in children with severe shock, and noninvasive blood pressure measurement may be inaccurate if perfusion is poor.

Components of General Management

General management of shock consists of the following (note that several of these interventions may be implemented by the team simultaneously):

- Positioning
- Airway and breathing
- Vascular access
- Fluid resuscitation
- Monitoring
- Frequent reassessment
- Laboratory studies
- Medication therapy
- Subspecialty consultation

Positioning

Initial management of shock includes positioning the critically ill or injured child. If the child is responsive and hemodynamically stable, allow the child to remain in the most comfortable position (e.g., sitting in the arms of a caregiver) to decrease anxiety and activity as you form your initial impression and conduct the primary assessment. If the child is hypotensive and breathing is not compromised, place the child in the Trendelenburg position (supine, head 30° below the feet).

Airway and Breathing

Maintain a patent airway and support breathing. Give a high concentration of supplementary O_2 to all children with shock. Usually this is best delivered by a high-flow O_2 delivery system. Sometimes O_2 delivery needs to be combined with ventilatory support if respirations are ineffective, mental status is impaired, or work of breathing is significantly increased. Appropriate interventions may include noninvasive positive airway pressure or mechanical ventilation after endotracheal intubation.

Vascular Access

Once the airway is patent and breathing is supported, obtain vascular access for fluid resuscitation and administration of medications. For compensated shock, initial attempts at peripheral venous cannulation are appropriate. For hypotensive shock, immediate vascular access is critical and is best accomplished by the IO route if peripheral IV access is not readily achieved. Depending on the provider's experience and expertise and clinical circumstances, central venous access may be useful. Gaining central venous access, however, typically takes longer than placement of an IO line.

For information on establishment of IO access, see "Intraosseous Access" in "Resources for Management of Circulatory Emergencies" at the end of this Part.

Fluid Resuscitation

Once vascular access is established, start fluid resuscitation immediately.

Monitoring

Assess effectiveness of fluid resuscitation and medication therapy by frequent or continuous monitoring of the following:

- O_2 saturation using pulse oximetry (SpO_2)
- Heart rate
- Blood pressure and pulse pressure
- Mental status
- Temperature
- Urine output

As soon as possible, start noninvasive monitoring (SpO_2, heart rate, blood pressure). Assess mental status. Measure temperature and measure urine output with an indwelling bladder catheter. Consider invasive monitoring (e.g., arterial and central venous catheterization), depending on the providers' experience and available resources.

Critical Concept **IO Access**	If peripheral vascular access cannot be readily obtained in a child with compensated or hypotensive shock, be prepared to establish IO access.

| **Critical Concept**
Fluid Resuscitation | Give isotonic crystalloid in a 20 mL/kg bolus over 5 to 20 minutes. Reassess* and repeat 20 mL/kg boluses to restore blood pressure and tissue perfusion.

*Repeat fluid boluses based on clinical signs of end-organ perfusion, including heart rate, capillary refill, level of consciousness, and urine output. Remember that if you suspect cardiogenic shock, use smaller fluid boluses of 5 to 10 mL/kg, given over 10 to 20 minutes. Carefully monitor for signs of pulmonary edema or worsening tissue perfusion. Stop the infusion if such signs occur. Be prepared to support oxygenation and ventilation as necessary. |

Critical Concept	The condition of a child in shock is dynamic. Continuous monitoring and frequent reassessment are essential to evaluate trends in the child's condition and determine response to therapy.
Monitor to Evaluate Trends	

Frequent Reassessment

Frequently reassess the child's respiratory, cardiovascular, and neurologic status to:

- Evaluate trends in the child's condition
- Determine response to therapy
- Plan the next interventions

A child in shock is in a dynamic clinical condition that can deteriorate at any moment and require lifesaving interventions, such as endotracheal intubation. Continue frequent reassessment until the child's condition becomes stable or the child is transferred to advanced care.

Laboratory Studies

Laboratory studies provide important information to help you

- Identify the etiology and severity of shock
- Evaluate organ dysfunction secondary to shock
- Identify metabolic derangements
- Evaluate response to therapy

See Part 11: "Postresuscitation Management" for additional information on evaluation of end-organ function. Also consider expert consultation in diagnosis and management of end-organ failure.

Table 1 outlines some laboratory studies that can help identify the etiology and severity of shock and guide therapy.

Table 1. Laboratory Studies to Evaluate Shock and Guide Therapy

Laboratory Study	Finding	Possible Etiology	Possible Interventions
CBC	Hgb/Hct decreased	• Hemorrhage • Fluid resuscitation (dilution) • Hemolysis	• Administer 100% O_2 • Control bleeding • Transfuse blood • Titrate fluid administration
	WBC count increased or decreased	• Sepsis	• Obtain appropriate cultures • Give antibiotics
	Platelets decreased	• Disseminated intravascular coagulation (DIC) • Decreased platelet production	• Transfuse platelets if child has serious bleeding • Obtain INR/PTT, fibrinogen, and D-dimers
Glucose	Increased or decreased	• Stress (usually increased but may be decreased in infants) • Sepsis • Decreased production (e.g., liver failure)	• If hypoglycemia is present, give dextrose bolus and start infusion of dextrose-containing solution if needed • Severe hyperglycemia may require treatment (per institutional protocols or obtain expert consultation)
Potassium	Increased or decreased	• Renal dysfunction • Acidosis (increases serum potassium concentration) • Diuresis (decreased)	• Treat hyperkalemia or hypokalemia • Correct acidosis
Calcium	Decreased (ionized calcium concentration)	• Sepsis • Transfusion of blood products	• Give calcium

(continued)

(continued)

Laboratory Study	Finding	Possible Etiology	Possible Interventions
Lactate	Increased as product of anaerobic metabolism from tissue hypoperfusion	• Tissue hypoxia • Increased glucose production (gluconeogenesis) • Decreased metabolism (e.g., liver failure)	• Improve tissue perfusion • Treat acidosis if end-organ function is impaired
ABG	pH decreased in acidosis; increased with alkalosis	• Lactic acid accumulation caused by tissue hypoperfusion • Renal failure • Inborn error of metabolism • DKA • Poisoning/overdose • Diarrhea or ileostomy losses • Hyper/hypoventilation (sepsis, poisoning) • Vomiting	• Give fluid • Support ventilation • Correct shock • Consider buffer • Evaluate anion gap to determine if acidosis is from increased unmeasured ions (increased anion gap) or is more likely from loss of bicarbonate (normal anion gap)
$ScvO_2$	Variable	• Low central venous O_2 saturation—inadequate O_2 delivery or increased consumption • High central venous O_2 saturation—maldistribution of blood flow or decreased O_2 utilization	• Attempt to maximize O_2 delivery and minimize O_2 demand

Abbreviations: ABG, arterial blood gas; CBC, complete blood cell count; DKA, diabetic ketoacidosis; Hct, hematocrit; Hgb, hemoglobin; PT/PTT, prothrombin time/partial thromboplastin time; $ScvO_2$, central venous oxygen saturation; WBC, white blood cell.

Medication Therapy

Medication therapy is used in the management of shock to affect myocardial contractility, heart rate, and vascular resistance. The choice of agent(s) is determined by the child's physiologic state.

Vasoactive agents are indicated when shock persists despite adequate volume resuscitation to optimize preload. For example, a child with septic shock who remains hypotensive with signs of vasodilation despite administration of fluids may benefit from a vasoconstrictor. In children with cardiogenic shock, vasoactive agents should be used early because fluid resuscitation is ineffective and may cause respiratory failure. Most children with cardiogenic shock benefit from a vasodilator (provided that blood pressure is adequate), to decrease SVR and increase cardiac output and tissue perfusion.

Inotropes, phosphodiesterase inhibitors (i.e., inodilators), vasodilators, and vasopressors are classes of pharmacologic agents commonly used in shock. Table 2 lists vasoactive medications by class and pharmacologic effects.

Table 2. Vasoactive Therapy Used in the Treatment of Shock

Class	Medication	Effect
Inotropes	• Dopamine • Epinephrine • Dobutamine	• Increase cardiac contractility • Increase heart rate • Produce variable effects on SVR *Note:* Includes agents with both α-adrenergic and β-adrenergic effects
Phosphodiesterase inhibitors (inodilators)	• Milrinone	• Decrease SVR • Improve coronary artery blood flow • Improve contractility
Vasodilators	• Nitroglycerin • Nitroprusside	• Decrease SVR and venous tone
Vasopressors (vasoconstrictors)	• Epinephrine (doses >0.3 mcg/kg per minute) • Norepinephrine • Dopamine (doses >10 mcg/kg per minute) • Vasopressin	• Increase SVR • Increase myocardial contractility (except vasopressin)

Abbreviation: SVR, systemic vascular resistance.
See Part 12: "Pharmacology" for dosing information.

Critical Concept **Colour-Coded Length-Based Tape**	Use a colour-coded length-based tape to determine the child's weight (if not known) for calculating drug doses and for selecting the correct sizes of resuscitation equipment. See "Resources for Management of Circulatory Emergencies" at the end of this Part for an example.

Critical Concept **Expert Consultation**	When treating the child in shock, providers must obtain consultation from appropriate experts as soon as possible.

Subspecialty Consultation

For specific categories of shock, lifesaving diagnostic and therapeutic interventions may be required that are beyond the scope of practice of many PALS providers. For example, a provider may not be trained to interpret an echocardiogram or perform a thoracostomy or pericardiocentesis. Recognize your own scope-of-practice limitations and call for help when needed. Early subspecialty consultation (e.g., pediatric critical care, pediatric cardiology, pediatric surgery) is an essential component of shock management and may influence outcome.

Summary: Initial Management Principles

Table 3 summarizes initial shock management principles discussed in this section.

Table 3. Fundamentals of Initial Shock Management

Position the child
• Stable—Allow to remain with caregiver in a position of comfort • Unstable—If hypotensive, place in Trendelenburg position unless breathing is compromised

Optimize arterial O₂ content
• Administer a high concentration of O₂ via a nonrebreathing mask • Consider blood transfusion in cases of blood loss or other causes of severe anemia • Consider use of CPAP, noninvasive positive airway pressure, or mechanical ventilation with PEEP

Support ventilation as indicated (invasive or noninvasive)

(continued)

(continued)

Establish vascular access

- Consider IO access early

Begin fluid resuscitation

- Give an isotonic crystalloid bolus of 20 mL/kg over 5 to 20 minutes; repeat 20 mL/kg boluses to restore blood pressure and tissue perfusion
- For trauma and hemorrhage, administer PRBCs if the child does not respond to isotonic crystalloid
- Modify volume and rate of bolus fluid therapy if you suspect cardiogenic shock or severe myocardial dysfunction

Monitor

- SpO$_2$
- Heart rate
- Blood pressure
- Level of consciousness
- Temperature
- Urine output

Perform frequent reassessment

- Evaluate trends
- Determine response to therapy

Conduct laboratory studies

- To identify shock etiology and severity
- To evaluate organ dysfunction secondary to shock
- To identify metabolic derangements
- To evaluate the response to therapy

Administer pharmacologic support—see Table 2: Vasoactive Therapy Used in the Treatment of Shock

- To improve or redistribute cardiac output (increase contractility, reduce or increase SVR, improve organ perfusion)
- To correct metabolic derangements
- To manage pain and anxiety

Obtain subspecialty consultation

Abbreviations: CPAP, continuous positive airway pressure; IO, intraosseous; PEEP, positive end-expiratory pressure; PRBC, packed red blood cells; SpO$_2$, O$_2$ saturation assessed by pulse oximetry; SVR, systemic vascular resistance.

Fluid Therapy

The primary objective of fluid therapy in shock is to restore intravascular volume and tissue perfusion. Rapid and aggressive fluid resuscitation is required for hypovolemic and distributive shock. Cardiogenic and obstructive shock, as well as special conditions such as severe poisonings or DKA, may dictate alternative approaches to fluid resuscitation.

Both isotonic crystalloid and colloid will expand intravascular volume. Blood and blood products are generally not used for volume expansion in children with shock unless shock is due to hemorrhage. Blood products may also be indicated for correction of some coagulopathies.

Isotonic Crystalloid Solutions

Isotonic crystalloid solutions, such as normal saline (NS) or lactated Ringer's (LR), are the preferred initial fluids for volume replacement in the management of shock. They are inexpensive, readily available, and do not cause sensitivity reactions.

Isotonic crystalloids are distributed throughout the extracellular compartment. They do not expand the intravascular (circulating) space efficiently because only about one fourth of their volume remains in the intravascular space; the remainder moves to the extravascular (interstitial) space. A large trial of volume resuscitation that compared isotonic saline with albumin found that about 1½ times more crystalloid than colloid was needed for equal effect.

Rapid infusion of a large volume of fluid may be well tolerated by a healthy child but may cause pulmonary and peripheral edema in a critically ill child with cardiac or renal disease.

Colloid Solutions

Colloid solutions (albumin, hydroxyethyl starch solutions, dextrans or gel solutions) contain relatively large molecules that remain in the intravascular compartment hours longer than isotonic crystalloids. As a result they are more efficient intravascular volume expanders than crystalloid solutions.

Colloid solutions, however, may have disadvantages for the acute resuscitation of a child in shock. They are less widely available than crystalloid solutions and may take time to prepare. Blood-derived colloid solutions may cause sensitivity reactions. Synthetic colloids may cause coagulopathies; their use is usually limited to 20 to 40 mL/kg. As with crystalloids, excessive administration of colloids can lead to pulmonary edema, particularly in children with cardiac or renal disease.

Critical Concept

Quantity of Crystalloid Solution

Because isotonic crystalloids are distributed throughout the extracellular space, a large quantity of crystalloid solution may be needed to restore intravascular volume for children in shock.

Fundamental Fact	For most children with shock, isotonic crystalloids are recommended as the initial resuscitation fluid.
Initial Resuscitation Fluid	

Crystalloid vs. Colloid

The results and analysis of decades of trials to compare crystalloid versus colloid solutions for shock have yielded contradictory results. In general, base the choice of resuscitation fluid on the child's condition and response to initial isotonic crystalloid resuscitation.

After administering multiple boluses of isotonic crystalloid, consider administration of colloid if additional fluid is indicated. Colloids may also be indicated in children with an underlying process that may be associated with decreased plasma oncotic pressure (e.g., malnutrition, hypoproteinemia, nephrotic syndrome).

Rate and Volume of Fluid Administration

Start fluid resuscitation for shock with 20 mL/kg of isotonic crystalloid administered as a bolus over 5 to 20 minutes. Repeat boluses of 20 mL/kg as needed to restore blood pressure and perfusion. The volume of fluid deficit is often difficult to predict from the child's history. Use clinical examination and supporting laboratory studies to identify the volume needed; it may be necessary to administer more than the estimated volume deficit. Reassess frequently.

Give fluid boluses rapidly for hypotensive and septic shock. Children with septic shock typically require at least 60 mL/kg of isotonic crystalloid solution during the first hour of therapy; 200 mL/kg or more may be required in the first 8 hours of therapy.

If myocardial dysfunction or obstructive shock is present or suspected, *give smaller volumes of fluid more slowly*. Administer boluses of 5 to 10 mL/kg over 10 to 20 minutes

and reassess frequently for signs of worsening respiratory status from pulmonary edema. Obtain further diagnostic testing and expert consultation (e.g., echocardiogram) to confirm suspicions and guide the next interventions. Be prepared to provide support of airway and ventilation with PEEP as needed if pulmonary edema develops.

Modification of fluid resuscitation is appropriate for children in shock associated with DKA, large burns, and some poisonings (particularly calcium channel blocker and β-adrenergic blocker overdoses). Children with DKA may be significantly dehydrated but often have high serum osmolality (caused by hyperglycemia). Rapid administration of crystalloid and reduction in serum osmolality may contribute to risk of cerebral edema. Children who have ingested calcium channel blockers or β-adrenergic blockers may have myocardial dysfunction and are less tolerant of rapid volume expansion.

Table 4 provides a general guide to fluid bolus volumes and rates of delivery based on the underlying cause of shock.

Rapid Fluid Delivery

IV fluid administration systems generally used for pediatric fluid therapy do not deliver fluid boluses as rapidly as required for management of some forms of shock. To facilitate rapid fluid delivery

- Place as large an IV catheter as possible, especially if blood or colloid administration is needed
- Place an in-line 3-way stopcock in the IV tubing system
- Deliver fluid by using a 30- to 60-mL syringe to push fluids through the stopcock, or use a pressure bag (beware of risk of air embolism) or a rapid infusion device

Table 4. Guide to Fluid Boluses and Rates of Delivery Based on Underlying Cause of Shock

Type of Shock	Volume of Fluid	Approximate Rate of Delivery
Hypovolemic shock (non-DKA) **Distributive shock**	20 mL/kg bolus (repeat PRN)	Over 5 to 10 minutes
Cardiogenic shock (nonpoisoning)	5 to 10 mL/kg bolus (repeat PRN)	Over 10 to 20 minutes
DKA with compensated shock	10 to 20 mL/kg	Over 1 hour
Poisonings (e.g., calcium channel blocker or β-adrenergic blocker)	5 to 10 mL/kg (repeat PRN)	Over 10 to 20 minutes

Abbreviations: DKA, diabetic ketoacidosis; PRN, as needed.

Note: Standard infusion pumps—even if set at the maximum infusion rate—do not provide a sufficiently rapid rate of fluid delivery, especially in larger children. For example, a 50-kg patient with septic shock should ideally receive 1 L of crystalloid in 5 to 10 minutes rather than the hour required by an infusion pump.

Frequent Reassessment During Fluid Resuscitation

Frequent reassessment is essential during fluid resuscitation to manage shock effectively. Such reassessment should

- Assess the physiologic response to therapy after each fluid bolus
- Determine the need for further fluid boluses
- Assess for signs of detrimental effects (e.g., pulmonary edema) during and after fluid resuscitation

Signs of physiologic improvement include improved perfusion, increase in blood pressure, slowing of heart rate (toward normal), decreased respiratory rate (toward normal), increased urine output, and improved mental status. If the child's condition does not improve or worsens after fluid boluses, try to identify the cause of the shock to help determine the next interventions. For example, persistently delayed capillary refill despite initial fluid administration may indicate ongoing hemorrhage or other fluid loss. Deterioration of the child's condition after fluid therapy may signal cardiogenic or obstructive shock. Increased work of breathing may indicate pulmonary edema.

Indication for Blood Products

Blood is recommended for replacement of traumatic volume loss if the child's perfusion is inadequate despite administration of 2 to 3 boluses of 20 mL/kg of isotonic crystalloid. Under these circumstances administer 10 mL/kg PRBCs as soon as available.

Fully crossmatched blood is generally not available in emergencies because most blood banks require about 1 hour for the crossmatching process. Crossmatched blood may become available for children who are stabilized with crystalloid but have ongoing blood losses. Priorities for the type of blood or blood products used in order of preference are

- Crossmatched
- Type specific
- Type O-negative (O– preferred for females and either O+ or O– for males)

Unmatched, type-specific blood may be used if ongoing blood loss results in hypotension despite administration of crystalloid. Most blood banks can supply type-specific blood within 10 minutes. Type-specific blood is ABO and Rh compatible, but, unlike fully crossmatched blood, incompatibilities of other antibodies may exist.

Use type O blood if there is an immediate need for blood to prevent cardiopulmonary arrest, because it can be administered to children of any blood type. O-negative blood is preferred in females of childbearing age to avoid Rh sensitization. Either O-negative or O-positive blood may be administered to males.

Complications of Rapid Administration of Blood Products

Rapid infusion of cold blood or blood products, particularly in large volume, may produce several complications, including

- Hypothermia
- Myocardial dysfunction
- Ionized hypocalcemia

Hypothermia may adversely affect cardiovascular function and coagulation and may compromise several metabolic functions, including metabolism of citrate, which is present in stored blood. Inadequate citrate clearance in turn causes ionized hypocalcemia. The combined effects of hypothermia and ionized hypocalcemia can result in significant myocardial dysfunction and hypotension.

To minimize these problems, warm blood and blood products if possible with an approved commercial blood-warming device before or during rapid IV administration. Prepare calcium for administration if the child becomes hypotensive during rapid transfusion; in some cases it may be beneficial to administer calcium empirically to prevent hypocalcemia.

Recent battlefield experience has demonstrated improved survival in trauma patients receiving massive transfusion (blood volume administered exceeds the patient's blood volume) when plasma is transfused in approximately a 1:1 ratio to red cells.

Glucose

Monitor blood glucose concentration as a component of shock management. Hypoglycemia is a common finding in critically ill children. It can result in brain injury if not rapidly identified and effectively treated. In one pediatric study, hypoglycemia was present in 18% of children who received resuscitative care in an emergency department for decreased level of consciousness, status epilepticus, respiratory failure, cardiopulmonary failure, or cardiac arrest. For more details see Losek, 2000 (full reference in the Suggested Reading List at the end of this Part).

Critical Concept Identify Hypoglycemia	In all critically ill or injured children, perform a rapid glucose test to rule out hypoglycemia as a cause of or a contributing factor to shock or decreased level of consciousness.

Glucose Monitoring

Measure serum glucose concentration in all infants and children with evidence of neurologic dysfunction (e.g., seizures, coma), shock, or respiratory failure. The serum glucose concentration can be measured from capillary, venous, or arterial blood samples with a point-of-care device or by laboratory analysis. Small infants and chronically ill children have higher glucose utilization rates and limited stores of glycogen. This limited supply may be rapidly depleted during episodes of physiologic stress, resulting in hypoglycemia. Infants receiving non–glucose-containing IV fluids are at increased risk for developing hypoglycemia.

Hyperglycemia, also frequently present in seriously ill or injured children, may result from a relative insulin-resistant state induced by high levels of endogenous catecholamines and cortisol. Although controlling serum glucose concentration by using an insulin infusion improved outcome in studies of critically ill adult patients, there are insufficient data to support routine use of this treatment in critically ill children. It is best to avoid hyperglycemia if possible. Consider treating hyperglycemia in high-risk groups, such as brain-injured children, while monitoring closely to prevent hypoglycemia.

Diagnosis of Hypoglycemia

Hypoglycemia may be difficult to recognize clinically because some children may have no outward signs or symptoms (i.e., asymptomatic hypoglycemia). Others may show nonspecific clinical signs (e.g., poor perfusion, diaphoresis, tachycardia, hypothermia, irritability or lethargy, hypotension). These clinical signs are also common to many other conditions, including hypoxemia, ischemia, or shock.

Although single threshold values are not applicable to every patient, the following lowest acceptable glucose concentrations can be used to define hypoglycemia:

Age	Consensus Definition of Hypoglycemia
Preterm neonates **Term neonates**	<2.5 mmol/L
Infants **Children** **Adolescents**	<3.3 mmol/L

The reported low range of normal glucose is typically related to sample measurements obtained in nonstressed, fasting infants and children. It is difficult to extrapolate these thresholds to the glucose concentration required by a stressed, critically ill, or injured child.

Management of Hypoglycemia

If the glucose concentration is low and the child has minimal symptoms and normal mental status, you may administer glucose orally (e.g., orange juice or other glucose-containing fluid). If the concentration is very low or the child is symptomatic, you should give IV glucose at a dose of 0.5 to 1 g/kg. IV dextrose is commonly administered as $D_{25}W$ (2 to 4 mL/kg) or $D_{10}W$ (5 to 10 mL/kg). Dextrose is the same substance as glucose. Reassess the serum glucose concentration after dextrose administration. Provide a continuous infusion of glucose-containing IV fluid to prevent recurrent hypoglycemia.

Do not routinely infuse dextrose-containing fluids for volume resuscitation of shock. This can cause hyperglycemia, increase the serum osmolality, and produce an osmotic diuresis that will further exacerbate hypovolemia and shock. Electrolyte imbalances (e.g., hyponatremia) can also develop.

Management According to Type of Shock

Effective management of shock targets treatment to the etiology of the shock. For the purposes of the PALS Provider Course, shock is categorized into 4 types, based on the underlying cause. This classification method, however, oversimplifies the physiologic state seen in individual patients. Some children with shock have elements of hypovolemic, distributive, and cardiogenic shock, with one type being dominant. Any child with severe shock may develop characteristics of myocardial dysfunction and maldistribution of blood flow. For a more comprehensive discussion of shock by etiology, see Part 6: "Recognition of Shock."

Management of the following types of shock is discussed in this section:

- Hypovolemic
- Distributive
- Cardiogenic
- Obstructive

Critical Concept	It is important to provide rapid, adequate fluid resuscitation for hypovolemic shock.
Timely Fluid Resuscitation in Hypovolemic Shock	Avoid the common errors of inadequate or delayed administration of fluid resuscitation.

Management of Hypovolemic Shock

Fluid resuscitation is the primary therapy for hypovolemic shock. Children with hypovolemic shock who receive an appropriate volume of fluid within the first hour of resuscitation have the best chance for survival and recovery. Timely administration of fluid is key to preventing deterioration from compensated hypovolemic shock to refractory hypotensive shock.

Other components in effective management of hypovolemic shock are

- Identify the type of volume loss (nonhemorrhagic versus hemorrhagic)
- Replace volume deficit
- Prevent and replace ongoing losses (e.g., bleeding, GI losses)
- Restore acid-base balance
- Correct metabolic derangements

Determining Adequate Fluid Resuscitation

Adequate fluid resuscitation in hypovolemic shock is determined by the

- Extent of volume depletion
- Type of volume loss (e.g., blood, electrolyte-containing fluid, or electrolyte-and-protein–containing fluid)

The extent of volume depletion may be underestimated and undertreated. In many cases volume loss is compounded by inadequate fluid intake. The clinical parameters used to help determine the percentage of dehydration include

- General appearance
- Presence or absence of tears and appearance of eyes (normal vs. sunken)
- Moisture of mucous membranes
- Skin elasticity
- Respiratory rate and depth

- Heart rate
- Blood pressure
- Capillary refill time
- Urinary output
- Mental status

Clinically significant dehydration in children is generally associated with at least 5% volume depletion (i.e., ≥5% loss in body weight) corresponding to a fluid deficit of ≥50 mL/kg. Therefore, treating a child with clinically evident dehydration with administration of a single 20 mL/kg bolus of isotonic crystalloid may be insufficient. Conversely, it is usually unnecessary to completely correct the estimated deficit within the first hour. After perfusion is restored and the child is no longer in shock, the total fluid deficit may be corrected over the next 24 to 48 hours.

Although all forms of hypovolemic shock are initially treated with rapid infusion of isotonic crystalloid, early identification of the type of volume loss can optimize further treatment. Fluid losses may be classified as hemorrhagic and nonhemorrhagic. Nonhemorrhagic losses include electrolyte-containing fluids (e.g., diarrhea, vomiting, osmotic diuresis associated with DKA) and protein-and-electrolyte–containing fluids (e.g., losses associated with burns and peritonitis).

Nonhemorrhagic Hypovolemic Shock

Common sources of nonhemorrhagic fluid loss are gastrointestinal (i.e., vomiting and diarrhea), urinary (e.g., DKA), and capillary leak (e.g., burns). Hypovolemia caused by nonhemorrhagic fluid loss is generally classified in terms of percent loss of body weight (Table 5). Correlation of blood pressure and fluid deficits is imprecise. As a general rule, however, hypotensive shock may be observed in children with fluid deficits of 50 to 100 mL/kg but is more consistently observed with deficits ≥100 mL/kg.

Table 5. Stages and Signs of Dehydration

Severity of Dehydration	Infant EWL (mL/kg)	Adolescent EWL (mL/kg)	Clinical Signs	Problems in Assessment
Mild	5% (50)	3% (30)	• Dry mucous membranes • Oliguria	• Frequency and amount of urine are difficult to assess during diarrhea, especially infants in diapers
Moderate	10% (100)	5% to 6% (50 to 60)	• Poor skin turgor • Sunken fontanel • Marked oliguria • Tachycardia • Quiet tachypnea	• Increased sodium concentration helps maintain intravascular volume • Fontanel open only in infants • Degree of oliguria is affected by fever, sodium concentration, underlying disease
Severe	15% (150)	7% to 9% (70 to 90)	• Marked tachycardia • Weak to absent distal pulses • Narrow pulse pressure • Increased respiratory rate • Hypotension and decreased level of consciousness (late findings)	• Clinical signs are affected by fever, sodium concentration, underlying disease

Abbreviation: EWL, estimated weight loss.
mL/kg refers to the estimated corresponding fluid deficit normalized to body weight.

Infuse 20 mL/kg boluses of isotonic crystalloid rapidly to effectively treat children with hypovolemic shock secondary to dehydration. Failure to improve after at least 3 boluses (i.e., 60 mL/kg) of isotonic crystalloid indicates that

- The extent of fluid losses may be underestimated
- The type of fluid replacement may need to be altered (e.g., need for colloid or blood)
- There are ongoing fluid losses (e.g., occult bleeding)
- Your initial assumption about the etiology of the shock may be incorrect (i.e., consider alternative or combined types of shock)

Ongoing fluid losses (e.g., diarrhea, DKA, burns) must be replaced in addition to correcting existing fluid deficits. Colloid is not routinely indicated as the initial treatment of hypovolemic shock. Albumin and other colloids, however, have been used successfully for volume replacement in children with large "third-space" losses or albumin deficits.

Hemorrhagic Hypovolemic Shock

Hemorrhagic hypovolemic shock is classified according to an estimated percentage of total blood volume loss (Table 6). In children the dividing line between mild and compensated versus moderate or severe and hypotensive hemorrhagic shock correlates with a loss of blood volume of about 30%. The estimated total blood volume of a child is 75 to 80 mL/kg; a 30% blood volume loss therefore represents a blood loss of about 25 mL/kg.

Critical Concept	For fluid resuscitation in hemorrhagic shock, give about 3 mL of crystalloid for every 1 mL of blood lost.
3 mL to 1 mL Rule	

Table 6. Systemic Responses to Blood Loss in Pediatric Patients

System	Mild Blood Volume Loss (<30%)	Moderate Blood Volume Loss (30%-45%)	Severe Blood Volume Loss (>45%)
Cardiovascular	Increased heart rate; weak, thready peripheral pulses; normal systolic blood pressure (80-90 + 2 × age in years); normal pulse pressure	Markedly increased heart rate; weak, thready central pulses; absent peripheral pulses; low normal systolic blood pressure (70-80 + 2 × age in years); narrowed pulse pressure	Tachycardia followed by bradycardia; very weak or absent peripheral pulses; hypotension (<70 + 2 × age in years); undetectable diastolic blood pressure (or widened pulse pressure)
Central nervous system	Anxious; irritable; confused	Lethargic; dulled response to pain*	Comatose
Skin	Cool, mottled; prolonged capillary refill	Cyanotic; markedly prolonged capillary refill	Pale and cold
Urine output†	Low to very low	Minimal	None

*The child's dulled response to pain with this degree of blood loss (30%-45%) may be indicated by a decreased response to IV catheter insertion.

†After initial decompression by urinary catheter. Low normal is 2 mL/kg per hour (infant), 1.5 mL/kg per hour (younger child), 1 mL/kg per hour (older child), and 0.5 mL/kg per hour (adolescent). Intravenous contrast can falsely elevate urinary output.

Modified from American College of Surgeons Committee on Trauma. *Advanced Trauma Life Support® for Doctors: ATLS Student Course Manual.* 8th ed. Chicago, IL: American College of Surgeons; 2008.

Fluid resuscitation in hemorrhagic shock begins with rapid infusion of isotonic crystalloid in boluses of 20 mL/kg. Because isotonic crystalloids are distributed throughout the extracellular space, it may be necessary to give up to 3 boluses of 20 mL/kg (60 mL/kg) of fluid to replace a 25% loss of blood volume; approximately 3 mL of crystalloid is needed for every 1 mL of blood lost. If the child remains hemodynamically unstable despite 2 to 3 boluses of 20 mL/kg isotonic crystalloid, consider a transfusion of PRBCs.

For blood replacement, use PRBCs in 10 mL/kg boluses. Whole blood (20 mL/kg) can be given in place of PRBCs, but it is harder and more time-consuming to obtain. Also the risk of transfusion reaction is significantly increased if the blood is not crossmatched. To minimize adverse effects, warm the blood if a blood-warming device is available, especially when transfusing rapidly.

Indications for transfusion in hemorrhagic shock include

- Crystalloid-refractory hypotension or poor perfusion
- Known significant blood loss

Crystalloid-refractory hemorrhagic shock is defined as persistent hypotension despite administration of 40 to 60 mL/kg crystalloid. Children with rapid hemorrhage may demonstrate a normal or low initial hemoglobin concentration. Transfuse blood for a low hemoglobin concentration because anemia increases the risk of tissue hypoxia from inadequate O_2 content and delivery.

Medication Therapy

Vasoactive agents are not routinely indicated for the management of hypovolemic shock. Moribund children with profound hypovolemic shock and hypotension may require short-term administration of vasoactive agents such as epinephrine to restore cardiac contractility and vascular tone until adequate fluid resuscitation is provided.

Acid-Base Balance

Early in the progression of hypovolemic shock, the child may develop tachypnea and respiratory alkalosis. However, the alkalosis does not completely correct the metabolic (lactic) acidosis produced by hypovolemic shock. A child with long-standing or severe shock may have severe acidosis because the child eventually develops fatigue or cardiorespiratory failure. Injured children with head or chest injuries may not demonstrate compensatory tachypnea.

Persistent acidosis and poor perfusion are indications of inadequate resuscitation or, in hemorrhagic shock, of ongoing blood loss. Sodium bicarbonate is not recommended for the treatment of metabolic acidosis secondary to hypovolemic shock. As long as fluid resuscitation improves perfusion and end-organ function, metabolic acidosis is well tolerated and will correct gradually. Bicarbonate is indicated if the metabolic acidosis is caused by significant bicarbonate losses from renal or gastrointestinal losses (i.e., a non–anion gap metabolic acidosis) because it is difficult to compensate for an ongoing bicarbonate loss.

Specific Treatment Considerations

Follow the initial management principles (Table 3) in addition to the considerations specific to hypovolemic shock shown in Table 7.

Table 7. Management of Hypovolemic Shock: Specific Treatment Considerations

Initiate fluid resuscitation as quickly as possible.
In all patients rapidly infuse isotonic crystalloid (NS or LR) in 20 mL/kg boluses; repeat as needed. • In patients with crystalloid-refractory hemorrhagic shock, give a transfusion of PRBCs 10 mL/kg. • If loss of protein-containing fluids is documented or suspected (low albumin concentration), consider administration of colloid-containing fluids if the child fails to respond to crystalloid resuscitation.
Correct metabolic derangements.
Identify the type of volume loss (hemorrhagic or nonhemorrhagic) to determine best treatment.
Control any external hemorrhage with direct pressure; measure and replace ongoing losses (e.g., continued diarrhea).
Consider other studies: • CBC • Type and crossmatch • ABG with particular attention to the base deficit • Electrolyte panel to calculate anion gap, glucose, and ionized calcium • Serum or plasma lactate concentration • Diagnostic imaging to identify the source of bleeding or volume loss

Abbreviations: ABG, arterial blood gas; CBC, complete blood cell count; LR, lactated Ringer's; NS, normal saline; PRBC, packed red blood cell.

Management of Distributive Shock

Initial management of distributive shock focuses on expanding intravascular volume to correct hypovolemia and fill the expanded dilated vascular space. Use vasoactive agents if the child remains hypotensive or poorly perfused despite rapid bolus fluid administration or if the diastolic pressure remains low with a wide pulse pressure.

This section discusses management of the following types of distributive shock:

• Septic shock
• Anaphylactic shock
• Neurogenic shock

Management of Septic Shock

The clinical, hemodynamic, and metabolic changes observed in septic shock result from the host's response to an infection, including the release or activation of inflammatory mediators. The primary goals in the initial management of septic shock are

• Restoration of hemodynamic stability
• Identification and control of infection

Fundamental principles of management include increasing tissue O_2 delivery by optimizing cardiac output and arterial O_2 content and minimizing O_2 consumption.

Overview of Pediatric Septic Shock Algorithm

The recommended treatment approach to restore hemodynamic stability for septic shock in children is presented in the Pediatric Septic Shock Algorithm (Figure 1). It outlines a 3-tiered treatment plan:

• Give O_2, support ventilation, monitor respiratory rate, O_2 saturation, heart rate, blood pressure, and temperature, and establish vascular access.
• Initiate aggressive isotonic bolus fluid administration during the first hour with frequent reassessment of perfusion and monitoring for evidence of pulmonary edema or hepatomegaly.
• Treat fluid-refractory septic shock with vasoactive agents.
• Anticipate adrenal insufficiency and administer stress-dose hydrocortisone if the child does not readily respond to vasoactive medications.

Identify and Intervene **Septic Shock**	Early identification of septic shock is key to initiating resuscitation and preventing cardiac arrest. Hemodynamic support to maintain O_2 delivery can reduce pediatric morbidity and mortality from septic shock.

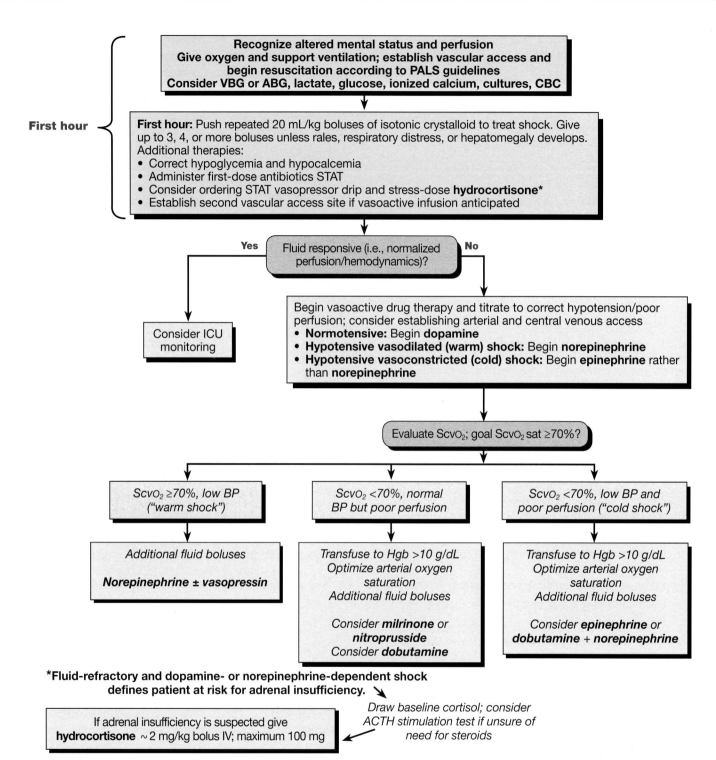

First hour

Recognize altered mental status and perfusion
Give oxygen and support ventilation; establish vascular access and
begin resuscitation according to PALS guidelines
Consider VBG or ABG, lactate, glucose, ionized calcium, cultures, CBC

First hour: Push repeated 20 mL/kg boluses of isotonic crystalloid to treat shock. Give up to 3, 4, or more boluses unless rales, respiratory distress, or hepatomegaly develops. Additional therapies:
• Correct hypoglycemia and hypocalcemia
• Administer first-dose antibiotics STAT
• Consider ordering STAT vasopressor drip and stress-dose **hydrocortisone***
• Establish second vascular access site if vasoactive infusion anticipated

Fluid responsive (i.e., normalized perfusion/hemodynamics)?

Yes — Consider ICU monitoring

No — Begin vasoactive drug therapy and titrate to correct hypotension/poor perfusion; consider establishing arterial and central venous access
• **Normotensive:** Begin **dopamine**
• **Hypotensive vasodilated (warm) shock:** Begin **norepinephrine**
• **Hypotensive vasoconstricted (cold) shock:** Begin **epinephrine** rather than **norepinephrine**

Evaluate $ScvO_2$; goal $ScvO_2$ sat ≥70%?

$ScvO_2$ ≥70%, low BP ("warm shock")

$ScvO_2$ <70%, normal BP but poor perfusion

$ScvO_2$ <70%, low BP and poor perfusion ("cold shock")

Additional fluid boluses

Norepinephrine ± vasopressin

*Transfuse to Hgb >10 g/dL
Optimize arterial oxygen saturation
Additional fluid boluses*

*Consider **milrinone** or **nitroprusside**
Consider **dobutamine***

*Transfuse to Hgb >10 g/dL
Optimize arterial oxygen saturation
Additional fluid boluses*

*Consider **epinephrine** or **dobutamine** + **norepinephrine***

***Fluid-refractory and dopamine- or norepinephrine-dependent shock defines patient at risk for adrenal insufficiency.**

Draw baseline cortisol; consider ACTH stimulation test if unsure of need for steroids

If adrenal insufficiency is suspected give **hydrocortisone** ~2 mg/kg bolus IV; maximum 100 mg

Figure 1. Pediatric Septic Shock Algorithm. Modified from Brierley J, Carcillo JA, Choong K, Cornell T, Decaen A, Deymann A, Doctor A, Davis A, Duff J, Dugas MA, Duncan A, Evans B, Feldman J, Felmet K, Fisher G, Frankel L, Jeffries H, Greenwald B, Gutierrez J, Hall M, Han YY, Hanson J, Hazelzet J, Hernan L, Kiff J, Kissoon N, Kon A, Irazuzta J, Lin J, Lorts A, Mariscalco M, Mehta R, Nadel S, Nguyen T, Nicholson C, Peters M, Okhuysen-Cawley R, Poulton T, Relves M, Rodriguez A, Rozenfeld R, Schnitzler E, Shanley T, Kache S, Skippen P, Torres A, von Dessauer B, Weingarten J, Yeh T, Zaritsky A, Stojadinovic B, Zimmerman J, Zuckerberg A. Clinical practice parameters for hemodynamic support of pediatric and neonatal septic shock: 2007 update from the American College of Critical Care Medicine. *Crit Care Med.* 2009;37(2):666-688.

Adequate treatment during the first hour is critical to maximize survival for the child in septic shock. Early intubation and mechanical ventilation may be indicated for a decreased level of consciousness or to reduce work of breathing. Initial components of management of septic shock are

- Rapid, aggressive bolus fluid administration
- Rapid administration of antibiotics after cultures are obtained if possible
- Rapid initiation of hemodynamic support, including vasopressors and possible stress-dose hydrocortisone
- Identification and correction of metabolic derangements
- Diagnostic tests (e.g., lactate concentration, base deficit, and central venous O_2 saturation) to identify the severity of shock and monitor response to fluid therapy

Rapid, aggressive bolus fluid administration is a priority. Inadequate intravascular volume rapidly leads to low stroke volume and hypotension. A child in septic shock typically requires a large volume of fluid to restore perfusion. *Rapidly infuse 3 or 4 boluses (20 mL/kg each) of isotonic crystalloid solution.* Titrate the volume and rate of fluid administration by ongoing assessment of tissue perfusion, heart rate, presence and quality of peripheral pulses, capillary refill, skin temperature, level of consciousness, and urine output.

Pulmonary edema may develop during fluid administration but is actually more frequent when fluid administration is inadequate. Generally fluid should be given rapidly despite an increase in capillary permeability and risk for pulmonary edema. If the pulmonary edema is cardiogenic (hepatomegaly, cardiomegaly, poor myocardial contractility), you may need to reduce the volume and rate of fluid administration. If significant noncardiogenic pulmonary edema develops, the child may require insertion of an advanced airway and mechanical ventilatory support with supplementary O_2 and PEEP.

Draw blood samples for culture. Administer the first dose of broad-spectrum antibiotics as soon as possible. For sepsis, do not delay antimicrobial therapy to wait for blood cultures or to perform other diagnostic tests such as lumbar puncture. When possible, also obtain arterial or central venous samples, or both, for blood gas analysis and measurement of lactate concentration. A central venous O_2 saturation and comparison with arterial O_2 saturation can provide an estimate of cardiac output.

Anticipate the possible need for vasopressors and stress-dose hydrocortisone. Order these drugs from the pharmacy early so that they will be at the bedside. They should be immediately available if the shock is fluid refractory or adrenal insufficiency is suspected.

Identify and correct metabolic derangements immediately. Hypoglycemia and ionized hypocalcemia are commonly seen in septic shock and may contribute to myocardial dysfunction.

Use diagnostic tests (e.g., lactate concentration, base deficit, and central venous O_2 saturation) to identify the severity of shock and monitor the response to fluid therapy.

After initial treatment, evaluate heart rate, blood pressure, and peripheral perfusion to determine the next intervention. If heart rate, blood pressure, and perfusion are returning to normal, arrange admission or transfer to an appropriate pediatric facility. If the child remains hypotensive or poorly perfused, proceed to the next level in the algorithm. Initiate consultation with a pediatric critical care unit or transport team. Continue resuscitation while preparing for admission or transfer.

Managing Fluid-Refractory Septic Shock

If severe shock persists despite rapid, aggressive administration of isotonic crystalloid in the first hour, start treatment for fluid-refractory septic shock as follows:

- Establish arterial and central venous access if not already obtained.
- Administer vasoactive therapy to improve tissue perfusion and blood pressure.
- Administer additional fluid boluses of 20 mL/kg isotonic crystalloid and consider giving a colloid-containing fluid.
- If the hemoglobin concentration is <10 g/dL, consider transfusion to increase O_2-carrying capacity.
- Consider early assisted ventilation with supplementary O_2 and PEEP as needed.

Medication therapy is directed by assessment of blood pressure (including pulse pressure), evaluation of vascular resistance (including peripheral pulses, temperature and perfusion), and $ScvO_2$ if available. It is not always clear from the physical examination whether a child has vasodilation or vasoconstriction. For example, some children with cool extremities may have vasodilation but be poorly perfused because of low stroke volume and poor cardiac function. The reasons for specific drug selection according to type of shock are described below.

"Warm" Shock

Norepinephrine is the vasoactive agent of choice for the child with fluid-refractory septic shock who presents in vasodilated ("warm") shock with poor perfusion or hypotension. Norepinephrine is chosen for its potent α-adrenergic vasoconstricting effects, which can raise diastolic blood pressure by increasing SVR. It is also chosen for its ability to increase cardiac contractility with little change in heart rate. This can restore blood pressure by increasing SVR, venous tone, and stroke volume.

A *vasopressin* infusion may be useful in the setting of norepinephrine-refractory shock. Vasopressin antagonizes the mechanisms of sepsis-mediated vasodilation. It acts synergistically with endogenous and exogenous catecholamines in stabilizing blood pressure but it has no effect on cardiac contractility.

Normotensive Shock

Dopamine is the preferred vasoactive agent for the child with fluid-refractory septic shock who presents with impaired perfusion but adequate blood pressure. Dopamine has variable effects that are dose-dependent. At low doses dopamine improves splanchnic and renal blood flow. At intermediate doses it improves cardiac contractility. At higher doses SVR is increased. If the child's perfusion does not rapidly improve with a dopamine infusion, start an epinephrine or norepinephrine infusion. On the basis of the child's pulse pressure and clinical examination, use epinephrine if the child has normal to high vascular resistance; use norepinephrine if the child has low vascular resistance.

Vasodilators may be useful for improving tissue perfusion in normotensive children who have high SVR despite fluid resuscitation and initiation of inotropic support.

If poor perfusion persists despite dopamine, consider adding milrinone or nitroprusside to the treatment regimen. Milrinone is a phosphodiesterase inhibitor that has both inotropic and vasodilating effects. Nitroprusside is a pure vasodilator.

You may also consider dobutamine. Dobutamine provides both inotropic and vasodilating effects, but it often causes significant tachycardia and may produce a substantial decrease in SVR, with resulting hypotension.

"Cold" Shock

Epinephrine is the preferred vasoactive agent to treat "cold" shock. It has potent inotropic effects that improve stroke volume. The epinephrine dose can be titrated to support blood pressure and systemic perfusion. At low infusion doses, epinephrine can lower SVR (from its β-adrenergic effects). At higher infusion rates, epinephrine can increase SVR (from its α-adrenergic action). An infusion dose of epinephrine in the range of ≥0.3 mcg/kg per minute usually produces a predominant α-adrenergic action. Epinephrine may increase lactate levels by stimulating lactate production in skeletal muscle.

A combination of dobutamine and norepinephrine may also be considered, based on its effectiveness in adults with septic shock. The norepinephrine infusion counterbalances the tendency of dobutamine to cause an excessive decline in SVR and appears to better restore splanchnic perfusion.

Correction of Adrenal Insufficiency

A child in septic shock who is fluid refractory and dopamine dependent or norepinephrine dependent may have adrenal insufficiency. If possible, obtain a baseline cortisol level. In the absence of prospective data defining adrenal insufficiency based on cortisol level, adrenal insufficiency may be present if a random cortisol level is <18 mcg/dL (496 nmol/L).

If you suspect or confirm adrenal insufficiency, give hydrocortisone 2 mg/kg IV bolus (maximum dose 100 mg).

Therapeutic End Points

Titrate vasoactive agents in septic shock to therapeutic end points, including

- Good distal pulses and perfusion
- Adequate blood pressure
- $ScvO_2$ ≥70%
- Correcting metabolic acidosis and lactate concentration

Strict adherence to end points is recommended to avoid excessive vasoconstriction in key organs.

Management of Anaphylactic Shock

Management of anaphylactic shock focuses on treatment of life-threatening cardiopulmonary problems and reversal or blockade of the mediators released as part of the uncontrolled allergic response. Because angioedema (tissue swelling resulting from a marked increase in capillary permeability) may result in complete upper airway obstruction, providers should anticipate the need for early airway intervention with assisted ventilation. Primary therapy is administration of epinephrine to reverse hypotension and release of histamine and other allergic mediators. Fluid resuscitation may also be helpful to restore blood pressure.

Fundamental Fact **Adrenal Insufficiency**	If the diagnosis of adrenal insufficiency is in doubt, perform a corticotropin stimulation test. An increase in cortisol of ≤9 mcg/dL (248 nmol/L) after a 30- or 60-minute corticotropin stimulation test is sufficient to suggest diagnosis of adrenal insufficiency.

Specific Treatment Considerations

Consider the initial general management of shock outlined in Table 3 in addition to the following specific treatments for anaphylactic shock as indicated (Table 8).

Table 8. Management of Anaphylactic Shock: Specific Treatment Considerations

> - Epinephrine
>   - IM epinephrine (1:1000) or epinephrine by autoinjector (pediatric or adult, depending on the child's size) is the most important agent for the treatment of anaphylaxis.
>   - A second dose or an epinephrine infusion may be needed after 10 to 15 minutes in severe anaphylaxis.
> - Administer isotonic crystalloid fluid boluses as needed to support circulation.
> - Salbutamol
>   - Administer salbutamol PRN for bronchospasm by metered dose inhaler, intermittent nebulizer, or continuous nebulizer.
> - Antihistamines
>   - H_1 blocker (i.e., diphenhydramine)
>   - Consider an H_2 blocker (i.e., ranitidine or famotidine).
>   - *Note:* The combination of both an H_1 and H_2 blocker may be more effective than either given alone.
> - Corticosteroids
>   - Methylprednisolone or equivalent corticosteroid
>
> For hypotension refractory to IM epinephrine and fluid, use vasopressors as indicated.
>
> - Epinephrine (1:10 000) infusion; titrate as needed. Frequently low doses (<0.05 mcg/kg per minute) are effective.

Observation is indicated for identification and treatment of late-phase symptoms. Late-phase symptoms may occur in 25% to 30% of children several hours after acute-phase symptoms. The likelihood of late-phase symptoms increases in proportion to the severity of acute-phase symptoms.

Management of Neurogenic Shock

Children with neurogenic shock typically present with hypotension, bradycardia, and sometimes hypothermia. Minimal response to fluid resuscitation is commonly observed. Blood pressure is characterized by a low diastolic blood pressure with a wide pulse pressure because of loss of vascular tone. Children with spinal shock may be more sensitive to variations in ambient temperature and may require supplementary warming or cooling.

Specific Treatment Considerations

The initial management principles for shock outlined in Table 3 may be considered in addition to the following specific treatments for neurogenic shock as indicated (Table 9).

Table 9. Management of Neurogenic Shock: Specific Treatment Considerations

Position the child flat or head-down to improve venous return.
Administer a trial of fluid therapy (isotonic crystalloid) and assess response.
For fluid-refractory hypotension, use vasopressors (e.g., norepinephrine, epinephrine) as indicated.
Provide supplementary warming or cooling as needed.

Management of Cardiogenic Shock

Cardiogenic shock is a condition of inadequate tissue perfusion that results from myocardial dysfunction. Initially cardiogenic shock may resemble hypovolemic shock, so identifying a cardiogenic etiology may be difficult. If you suspect cardiogenic shock, consider a slow administration (10- to 20-minute) fluid bolus (i.e., 5 to 10 mL/kg bolus) while carefully monitoring the child for response. Cardiogenic shock is probably present if the child does not improve, the child's respiratory function deteriorates, or the child develops signs of pulmonary edema. Evidence of venous congestion (e.g., distended jugular veins or hepatomegaly) and cardiomegaly (on chest x-ray) are also suggestive of a cardiac etiology of shock.

Main Objectives

A main objective in the management of cardiogenic shock is to improve the effectiveness of cardiac function and cardiac output by increasing the efficiency of ventricular ejection. Another main objective is to minimize metabolic demand.

Many children with cardiogenic shock have high preload and do not require additional fluid therapy. Others may require a cautious fluid bolus to increase preload. The most effective way to increase stroke volume is to reduce afterload (SVR) rather than give an inotropic agent. Inotropes may increase cardiac contractility but will also increase myocardial O_2 demand. Children who are already hypotensive, however, may require fluid therapy and inotropic support before they will tolerate afterload reduction. Specific management includes

- Cautious fluid administration and monitoring
- Laboratory and other diagnostic studies
- Medications
- Mechanical circulatory support

Consult a pediatric critical care or pediatric cardiology specialist at the earliest opportunity. This will help to facilitate a diagnosis (e.g., echocardiogram), guide ongoing therapy, and direct transfer to definitive care.

Cautious Fluid Administration and Monitoring

Large heart size on the chest x-ray in a child with evidence of shock and poor cardiac output is the hallmark of cardiogenic shock with adequate intravascular volume. Obtain an echocardiogram for more objective and accurate data about preload and cardiac function. If objective data or the child's history (e.g., vomiting and poor intake) is consistent with inadequate preload, you may give a fluid bolus *cautiously* (5 to 10 mL/kg over 10 to 20 minutes). Assess respiratory function frequently during fluid therapy. Watch for development of pulmonary edema and deterioration in pulmonary function. Give supplementary O_2. Be prepared to provide assisted ventilation. Noninvasive positive pressure may reduce the need for mechanical ventilation by decreasing the work of breathing and improving oxygenation.

Consider establishing central venous access to facilitate measurement of central venous pressure as an index of preload status and to provide access for multiple infusions. Central venous access also allows monitoring of central venous O_2 saturation as an objective measurement of the adequacy of O_2 delivery relative to metabolic demand. Invasive monitoring with a pulmonary artery catheter, an option in the pediatric intensive care unit, is not critical to the diagnosis of cardiogenic shock. However, in certain cases a pulmonary artery catheter may be helpful for guiding fluid resuscitation and vasoactive infusions, particularly if evaluation of left ventricular preload is needed.

Laboratory and Other Diagnostic Studies

Obtain laboratory studies to assess the impact of shock on end-organ function. No single laboratory study is completely sensitive or specific for cardiogenic shock. Appropriate studies often include

- An ABG to determine the magnitude of metabolic acidosis and adequacy of oxygenation and ventilation
- Hemoglobin concentration to ensure that O_2-carrying capacity is adequate
- Lactate concentration and central venous O_2 saturation as indicators of the adequacy of O_2 delivery relative to metabolic demand
- Cardiac enzymes and thyroid function tests

Other useful studies include the following:

Study	Use
Chest x-ray	Provides information about cardiac size, pulmonary vascular markings, pulmonary edema, and coexistent pulmonary pathology
ECG	May detect arrhythmia, myocardial injury, ischemic heart disease, or evidence of drug toxicity
Echocardiogram	May be diagnostic, revealing congenital heart disease, akinetic or dyskinetic ventricular wall motion, or valvular dysfunction; also provides objective measurement of ventricular chamber volume (i.e., preload) and function

Medications

If the child is normotensive, medication therapy consists of diuretics and vasodilators. Diuretics are indicated when the child has evidence of pulmonary edema or systemic venous congestion. Vasodilators are typically given by continuous infusion.

Children with cardiogenic shock may require medications to increase cardiac output by improving contractility. Most also require agents to reduce peripheral vascular resistance. This includes vasodilators, inotropes, and phosphodiesterase enzyme inhibitors (i.e., inodilators). Milrinone is the preferred drug in many centres. For a detailed discussion of these agents, see "Medication Therapy" in "General Management of Shock" in this Part.

Increased metabolic demand, particularly increased myocardial O_2 demand, plays a role in the vicious cycle of cardiogenic shock. Reducing metabolic demand is a critical component in the management of cardiogenic shock. Use ventilatory support and antipyretics to reduce metabolic demand. Analgesics and sedatives reduce O_2 consumption but also reduce the endogenous stress response. Give these agents in small doses. Monitor the child carefully for evidence of potential respiratory depression or hypotension.

Mechanical Circulatory Support

Children with cardiogenic shock who do not respond to medical therapy may benefit from mechanical circulatory support if the cause of shock is potentially reversible.

Extracorporeal life support (ECLS) can provide temporary maintenance of cardiac output, oxygenation, and ventilation while the underlying cause of cardiopulmonary failure is treated. Forms of ECLS include extracorporeal membrane oxygenation (ECMO) and ventricular assist devices. ECLS is usually available only in tertiary pediatric centres with the resources and expertise to manage children with acute cardiopulmonary failure.

Specific Treatment Considerations

Follow the initial management principles for shock outlined in Table 3 in addition to the following considerations specific to cardiogenic shock (Table 10).

Table 10. Management of Cardiogenic Shock: Specific Treatment Considerations

• Give 5 to 10 mL/kg isotonic crystalloid bolus slowly (over 10 to 20 min); repeat PRN. • Administer supplementary O_2 and consider need for noninvasive positive pressure or mechanical ventilation. • Assess frequently for pulmonary edema. • Be prepared to assist ventilation. • Obtain expert consultation early.
Order laboratory and other studies to determine degree of end-organ dysfunction.
Administer pharmacologic support (e.g., vasodilators, phosphodiesterase enzyme inhibitors, inotropes, analgesics, antipyretics).
Consider mechanical circulatory support.

Management of Obstructive Shock

Management of obstructive shock is specific to the type of obstruction. This section discusses management of

- Cardiac tamponade
- Tension pneumothorax
- Ductal-dependent congenital heart lesions
- Massive pulmonary embolism

Main Objectives

The early clinical presentation of obstructive shock may resemble hypovolemic shock. A reasonable initial approach may include administering a fluid challenge (10 to 20 mL/kg isotonic crystalloid). Rapid identification

of obstructive shock by the secondary assessment and diagnostic tests is critical to effective treatment. The main objectives in the management of obstructive shock are to

- Correct the cause of obstruction of cardiac output
- Restore tissue perfusion

General Management Principles

In addition to considerations specific to the etiology of the obstruction, follow the initial management principles outlined in the section "Fundamentals of Shock Management."

Specific Management of Cardiac Tamponade

Cardiac tamponade is caused by accumulation of fluid, blood, or air in the pericardial space. This accumulation limits systemic venous return, impairs ventricular filling, and reduces cardiac output. Favorable outcome requires rapid identification and immediate treatment. Children with cardiac tamponade may improve temporarily with fluid administration to augment cardiac output and tissue perfusion until pericardial drainage can be performed.

Consult appropriate specialists (e.g., pediatric critical care, pediatric cardiology, pediatric surgery) early. Elective pericardial drainage (pericardiocentesis), often guided by echocardiography or fluoroscopy, should be performed by specialists who are trained and skilled in the procedure. Emergency pericardiocentesis may be performed in the setting of impending or actual pulseless arrest when there is a strong suspicion of pericardial tamponade.

Specific Management of Tension Pneumothorax

Tension pneumothorax is characterized by the accumulation of air under pressure in the pleural space. This prevents the lung from expanding properly and applies pressure on the heart and great veins. Favorable outcome depends on immediate diagnosis and urgent treatment.

Treatment of a tension pneumothorax is immediate needle decompression followed by thoracostomy for chest tube placement as soon as possible. A trained provider can quickly perform an emergent needle decompression by inserting an 18- to 20-gauge over-the-needle catheter over the top of the child's third rib (second intercostal space) in the midclavicular line. A gush of air is a sign that needle decompression has been successful. This indicates relief of pressure buildup in the pleural space.

Identify and Intervene **Obstructive Shock**	Because children with obstructive shock can rapidly progress to cardiopulmonary failure and then cardiac arrest, immediate identification and correction of the underlying cause of the obstruction may be lifesaving.

Specific Management of Ductal-Dependent Lesions

Ductal-dependent lesions are a group of congenital cardiac abnormalities. These abnormalities result in pulmonary or systemic blood flow that must pass through a patent ductus arteriosus.

Ductal-dependent pulmonary blood flow usually includes a severe obstruction to pulmonary blood flow from the right ventricle, so all pulmonary blood flow comes from the aorta through the ductus arteriosus. When the ductus begins to close, the infant becomes profoundly cyanotic and hypoxemic.

Ductal-dependent systemic blood flow usually consists of an obstruction to outflow through or from the left side of the heart into the aorta. In such patients systemic blood flow must come from the right ventricle and pulmonary artery into the aorta. In these patients when the ductus starts to close (during the first days to weeks of life), signs of shock develop with severe deterioration in systemic perfusion.

For any infant with ductal-dependent pulmonary or systemic blood flow, immediate treatment with continuous infusion of prostaglandin E_1 (PGE_1) to restore ductal patency may be lifesaving.

An infusion of PGE_1 restores ductal patency.

Other management actions for ductal-dependent obstructive lesions are

- Ventilatory support with O_2 administration
- Echocardiography for diagnosis and expert consultation to direct therapy
- Administration of inotropic agents to improve myocardial contractility
- Judicious administration of fluids to improve cardiac output
- Correction of metabolic derangements, including metabolic acidosis

Specific Management of Massive Pulmonary Embolism

Massive pulmonary embolism is a sudden blockage in the main or large-branch pulmonary artery. This blockage is usually caused by a blood clot that has traveled to the lungs from another part of the body. The blockage also can result from other substances, including fat, air, amniotic fluid, catheter fragment, or injected matter. Blood flow through the pulmonary circulation to the left side of the heart is obstructed, resulting in decreased left-sided filling and inadequate cardiac output.

Initial treatment is supportive, including administration of O_2, ventilatory assistance, and fluid therapy if the child is poorly perfused. Consult a specialist who can perform echocardiography, a computed tomography (CT) scan with IV contrast, or angiography to confirm the diagnosis. Anticoagulants (e.g., heparin, enoxaparin) are the definitive treatment for most children with pulmonary embolism who are not in shock. Because anticoagulants do not act immediately to relieve obstruction, consider fibrinolytic agents (e.g., recombinant tissue plasminogen activator [rtPA]) in children with severe cardiovascular compromise.

CT angiography is the diagnostic test of choice because it can be rapidly obtained and does not require an invasive angiogram. Additional diagnostic studies that might be useful are an ABG, CBC, D-dimer, ECG, chest x-ray, ventilation-perfusion scan, and echocardiography.

Management of Shock Flowchart

Management of Shock Flowchart	
• Oxygen • Pulse oximetry • ECG monitor	• IV/IO access • BLS as indicated • Point-of-care glucose testing

Hypovolemic Shock **Specific Management for Selected Conditions**	
Nonhemorrhagic	**Hemorrhagic**
• 20 mL/kg NS/LR bolus, repeat as needed • Consider colloid	• Control external bleeding • 20 mL/kg NS/LR bolus, repeat 2 or 3× as needed • Transfuse PRBCs as indicated

Distributive Shock **Specific Management for Selected Conditions**		
Septic	**Anaphylactic**	**Neurogenic**
Management Algorithm: • Septic Shock	• IM epinephrine (or autoinjector) • Fluid boluses (20 mL/kg NS/LR) • Salbutamol • Antihistamines, corticosteroids • Epinephrine infusion	• 20 mL/kg NS/LR bolus, repeat PRN • Vasopressor

Cardiogenic Shock **Specific Management for Selected Conditions**	
Bradyarrhythmia/Tachyarrhythmia	**Other (e.g., CHD, Myocarditis, Cardiomyopathy, Poisoning)**
Management Algorithms: • Bradycardia • Tachycardia With Poor Perfusion	• 5 to 10 mL/kg NS/LR bolus, repeat PRN • Vasoactive infusion • Consider expert consultation

Obstructive Shock **Specific Management for Selected Conditions**			
Ductal-Dependent **(LV Outflow Obstruction)**	**Tension** **Pneumothorax**	**Cardiac** **Tamponade**	**Pulmonary** **Embolism**
• Prostaglandin E_1 • Expert consultation	• Needle decompression • Tube thoracostomy	• Pericardiocentesis • 20 mL/kg NS/LR bolus	• 20 mL/kg NS/LR bolus, repeat PRN • Consider thrombolytics, anticoagulants • Expert consultation

Figure 2. Management of Shock Flowchart.

Suggested Reading List

Akech S, Ledermann H, Maitland K. Choice of fluids for resuscitation in children with severe infection and shock: systematic review. *BMJ.* 2010;341:c4416.

Ben-Shoshan M, Clarke AE. Anaphylaxis: past, present and future. *Allergy.* 2011;66:1-14.

Carcillo JA. Choice of fluids for resuscitation in children with severe infection and shock. *BMJ.* 2010;341:c4546.

Choong K, Bohn D, Fraser DD, Gaboury L, Hutchison JS, Joffe AR, Litalien C, Menon K, McNamara P, Ward RE; Canadian Critical Care Trials Group. Vasopressin in pediatric vasodilatory shock: a multicenter randomized controlled trial. *Am J Respir Crit Care Med.* 2009;180:632-639.

Losek JD. Hypoglycemia and the ABC's (sugar) of pediatric resuscitation. *Ann Emerg Med.* 2000;35:43-46.

Stoner MJ, Goodman DG, Cohen DM, Fernandez SA, Hall MW. Rapid fluid resuscitation in pediatrics: testing the American College of Critical Care Medicine Guideline. *Ann Emerg Med.* 2007;50:601-607.

Septic Shock

Barton P, Garcia J, Kouatli A, Kitchen L, Zorka A, Lindsay C, Lawless S, Giroir B. Hemodynamic effects of I.V. milrinone lactate in pediatric patients with septic shock: a prospective, double-blinded, randomized, placebo-controlled, interventional study. *Chest.* 1996;109:1302-1312.

Brierley J, Carcillo JA, Choong K, Cornell T, Decaen A, Deymann A, Doctor A, Davis A, Duff J, Dugas MA, Duncan A, Evans B, Feldman J, Felmet K, Fisher G, Frankel L, Jeffries H, Greenwald B, Gutierrez J, Hall M, Han YY, Hanson J, Hazelzet J, Hernan L, Kiff J, Kissoon N, Kon A, Irazuzta J, Lin J, Lorts A, Mariscalco M, Mehta R, Nadel S, Nguyen T, Nicholson C, Peters M, Okhuysen-Cawley R, Poulton T, Relves M, Rodriguez A, Rozenfeld R, Schnitzler E, Shanley T, Kache S, Skippen P, Torres A, von Dessauer B, Weingarten J, Yeh T, Zaritsky A, Stojadinovic B, Zimmerman J, Zuckerberg A. Clinical practice parameters for hemodynamic support of pediatric and neonatal septic shock: 2007 update from the American College of Critical Care Medicine. *Crit Care Med.* 2009;37:666-688.

Carcillo JA, Davis AL Zaritsky A. Role of early fluid resuscitation in pediatric septic shock. *JAMA.* 1991;266:1242-1245.

Ceneviva, G, Paschall JA, Maffei F, Carcillo JA. Hemodynamic support in fluid-refractory pediatric septic shock. *Pediatrics.* 1998;102:e19.

de Oliveira CF, de Oliveira DS, Gottschald AF, Moura JD, Costa GA, Ventura AC, Fernandes JC, Vaz FA, Carcillo JA, Rivers EP, Troster EJ. ACCM/PALS haemodynamic support guidelines for paediatric septic shock: an outcomes comparison with and without monitoring central venous oxygen saturation. *Intensive Care Med.* 2008;34:1065-1075.

Goldstein B, Giroir B, Randolph A; International Consensus Conference on Pediatric Sepsis. International pediatric sepsis consensus conference: definitions for sepsis and organ dysfunction in pediatrics. *Pediatr Crit Care Med.* 2005;6:2-8.

Lindsay CA, Barton P, Lawless S, Kitchen L, Zorka A, Garcia J, Kouatli A, Giroir B. Pharmacokinetics and pharmacodynamics of milrinone lactate in pediatric patients with septic shock. *J Pediatr.* 1998;132:329-334.

Lipiner-Friedman D, Sprung CL, Laterre PF, Weiss Y, Goodman SV, Vogeser M, Briegel J, Keh D, Singer M, Moreno R, Bellissant E, Annane D. Adrenal function in sepsis: the retrospective Corticus cohort study. *Crit Care Med.* 2007;35:1012-1018.

Pizarro CF, Troster EJ, Damiani D, Carcillo JA. Absolute and relative adrenal insufficiency in children with septic shock. *Crit Care Med.* 2005;33:855-859.

Sprung CL, Annane D, Keh D, Moreno R, Singer M, Freivogel K, Weiss YG, Benbenishty J, Kalenka A, Forst H, Laterre PF, Reinhart K, Cuthbertson BH, Payen D, Briegel J. Hydrocortisone therapy for patients with septic shock. *N Engl J Med.* 2008;358:111-124.

Extracorporeal Cardiopulmonary Resuscitation (ECPR)

See the "Extracorporeal Life Support (ECLS)/Extracorporeal Cardiopulmonary Resuscitation (ECPR)" section in the Suggested Reading List for Part 10: "Recognition and Management of Cardiac Arrest."

Resources for Management of Circulatory Emergencies

Intraosseous Access

Intraosseous (IO) cannulation is a relatively simple and effective method of rapidly establishing vascular access for emergency fluids or medications. It provides access to a noncollapsible marrow venous plexus, which serves as a rapid, safe, and reliable route for administration of drugs, crystalloids, colloids, and blood during resuscitation. IO access can be achieved in children of all ages, often in about 30 to 60 seconds. In certain circumstances (e.g., cardiac arrest or severe shock with severe vasoconstriction), it may be the *initial* vascular access attempted. Fluids and medications can reach the central circulation within seconds when delivered via an IO route. If peripheral vascular access cannot be readily obtained in a child with compensated or hypotensive shock, be prepared to establish IO access as soon as it is needed.

Sites for IO Access

Many sites are appropriate for IO infusion. The proximal tibia, just below the growth plate, is often used. Other sites are the distal tibia just above the medial malleolus, the distal femur, and the anterior-superior iliac spine. Newer devices, such as the IO drill, are approved for use in the humerus in older children, adolescents, and adults.

Contraindications

Contraindications to IO access include

- Fractures and crush injuries near the access site
- Conditions with fragile bones (e.g., osteogenesis imperfecta)
- Previous attempts to establish access in the same bone

Avoid IO cannulation if infection is present in the overlying tissues.

Procedure (Proximal Tibia)

Use the following procedure to establish IO access.

Step	Action
1	• To establish access in the proximal tibia, position the leg with slight external rotation. • Identify the tibial tuberosity just below the knee joint. The insertion site is the flat part of the tibia, about 1 to 3 cm (about 1 finger's width) below and medial to this bony prominence (Figure 1). Always use universal precautions when attempting vascular access. Disinfect the overlying skin and surrounding area.
2	• Leave the stylet in the needle during insertion to prevent the needle from becoming clogged with bone or tissue. • Stabilize the leg on a firm surface. Do not place your hand behind the leg. *Note:* If a standard IO needle or bone marrow needle is not available, a large-bore (at least 18-gauge) standard hypodermic needle can be substituted, but the lumen may become clogged with bone or bone marrow during insertion. Short, wide-gauge spinal needles with internal stylets can be used in an emergency, but they tend to bend easily. A hemostat can be used to help stabilize the needle during insertion.
3	• Insert the needle through the skin over the anteromedial surface of the tibia perpendicular to the tibia. This avoids injury to the growth plate. • Use a twisting motion with gentle but firm pressure. • Continue inserting the needle through the cortical bone until there is a sudden decrease in resistance as the needle enters the marrow space. If the needle is placed correctly, it should stand easily without support.

(continued)

(continued)

Step	Action

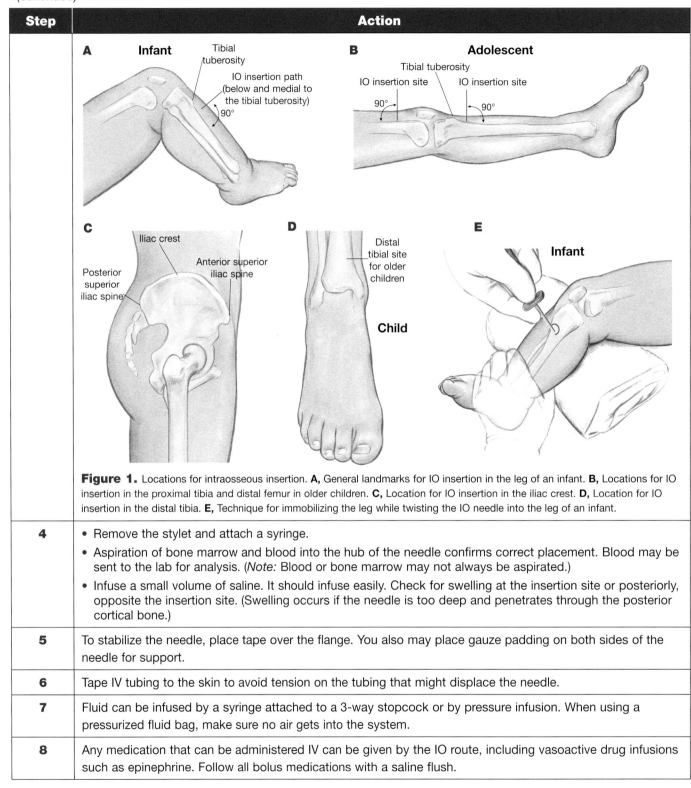

Figure 1. Locations for intraosseous insertion. **A,** General landmarks for IO insertion in the leg of an infant. **B,** Locations for IO insertion in the proximal tibia and distal femur in older children. **C,** Location for IO insertion in the iliac crest. **D,** Location for IO insertion in the distal tibia. **E,** Technique for immobilizing the leg while twisting the IO needle into the leg of an infant.

Step	Action
4	• Remove the stylet and attach a syringe. • Aspiration of bone marrow and blood into the hub of the needle confirms correct placement. Blood may be sent to the lab for analysis. (*Note:* Blood or bone marrow may not always be aspirated.) • Infuse a small volume of saline. It should infuse easily. Check for swelling at the insertion site or posteriorly, opposite the insertion site. (Swelling occurs if the needle is too deep and penetrates through the posterior cortical bone.)
5	To stabilize the needle, place tape over the flange. You also may place gauze padding on both sides of the needle for support.
6	Tape IV tubing to the skin to avoid tension on the tubing that might displace the needle.
7	Fluid can be infused by a syringe attached to a 3-way stopcock or by pressure infusion. When using a pressurized fluid bag, make sure no air gets into the system.
8	Any medication that can be administered IV can be given by the IO route, including vasoactive drug infusions such as epinephrine. Follow all bolus medications with a saline flush.

After IO Insertion

After IO needle/catheter insertion do the following:

• Check the site frequently for signs of swelling and needle displacement; fluids or drugs delivered via a displaced needle can cause severe complications (e.g., tissue necrosis, compartment syndrome).

• IO needles are intended for short-term use, generally <24 hours. Replacement with long-term vascular access is usually accomplished in an intensive care setting.

Colour-Coded Length-Based Resuscitation Tape

Use a colour-coded length-based tape to select the correct size of resuscitation supplies and to determine the child's weight (if not known) for calculating drug doses.

Table 1. Colour-Coded Length-Based Resuscitation Tape

Equipment	GRAY* 3-5 kg	PINK Small Infant 6-7 kg	RED Infant 8-9 kg	PURPLE Toddler 10-11 kg	YELLOW Small Child 12-14 kg	WHITE Child 15-18 kg	BLUE Child 19-23 kg	ORANGE Large Child 24-29 kg	GREEN Adult 30-36 kg
Resuscitation bag		Infant/child	Infant/child	Child	Child	Child	Child	Child	Adult
Oxygen mask (NRB)		Pediatric	Pediatric	Pediatric	Pediatric	Pediatric	Pediatric	Pediatric	Pediatric/ adult
Oral airway (mm)		50	50	60	60	60	70	80	80
Laryngoscope blade (size)		1 Straight	1 Straight	1 Straight	2 Straight	2 Straight	2 Straight or curved	2 Straight or curved	3 Straight or curved
ET tube (mm)†		3.5 Uncuffed 3.0 Cuffed	3.5 Uncuffed 3.0 Cuffed	4.0 Uncuffed 3.5 Cuffed	4.5 Uncuffed 4.0 Cuffed	5.0 Uncuffed 4.5 Cuffed	5.5 Uncuffed 5.0 Cuffed	6.0 Cuffed	6.5 Cuffed
ET tube insertion length (cm)	3 kg 9-9.5 4 kg 9.5-10 5 kg 10-10.5	10.5-11	10.5-11	11-12	13.5	14-15	16.5	17-18	18.5-19.5
Suction catheter (F)		8	8	10	10	10	10	10	10-12
BP cuff	Neonatal #5/infant	Infant/child	Infant/child	Child	Child	Child	Child	Child	Small adult
IV catheter (ga)		22-24	22-24	20-24	18-22	18-22	18-20	18-20	16-20
IO (ga)		18/15	18/15	15	15	15	15	15	15
NG tube (F)		5-8	5-8	8-10	10	10	12-14	14-18	16-18
Urinary catheter (F)	5	8	8	8-10	10	10-12	10-12	12	12
Chest tube (F)		10-12	10-12	16-20	20-24	20-24	24-32	28-32	32-38

Abbreviations: BP, blood pressure; ET, endotracheal; F, French; IO, intraosseous; IV, intravenous; NG, nasogastric; NRB, nonrebreathing.

*For Gray column, use Pink or Red equipment sizes if no size is listed.

†Per *2010 Guidelines*, in the hospital cuffed or uncuffed tubes may be used (see below for sizing of cuffed tubes).

Adapted from *Broselow™ Pediatric Emergency Tape*. Distributed by Armstrong Medical Industries, Lincolnshire, IL. Copyright 2007 Vital Signs, Inc. All rights reserved.

Part 8

Recognition and Management of Bradycardia

Overview

This Part discusses the recognition and management of bradycardia (slow heart rate) with a pulse in infants and children.

Learning Objectives

After studying this Part you should be able to

- Describe when bradycardia requires immediate intervention
- Describe initial steps to stabilize a child with cardiopulmonary compromise
- Know when to start CPR in a child with bradycardia
- Manage a child as outlined in the Pediatric Bradycardia With a Pulse and Poor Perfusion Algorithm
- Select appropriate medications for treatment of symptomatic bradycardia

Preparation for the Course

You will be expected to recognize bradycardic rhythms and manage a child as outlined in the Pediatric Bradycardia With a Pulse and Poor Perfusion Algorithm.

Definitions

Bradycardia is a heart rate that is slow in comparison with a normal heart rate range for the child's age and level of activity. See Part 2, Table 2: Normal Heart Rates (per Minute) by Age.

Bradycardia is an ominous sign of impending cardiac arrest in infants and children, especially if it is associated with hypotension or evidence of poor tissue perfusion. If, despite adequate oxygenation and ventilation, the heart rate is <60/min in an infant or child with signs of poor tissue perfusion, begin CPR.

Critical Concept **Symptomatic Bradycardia and Cardiopulmonary Compromise**	*Symptomatic bradycardia* is a heart rate slower than normal for the child's age (usually <60/min) associated with cardiopulmonary compromise. *Cardiopulmonary compromise* is defined as signs of shock (e.g., poor systemic perfusion, hypotension, altered mental status [i.e., decreased level of consciousness]) combined with respiratory distress or failure.

Fundamental Fact **Evaluating Heart Rate and Rhythm**	Consider the following when evaluating the heart rate and rhythm in any seriously ill or injured child: • The child's typical heart rate and baseline rhythm • The child's level of activity and clinical condition (including baseline cardiac function) Children with congenital heart disease may have underlying conduction abnormalities. Interpret the child's heart rate and rhythm by comparing them to the child's baseline heart rate and rhythm. Children with poor cardiac function are more likely to become symptomatic from arrhythmias than children with good cardiac function.

Tissue hypoxia is the leading cause of symptomatic bradycardia in children. Therefore, symptomatic bradycardia in children is usually the result of (and not the reason for) progressive hypoxemia and respiratory failure. Priorities in initial assessment and management should be to support the airway and provide adequate oxygenation and ventilation.

Bradycardia may be classified as

- Primary bradycardia
- Secondary bradycardia

Primary bradycardia is the result of congenital or acquired heart conditions that slow the spontaneous depolarization rate of the heart's normal pacemaker cells or slow conduction through the heart's conduction system. Causes of primary bradycardia include

- Congenital abnormality of the heart pacemaker or conduction system
- Surgical injury to the pacemaker or conduction system
- Cardiomyopathy
- Myocarditis

Secondary bradycardia is the result of noncardiac conditions that alter the normal function of the heart (i.e., slow the sinus node pacemaker or slow conduction through the atrioventricular [AV] junction). Causes of secondary bradycardia include

- Hypoxia
- Acidosis
- Hypotension
- Hypothermia
- Drug effects

Recognition of Bradycardia
Signs and Symptoms of Bradycardia

Cardiac output (the volume of blood pumped by the heart per minute) is the product of stroke volume (the volume of blood pumped with each beat) and heart rate (number of beats per minute):

Cardiac Output = Stroke Volume × Heart Rate

When heart rate decreases, cardiac output can only be maintained by an increase in stroke volume. Because the heart's ability to increase stroke volume is limited (especially in infants), cardiac output typically declines with bradycardia. An extremely slow heart rate results in critically low cardiac output that can be life threatening and lead to cardiopulmonary compromise. The signs of cardiopulmonary compromise associated with bradycardia are

- Hypotension
- Decreased level of consciousness
- Shock

- Poor end-organ perfusion
- Respiratory distress or failure
- Sudden collapse

ECG Characteristics of Bradycardia

The ECG characteristics of bradycardia include

Heart rate	Slow compared with normal heart rate for age
P waves	May or may not be visible
QRS complex	Narrow or wide (depending on the origin of the pacemaker and/or location of injury to the conduction system)
P wave and QRS complex	May be unrelated (i.e., atrioventricular [AV] dissociation)

See "Rhythm Recognition Review" in the Appendix for examples.

Types of Bradyarrhythmias

Bradycardia that is associated with a rhythm disturbance (arrhythmia) is called a bradyarrhythmia. Two common types of bradyarrhythmia in children are sinus bradycardia and AV block. These are discussed in detail in the next section. Other types of bradyarrhythmias are sinus node arrest with atrial, junctional, or ventricular escape rhythms. These are more complex rhythms and are not discussed in the PALS Provider Course.

Sinus Bradycardia

Sinus bradycardia is a sinus node discharge rate slower than normal for the child's age (see Part 2, Table 2: Normal Heart Rates [per Minute] by Age). Sinus bradycardia is not necessarily problematic. It is often present in healthy children at rest when metabolic demands of the body are relatively low (e.g., during sleep). Well-conditioned athletes often have sinus bradycardia because they have high stroke volume and increased vagal tone. However, sinus bradycardia can also develop in response to hypoxia, hypotension, and acidosis. As discussed above, it is often the result of progressive respiratory failure and may be the sign of impending cardiac arrest. Sinus bradycardia also may result from drug effects. Therefore, evaluation of sinus bradycardia always must involve assessment of the clinical status of the child.

Rarely, children with primary bradycardia have an intrinsic disorder of the sinus node that impairs the ability of the sinus node to depolarize sufficiently. These children usually have a history of surgery for complex congenital heart disease. Additional causes of sinus node disorders include congenital abnormalities of the conduction system, cardiomyopathy, and myocarditis.

AV Block

AV block is a disturbance of electrical conduction through the AV node. AV block is classified as follows:

- *First degree*: A prolonged PR interval representing slowed conduction through the AV node (Figure 1A)
- *Second degree*: Block of some but not all atrial impulses before they reach the ventricles. This block can be further classified as Mobitz type I or Mobitz type II second-degree AV block.
  - Mobitz type I AV block (also known as *Wenckebach phenomenon*) typically occurs at the AV node. It is characterized by progressive prolongation of the PR interval until an atrial impulse is not conducted to the ventricles (Figure 1B). The P wave corresponding to that atrial impulse is not followed by a QRS complex. The cycle often repeats.
  - Mobitz type II second-degree AV block (Figure 1C) occurs below the level of the AV node. It is characterized by nonconduction of some atrial impulses to the ventricle without any change in the PR interval of conducted impulses. Often there is a consistent ratio of atrial to ventricular depolarizations, typically 2 atrial depolarizations to 1 ventricular depolarization.
- *Third degree*: None of the atrial impulses conducts to the ventricles. This block may also be referred to as *complete heart block* or *complete AV block* (Figure 1D).

Type	Causes	Characteristics	Symptoms
First degree	• *Note:* May be present in healthy children • Intrinsic AV nodal disease • Enhanced vagal tone • Myocarditis • Electrolyte disturbances (e.g., hyperkalemia) • Hypoxemia • Myocardial infarction • Cardiac surgery • Drugs (e.g., calcium channel blockers, β-adrenergic blockers, digoxin) • Acute rheumatic fever	Prolonged PR interval	Asymptomatic
Second-degree Mobitz type I (Wenckebach phenomenon)	• *Note:* May be present in healthy children • Drugs (e.g., calcium channel and β-adrenergic blockers, digoxin) • Any condition that stimulates vagal (parasympathetic) tone • Myocardial infarction	Progressive prolongation of the PR interval until a P wave is not conducted; the cycle often repeats	May cause occasional light-headedness (feeling faint)
Second-degree Mobitz type II	• Typically results from intrinsic conduction system abnormalities • Rarely caused by increased parasympathetic tone or drugs • Cardiac surgery • Myocardial infarction	Some but not all P waves are blocked before they reach the ventricle (PR interval is constant); often, every other P wave is conducted (2:1 block)	May cause • Sensed irregularities of heartbeat (palpitations) • Presyncope (light-headedness) • Syncope

(continued)

(continued)

Type	Causes	Characteristics	Symptoms
Third degree	• Extensive conduction system disease or injury, including myocarditis • Cardiac surgery • Congenital complete heart block • Myocardial infarction • Can also result from increased parasympathetic tone, toxic drug effects, or severe hypoxia/acidosis	• No relationship between P waves and QRS complexes • No atrial impulses reach ventricles • Ventricular rhythm maintained by a lower pacemaker	Most frequent symptoms are • Fatigue • Light-headedness • Syncope

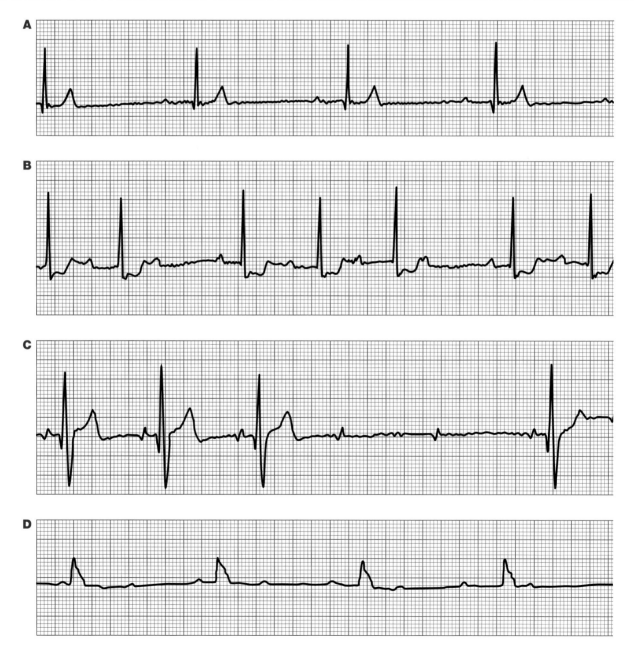

Figure 1. AV blocks. **A,** Sinus bradycardia with first-degree AV block. **B,** Second-degree AV block Mobitz type I (Wenckebach phenomenon). **C,** Second-degree AV block Mobitz type II. **D,** Third-degree AV block.

Management: Pediatric Bradycardia With a Pulse and Poor Perfusion Algorithm

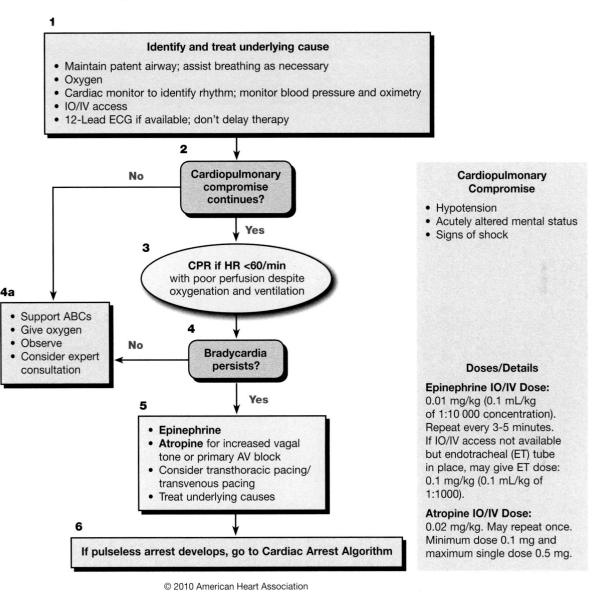

1

Identify and treat underlying cause
- Maintain patent airway; assist breathing as necessary
- Oxygen
- Cardiac monitor to identify rhythm; monitor blood pressure and oximetry
- IO/IV access
- 12-Lead ECG if available; don't delay therapy

2

No

Cardiopulmonary compromise continues?

Yes

3

CPR if HR <60/min with poor perfusion despite oxygenation and ventilation

4a
- Support ABCs
- Give oxygen
- Observe
- Consider expert consultation

4

No

Bradycardia persists?

Yes

5
- **Epinephrine**
- **Atropine** for increased vagal tone or primary AV block
- Consider transthoracic pacing/ transvenous pacing
- Treat underlying causes

6

If pulseless arrest develops, go to Cardiac Arrest Algorithm

Cardiopulmonary Compromise
- Hypotension
- Acutely altered mental status
- Signs of shock

Doses/Details

Epinephrine IO/IV Dose:
0.01 mg/kg (0.1 mL/kg of 1:10 000 concentration). Repeat every 3-5 minutes. If IO/IV access not available but endotracheal (ET) tube in place, may give ET dose: 0.1 mg/kg (0.1 mL/kg of 1:1000).

Atropine IO/IV Dose:
0.02 mg/kg. May repeat once. Minimum dose 0.1 mg and maximum single dose 0.5 mg.

© 2010 American Heart Association

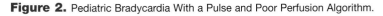

Figure 2. Pediatric Bradycardia With a Pulse and Poor Perfusion Algorithm.

The Pediatric Bradycardia Algorithm (Figure 2) outlines the steps for evaluation and management of the child presenting with symptomatic bradycardia (bradycardia with a pulse and poor perfusion). See the Critical Concept box in the "Definitions" section above for more information about symptomatic bradycardia and cardiopulmonary compromise. In the text that follows, box numbers refer to the corresponding boxes in this algorithm.

Identify and Treat Underlying Cause (Box 1)

Once you identify symptomatic bradycardia with cardiopulmonary compromise, initial management may include the following, but priorities are immediate oxygenation and ventilation:

Airway	Support the airway (position child or allow child to assume a position of comfort) or open the airway (perform manual airway maneuver) if needed.
Breathing	• Give O_2 in high concentration—use a nonrebreathing mask if available. • Assist ventilation as indicated (e.g., bag-mask ventilation). • Attach a pulse oximeter to assess oxygenation.
Circulation	• Monitor blood pressure and assess perfusion. • Attach a monitor/defibrillator (with transcutaneous pacing capability if available). • Establish vascular access (IV or IO). • Check electrode pad position and skin contact to ensure that there are no artifacts and that the ECG tracing is accurate. • Record a 12-lead ECG if available (do not delay therapy). • Obtain appropriate laboratory studies (e.g., potassium, glucose, ionized calcium, magnesium, blood gas for pH, toxicology screen).

A child with primary bradycardia may benefit from evaluation by a pediatric cardiologist. However, do not delay initiation of emergency treatment, including high-quality CPR, if symptoms are present.

Reassess (Box 2)

Reassess to determine if bradycardia and cardiopulmonary compromise continue despite adequate ventilation and oxygenation.

Bradycardia and cardiopulmonary compromise?	Management
No	Go to Box 4a. Support ABCs as needed, administer supplementary O_2, and perform frequent reassessments. Consider expert consultation.
Yes	Go to Box 3. Perform CPR if heart rate is <60/min with continued signs of poor perfusion despite adequate oxygenation and ventilation.

If Adequate Respiration and Perfusion (Box 4a)

If pulses, perfusion, and respirations are adequate, no emergency treatment is needed. Monitor and continue evaluation.

If Bradycardia and Cardiopulmonary Compromise Persist: Perform CPR (Box 3)

If bradycardia is associated with cardiopulmonary compromise (Critical Concept box) and if heart rate is <60/min despite effective oxygenation and ventilation, perform chest compressions and ventilations (CPR). If the bradycardia persists, proceed with medication therapy and possible pacing (Box 5). Reassess the child frequently in response to the therapy you are providing.

Critical Concept Reassess for Cardiopulmonary Compromise	Reassess the child for signs of cardiopulmonary compromise, including • Hypotension • Acutely decreased level of consciousness • Signs of poor perfusion

Fundamental Fact Perform High-Quality CPR	During CPR, push fast (at least 100 compressions/min); push hard (at least one third of the anterior-posterior diameter of the chest); allow complete chest recoil after each compression; minimize interruptions in chest compressions; and avoid excessive ventilation.

Reassess Rhythm (Box 4)

Reassess to determine if bradycardia and cardiopulmonary compromise continue despite provision of oxygenation, ventilation, and CPR.

Bradycardia and cardiopulmonary compromise?	Management
No	Go to Box 4a. Support ABCs as needed, administer supplementary O₂, and perform frequent reassessments. Consider expert consultation.
Yes	Go to Box 5. Administer medications and consider cardiac pacing.

Administer Medications (Box 5)

If bradycardia and cardiopulmonary compromise continue despite oxygenation, ventilation, and CPR, administer epinephrine. Consider atropine.

Epinephrine

Epinephrine is indicated for symptomatic bradycardia that persists despite effective oxygenation and ventilation. Epinephrine has both α- and β-adrenergic activity. β-Adrenergic activity increases heart rate and cardiac output, and α-adrenergic activity causes vasoconstriction. The efficacy of epinephrine and other catecholamines may be reduced by acidosis and hypoxia. This makes support of the airway, ventilation, oxygenation, and perfusion (with chest compressions) essential.

IV/IO	0.01 mg/kg (1:10 000: 0.1 mL/kg)
ET	0.1 mg/kg (1:1000: 0.1 mL/kg)
Repeat every 3 to 5 minutes as needed.	

For persistent bradycardia, consider a continuous infusion of epinephrine (0.1 to 0.3 mcg/kg per minute). A continuous epinephrine infusion may be useful, particularly if the child has responded to a bolus of epinephrine. Titrate the infusion dose to clinical response.

Atropine

Atropine sulfate is a parasympatholytic (or anticholinergic) drug that accelerates sinus or atrial pacemakers and enhances AV conduction. Administer atropine instead of epinephrine for bradycardia caused by increased vagal tone, cholinergic drug toxicity (e.g., organophosphates), or complete AV block. Atropine (and pacing) are preferred over epinephrine as the first-choice treatment of symptomatic AV block due to

primary bradycardia. The rationale for using atropine rather than epinephrine in these situations is that epinephrine can cause ventricular arrhythmias if the myocardium is chronically abnormal or hypoxic/ischemic. If the child does not respond to atropine in these situations, use epinephrine. Atropine is not indicated for AV block from secondary bradycardia (i.e., treatable causes such as hypoxia or acidosis).

Atropine may be used for the treatment of second-degree AV block (Mobitz types I and II) and third-degree AV block. The healthcare provider should recognize, however, that symptomatic AV block may not respond to atropine and the child may require pacing.

Atropine or atropine-like drugs are often used prophylactically in young children to prevent vagally mediated bradycardia during endotracheal intubation attempts.

Atropine	
Route	**Dose**
IV/IO	First dose 0.02 mg/kg; minimum 0.1 mg (maximum single dose 0.5 mg) May repeat dose in 5 minutes (maximum single dose 0.5 mg) *Note:* Larger doses may be required for organophosphate poisoning.
ET *Note:* IV/IO administration is preferred, but if it is not available, atropine can be administered by ET tube. Because absorption of atropine given by the endotracheal route is unreliable, a larger dose (2 to 3 times the IV dose) may be required.	0.04 to 0.06 mg/kg

Note that small doses of atropine may produce paradoxical bradycardia; for this reason, a minimum dose of 0.1 mg is recommended. Tachycardia may follow administration of atropine, but atropine-induced tachycardia is generally well tolerated in the pediatric patient.

Consider Cardiac Pacing (Box 5)

Temporary cardiac pacing may be lifesaving in selected cases of bradycardia caused by complete heart block or abnormal sinus node function. For example, pacing is indicated for AV block after surgical correction of congenital heart disease.

Treat Underlying Causes (Box 5)

Identify and treat potentially reversible causes and special circumstances that can cause bradycardia. The 2 most common potentially reversible causes of bradycardia are hypoxia and increased vagal tone. Be aware that after heart transplantation, sympathetic nerve fibers are no longer attached to the heart, so the response to sympathomimetic drugs may be unpredictable. For the same reason, anticholinergic drugs such as atropine may be ineffective. Early cardiac pacing may be indicated in such patients.

Treat potentially reversible causes of bradycardia as follows:

Reversible Cause	Treatment
Hypoxia	Give high-concentration supplementary O_2 with assisted ventilation as necessary.
Hydrogen ion (acidosis)	Provide ventilation to treat respiratory acidosis secondary to hypercarbia. Consider sodium bicarbonate in severe metabolic acidosis.
Hyperkalemia	Restore normal potassium concentration.
Hypothermia	Warm, but avoid hyperthermia if the patient has experienced a cardiac arrest.
Heart block	For AV block, consider atropine, chronotropic drugs, and electrical pacing. Obtain expert consultation.
Toxins/ poisons/ drugs	Treat with a specific antidote and provide supportive care. Some toxicologic causes of bradyarrhythmias are • Cholinesterase inhibitors (organophosphates, carbamates, and nerve agents) • Calcium channel blockers • β-Adrenergic blockers • Digoxin and other cardiac glycosides • Clonidine and other centrally acting α_2-adrenergic agonists • Opioids • Succinylcholine

(continued)

(continued)

Reversible Cause	Treatment
Trauma	Head trauma: Bradycardia in a child with head trauma is an ominous sign of high intracranial pressure (ICP). Provide oxygenation and ventilation, and hyperventilate if signs of impending herniation develop. Obtain immediate expert assistance for relief of increased ICP.

Pulseless Arrest (Box 6)

If pulseless cardiac arrest develops, start CPR. Proceed according to the Pediatric Cardiac Arrest Algorithm (see Part 10: "Recognition and Management of Cardiac Arrest").

Suggested Reading List

Donoghue A, Berg RA, Hazinski MF, Praestgaard AH, Roberts K, Nadkarni VM. Cardiopulmonary resuscitation for bradycardia with poor perfusion versus pulseless cardiac arrest. *Pediatrics*. 2009;124:1541-1548.

Drago F, Turchetta A, Calzolari A, Giannico S, Marianeschi S, Di Donato R, Di Carlo D, Ragonese P, Marcelletti C. Early identification of patients at risk for sinus node dysfunction after Mustard operation. *Int J Cardiol*. 1992;35:27-32.

Kugler JD. Sinus node dysfunction. In: Gillette PC, Garson AR Jr, eds. *Pediatric Arrhythmias, Electrophysiology and Pacing.* Philadelphia, PA: WB Saunders Co; 1990:250-300.

Rein AJ, Simcha A, Ludomirsky A, Appelbaum A, Uretzky G, Tamir I. Symptomatic sinus bradycardia in infants with structurally normal hearts. *J Pediatr*. 1985;107:724-727.

Ross BD. First and second degree atrioventricular block. In: Gillette PC, Garson AR Jr, eds. *Pediatric Arrhythmias, Electrophysiology and Pacing.* Philadelphia, PA: WB Saunders Co; 1990:301-305.

Walsh CK, Krongrad E. Terminal cardiac electrical activity in pediatric patients. *Am J Cardiol*. 1983;51:557-561.

Yabek SM, Dillon T, Berman W Jr, Vliand CJ. Symptomatic sinus node dysfunction in children without structural heart disease. *Pediatrics*. 1982;69:590-593.

Part 9

Recognition and Management of Tachycardia

Overview

This Part discusses the recognition and management of tachycardias (fast heart rates) with a palpable pulse and adequate or inadequate perfusion in infants and children. Providers should quickly treat symptomatic tachyarrhythmias before they result in shock or cardiac arrest.

Learning Objectives

After studying this Part you should be able to

- Differentiate supraventricular tachycardia (SVT) from sinus tachycardia (ST)
- Recognize and manage a child as outlined in the Pediatric Tachycardia With a Pulse and Poor Perfusion Algorithm
- Recognize and manage a child as outlined in the Pediatric Tachycardia With a Pulse and Adequate Perfusion Algorithm
- Describe when and how to use vagal maneuvers, adenosine, and synchronized cardioversion for the treatment of SVT
- Select appropriate interventions and contact expert consultation for treatment of unstable tachycardias

Preparation for the Course

You will be expected to recognize tachyarrhythmias and manage a child as outlined in the algorithms for tachycardia with a pulse and poor perfusion and tachycardia with a pulse and adequate perfusion.

Tachyarrhythmias

Tachycardia is a heart rate that is fast compared with the normal heart rate for the child's age. See Part 2, Table 2: Normal Heart Rates (per Minute) by Age. Sinus tachycardia is a normal response to stress or fever.

Tachyarrhythmias are fast abnormal rhythms originating either in the atria or the ventricles of the heart. Tachyarrhythmias can be tolerated without symptoms for a variable period of time. However, tachyarrhythmias can also cause acute hemodynamic compromise such as shock or deterioration to cardiac arrest.

Recognition of Tachyarrhythmias
Signs and Symptoms

Tachyarrhythmias may cause nonspecific signs and symptoms that differ according to the age of the child. Clinical findings may include palpitations, light-headedness, and syncope. In infants who are at home, the tachyarrhythmia may be undetected for long periods (e.g., for hours or days) until cardiac output is significantly compromised and the infant develops signs of congestive heart failure such as irritability, poor feeding, and rapid breathing. Episodes of extremely rapid heart rate may be life threatening if cardiac output is compromised.

Signs of hemodynamic instability associated with tachyarrhythmias are

- Respiratory distress/failure
- Signs of shock (poor end-organ perfusion) with or without hypotension
- Altered mental status (i.e., decreased level of consciousness)
- Sudden collapse with rapid, weak pulses

Effect on Cardiac Output

An increased heart rate can produce increased cardiac output, up to a point. If that point is exceeded (i.e., the heart rate is extremely rapid), stroke volume decreases because diastole is shortened and there is insufficient time for filling of the ventricles during diastole. Cardiac output then decreases substantially. In addition, coronary perfusion (blood flow to heart muscle) occurs chiefly during diastole; the decrease in duration of diastole that occurs with a very rapid heart rate reduces coronary perfusion. Finally, a fast heart rate increases myocardial O_2 demand. In infants prolonged episodes of rapid heart rate (SVT) can cause myocardial dysfunction, leading to congestive heart failure (CHF). In any child an extremely rapid heart rate can result in inadequate cardiac output and, ultimately, cardiogenic shock.

Classification of Tachycardia and Tachyarrhythmias

Tachycardia and tachyarrhythmias are classified according to the width of the QRS complex; the arrhythmias are divided into those with narrow versus wide QRS complexes:

Narrow Complex (≤0.09 second)	Wide Complex (>0.09 second)
• Sinus tachycardia (ST) • Supraventricular tachycardia (SVT) • Atrial flutter	• Ventricular tachycardia (VT) • Supraventricular tachy-cardia (SVT) with aberrant intraventricular conduction

Sinus Tachycardia

Sinus tachycardia (ST) is a sinus node discharge rate faster than normal for the child's age. It typically develops in response to the body's need for increased cardiac output or O_2 delivery. ST is a normal physiologic response and is not considered an arrhythmia (Figure 1). In ST the heart rate is not fixed but varies with activity and other factors (e.g., the child's temperature) that influence O_2 demand.

Common causes of ST include exercise, pain, anxiety, tissue hypoxia, hypovolemia (hemorrhagic and nonhemorrhagic fluid loss), shock, fever, metabolic stress, injury, toxins/poisons/drugs, and anemia. Cardiac tamponade, tension pneumothorax, and thromboembolism are less common causes of ST.

ECG Characteristics of ST

The ECG characteristics of ST include the following:

Heart rate	Beat-to-beat variability with changes in activity or stress level • Usually <220/min in infants • Usually <180/min in children
P waves	Present/normal
PR interval	Constant, normal duration
R-R interval	Variable
QRS complex	Narrow (≤0.09 second)

Supraventricular Tachycardia

Supraventricular tachycardia (SVT) is an abnormally fast rhythm originating above the ventricles. It is most commonly caused by a reentry mechanism that involves an accessory pathway or the AV conduction system. SVT is the most common tachyarrhythmia that causes cardiovascular compromise during infancy. Mechanisms that can cause SVT are accessory pathway reentry, AV nodal reentry, or ectopic atrial focus.

Two outdated terms for SVT are *paroxysmal atrial tachycardia* and *paroxysmal supraventricular tachycardia*. SVT was labeled "paroxysmal" because it occurs episodically (in paroxysms). The rapid rhythm starts and stops suddenly, often without warning.

Clinical Presentation of SVT

SVT (Figure 2) is a rapid, regular rhythm that often appears abruptly and may be episodic. During episodes of SVT, cardiopulmonary function is influenced by the child's age, duration of the tachycardia, prior ventricular function, and ventricular rate. In infants, SVT may be present but undetected for long periods until cardiac output is significantly impaired. If baseline myocardial function is impaired (e.g., in a child with congenital heart disease or cardiomyopathy), SVT can produce signs of shock in a short time.

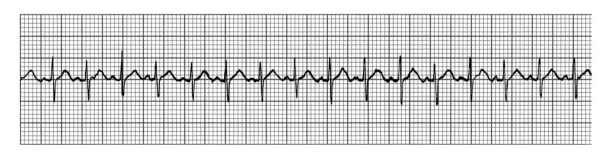

Figure 1. Sinus tachycardia (heart rate 180/min) in a febrile 10-month-old infant.

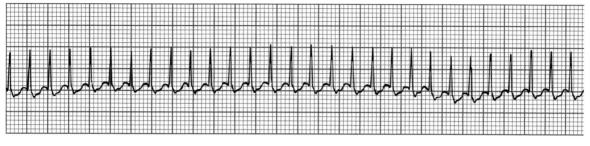

Figure 2. SVT in a 10-month-old infant.

In infants, SVT is often diagnosed when symptoms of CHF develop. *Common signs and symptoms of SVT in infants* include irritability, poor feeding, rapid breathing, unusual sleepiness, vomiting, and pale, mottled, gray, or cyanotic skin. *Common signs and symptoms of SVT in older children* include palpitations, shortness of breath, chest pain or discomfort, dizziness, light-headedness, and fainting.

SVT is initially well tolerated in most infants and older children. However, it can lead to CHF and clinical evidence of shock when baseline myocardial function is impaired (e.g., in a child with congenital heart disease or cardiomyopathy) or in an infant having prolonged episodes over hours to days. Ultimately SVT can cause cardiovascular collapse.

Signs

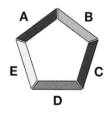

SVT may be recognized by its effect on systemic perfusion. SVT with cardiopulmonary compromise can produce the following signs and symptoms:

Airway	Usually patent unless level of consciousness is significantly impaired
Breathing	• Tachypnea • Increased work of breathing • Crackles (or "wheezing" in infants) if CHF develops • Grunting if CHF develops

(continued)

(continued)

Circulation	• Tachycardia beyond the typical range for sinus tachycardia and characterized by fixed rate and/or abrupt onset • Delayed capillary refill time • Weak peripheral pulses • Cool extremities • Diaphoretic, pale, mottled, gray, or cyanotic skin • Hypotension • Jugular venous distention (difficult to observe in young children) if CHF develops
Disability	• Altered mental status (i.e., decreased level of consciousness) • Sleepiness or lethargy • Irritability
Exposure	Defer evaluation of temperature until ABCs are supported

ECG Characteristics of SVT

The ECG characteristics of SVT include

Heart rate	No beat-to-beat variability with activity • Usually ≥220/min in infants • Usually ≥180/min in children
P waves	Absent or abnormal (may appear after the QRS complex)
PR interval	Because P waves are usually absent, PR interval cannot be determined; in ectopic atrial tachycardia a short PR interval may be seen
R-R interval	Often constant
QRS complex	Usually narrow; wide complex uncommon

Narrow-Complex SVT

In >90% of children with SVT, the QRS complex is narrow (Figure 2), i.e., ≤0.09 second.

Wide-Complex SVT

SVT with aberrant conduction (uncommon in the pediatric age group) produces a wide QRS complex (i.e., >0.09 second). This form of SVT most often occurs as a result of rate-related bundle branch block (within the ventricles) or preexisting bundle branch block. It also may be caused by an accessory pathway in which electrical impulses are conducted from the atria to the ventricles through the accessory pathway rather than through the AV node. The impulse then returns to the atria through the AV node (or through a different accessory pathway).

It can be difficult to differentiate SVT with aberrant conduction from ventricular tachycardia (VT). This requires careful analysis of at least one 12-lead ECG. Both can cause similar hemodynamic instability, have similar rates, and have a wide QRS complexes (>0.09 second). In the pediatric age group, unless patient history or previous ECGs suggest the likelihood of SVT with aberrant conduction (e.g., preexisting bundle branch block), assume that a tachycardia with a wide QRS is due to VT.

Comparison of ST and SVT

It may be difficult to differentiate SVT with shock from shock from another etiology with compensatory ST. The following characteristics may aid in differentiating ST from SVT. Note that signs of heart failure and other signs and symptoms of poor perfusion may be absent early after the onset of SVT.

Characteristic	ST	SVT
History	Gradual onset Compatible with ST (e.g., history of fever, pain, dehydration, hemorrhage)	Abrupt onset or termination or both Infant: Symptoms of CHF Child: Sudden onset of palpitations
Physical examination	Signs of underlying cause of ST (e.g., fever, hypovolemia, anemia)	Infant: Signs of CHF (e.g., crackles, hepatomegaly, edema)
Heart rate	Infant: Usually <220/min Child: Usually <180/min	Infant: Usually ≥220/min Child: Usually ≥180/min
Monitor	Variability in heart rate with changes in level of activity or stimulation; slowing of heart rate with rest or treatment of underlying cause (e.g., administration of IV fluids for hypovolemia)	Minimal variability in heart rate with changes in level of activity or stimulation
ECG	P waves present/normal/upright in leads I/aVF	P waves absent/abnormal/inverted (negative) in leads II/III/aVF, usually following the QRS complex
Chest x-ray	Usually small heart and clear lungs unless ST is caused by pneumonia, pericarditis, or underlying heart disease	Signs of CHF (e.g., enlarged heart, pulmonary edema) may be present

P waves may be difficult to identify in both ST and SVT once the ventricular rate exceeds 200/min.

Atrial Flutter

Atrial flutter is a narrow-complex tachyarrhythmia that can develop in newborn infants with normal hearts. It also can develop in children with congenital heart disease, especially following cardiac surgery. A reentrant pathway typically is present in children with enlarged atria or with anatomical barriers resulting from cardiac surgery (e.g., atriotomy scars or surgical anastomoses). A reentry circuit within the atria allows a wave of depolarization to travel in a circle within the atria. Because the AV node is not part of the circuit, AV conduction may be variable. The atrial rate can exceed 300/min, whereas the ventricular rate is slower and may be irregular. Classically a "sawtooth" pattern of the P waves is present on the ECG.

Ventricular Tachycardia

VT is a wide-complex tachyarrhythmia generated within the ventricles (Figure 3). VT is uncommon in children. When VT with pulses is present, the ventricular rate may vary from near normal to >200/min. Rapid ventricular rates compromise ventricular filling, stroke volume and cardiac output and may deteriorate into pulseless VT or ventricular fibrillation (VF).

Most children who develop VT have underlying heart disease (or have had surgery for heart disease), long QT syndrome, or myocarditis/cardiomyopathy. They may have a family history of a sudden, unexplained death in a child or young adult, suggesting cardiomyopathy or an inherited cardiac ion "channelopathy." Other causes of VT in children include electrolyte disturbances (e.g., hyperkalemia, hypocalcemia, hypomagnesemia) and drug toxicity (e.g., tricyclic antidepressants, cocaine, methamphetamines).

ECG Characteristics of VT

The ECG characteristics of VT include the following:

Ventricular rate	At least 120/min and regular
QRS complex	Wide (>0.09 second)
P waves	Often not identifiable; when present, may not be related to QRS (AV dissociation); at slower rates, atria may be depolarized in a retrograde manner, resulting in a 1:1 ventricular-to-atrial association
T waves	Typically opposite in polarity from QRS

It may be difficult to differentiate SVT with aberrant conduction from VT. Fortunately, aberrant conduction is present in <10% of children with SVT. In general the healthcare provider should initially assume that a wide-complex rhythm is VT unless the child is known to have aberrant conduction or previous episodes of wide QRS complex SVT.

Polymorphic VT, Including Torsades de Pointes

Pulseless VT may be monomorphic (QRS complexes are uniform in appearance) or polymorphic (QRS complexes vary in appearance). Torsades de pointes is a distinctive form of polymorphic VT. The term *torsades de pointes* is French and means "turning on a point." In torsades de pointes the QRS complexes change in polarity and amplitude, appearing to rotate around the ECG isoelectric line (Figure 3B). The ventricular rate can range from 150 to 250/min. Torsades de pointes can be seen in conditions

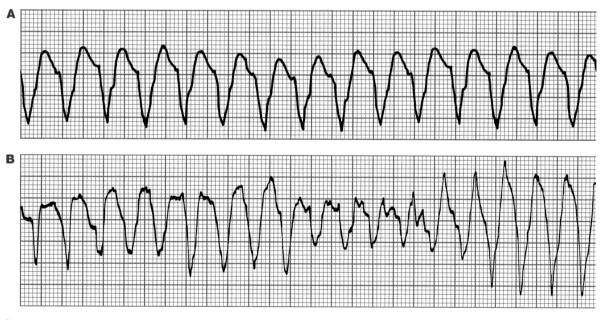

Figure 3. Ventricular tachycardia. **A,** Monomorphic. **B,** Polymorphic (torsades de pointes).

associated with a prolonged QT interval, including congenital long QT syndrome and drug toxicity. The prolonged QT interval is identified during sinus rhythm; it cannot be evaluated during the tachycardia. A rhythm strip may show the child's baseline QT prolongation because torsades de pointes sometimes occurs in bursts that convert spontaneously to sinus rhythm.

Conditions and agents that predispose to torsades de pointes include

- Long QT syndromes (often congenital and inherited)
- Hypomagnesemia
- Hypokalemia
- Antiarrhythmic drug toxicity (i.e., Class IA, quinidine, procainamide, diisopyramide; Class IC, encainide, flecainide; Class III, sotalol, amiodarone)
- Other drug toxicities (e.g., tricyclic antidepressants, calcium channel blockers, phenothiazines)

It is important to recognize that VT, including torsades de pointes, can deteriorate to VF. The long QT syndromes and other inherited arrhythmia syndromes (i.e., channelopathies) are associated with sudden death due to either primary VF or torsades de pointes. Polymorphic VT not associated with a prolonged QT interval during sinus rhythm is treated as generic VT.

Management of Tachyarrhythmias
Initial Management Questions

Answer the following questions to direct your initial management of a critically ill or injured child with a rapid heart rate:

Does the child have a pulse (or signs of circulation)?

Pulse or Signs of Circulation	Management
Absent	Initiate the Pediatric Cardiac Arrest Algorithm (see Part 10). *Note:* Because the accuracy of a pulse check is poor, recognition of cardiac arrest may require that you identify the absence of signs of circulation (i.e., the child is unresponsive, is not breathing other than agonal gasps). With invasive monitoring of arterial pressure, absence of arterial waveform is observed.
Present	Proceed with the tachycardia algorithms.

Is perfusion adequate or poor?

Perfusion	Management
Poor	Follow the Pediatric Tachycardia With a Pulse and Poor Perfusion Algorithm for emergency treatment.
Adequate	Follow the Pediatric Tachycardia With a Pulse and Adequate Perfusion Algorithm. Consider consulting a pediatric cardiologist.

Is the QRS complex narrow or wide?

Rhythm	Management
Narrow complex	Consider the differential of ST versus SVT.
Wide complex	Consider the differential of SVT versus VT, but treat as presumed VT unless the child has known aberrant conduction.

Initial Management Priorities

As soon as you recognize a tachyarrhythmia in an infant or child, assess for signs of shock or life-threatening hemodynamic instability. Initial management priorities include the following:

- Support the ABCs and oxygenation as needed.
- Establish monitoring: attach monitor/defibrillator and pulse oximeter.
- Establish vascular access.
- Obtain a 12-lead ECG. (But do not delay urgent intervention.)
- Obtain laboratory studies (e.g., potassium, glucose, ionized calcium, magnesium, blood gas to assess pH and cause of pH changes) as appropriate (do not delay urgent intervention for these studies).
- Assess neurologic status.
- Anticipate the need for medications depending on the type of rhythm disturbance (i.e., supraventricular versus ventricular).
- Simultaneously try to identify and treat reversible causes.

Emergency Interventions

Specific emergency interventions used to treat tachyarrhythmias with pulses are dictated by the severity of the child's condition. Treatments also vary based on the width of the observed QRS complex (narrow versus wide). Interventions may include the following:

- Vagal maneuvers (if the child with a narrow-complex tachycardia is stable or while preparations are made for synchronized cardioversion)

Critical Concept

Vagal Maneuvers

Ice to the face is a vagal maneuver that can be performed in infants and children of all ages (Figure 4). Fill a small plastic bag with a mixture of ice and water. Apply it to the upper half of the child's face for 15 to 20 seconds. Do not occlude the nose or mouth.

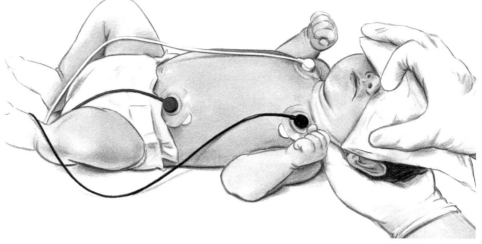

Figure 4. Vagal maneuvers. Ice water is applied to the upper half of the infant's face for vagal stimulation in an attempt to terminate SVT. Note that the bag of ice water does not cover the nose or mouth and does not obstruct ventilation.

- Children old enough to cooperate can perform a Valsalva maneuver by blowing through a narrow straw.
- Carotid sinus massage may also be performed safely and easily in older children.
- Do not use ocular pressure because it may produce retinal injury.

Fundamental Fact

Do Not Delay Emergency Treatment for Tachycardia

Seek expert consultation from a pediatric cardiologist for evaluation of children with tachyarrhythmias. However, do not delay emergency treatment.

- Cardioversion
- Medication therapy
- Other interventions

Vagal Maneuvers

In normal infants and children the heart rate decreases when the vagus nerve is stimulated. In patients with SVT, vagal stimulation may terminate the tachycardia by slowing conduction through the AV node. Several maneuvers can stimulate vagal activity. The success rates of these maneuvers in terminating tachyarrhythmias vary, depending on the child's age, level of cooperation, and underlying condition.

Be sure to support the child's airway, breathing, and circulation. If possible, obtain a 12-lead ECG before and after the maneuver; record and monitor the ECG continuously during the maneuver. *If the child is stable* and the rhythm does not convert, you may repeat the attempt. If the second attempt fails, select another method or provide medication therapy. *If the child is unstable,*

attempt vagal maneuvers only while making preparations for pharmacologic or electrical cardioversion. Do not delay definitive treatment to perform vagal maneuvers.

Cardioversion

Electrical cardioversion is painful. Whenever possible, establish vascular access and provide procedural sedation and analgesia before cardioversion, especially in a hemodynamically stable infant or child. If the child's condition is unstable, do not delay synchronized cardioversion to achieve vascular access. Sedation in the setting of an arrhythmia carries increased risk. When procedural sedation is given in this setting, providers must carefully select medications to minimize hemodynamic effects.

This section discusses the following important concepts regarding cardioversion:

- Definition of synchronized cardioversion
- Potential problems with synchronized shocks

- Indications for the use of synchronized cardioversion
- Energy doses

Synchronized Cardioversion

Defibrillators are capable of delivering unsynchronized and synchronized shocks. If the shock is unsynchronized, it is delivered at any time in the cardiac cycle. Unsynchronized shocks are used for defibrillation because the cardiac arrest rhythms have no QRS. Synchronized shocks are used for cardioversion from SVT and VT with a pulse. If the shock is synchronized, shock delivery is timed to coincide with the R wave of the patient's QRS complex. The goal is to prevent VF that could result from delivery of the shock during the vulnerable period of the T wave. When you press the SHOCK button, the defibrillator/cardioverter may seem to pause before it delivers a shock because it is waiting to synchronize shock delivery with the next QRS complex. See the Critical Concept box "Cardioversion" for a description of the procedure.

Potential Problems

In theory, synchronization is simple. The operator pushes the SYNC button on the defibrillator, charges the device, and delivers the shock. In practice, however, there can be potential problems, such as the following:

- In most units the SYNC button must be activated each time synchronized cardioversion is attempted. Most devices will default to an unsynchronized shock immediately after delivery of a synchronized shock.
- If the R waves of a tachycardia are undifferentiated or of low amplitude, the monitor sensors may be unable to identify them and therefore will not deliver the shock.

Critical Concept

Cardioversion (for Unstable SVT or VT With a Pulse)

Consider expert consultation for suspected VT.

1. Turn on defibrillator.

2. Set *lead switch* to *paddles* (or *lead I, II,* or *III* if monitor leads are used).

3. Select adhesive pads to paddles. Use the largest pads or paddles that can fit on the patient's chest without touching each other.

4. If using paddles, apply conductive gel or paste. Be sure cables are attached to defibrillator.

5. Consider sedation.

6. Select **synchronized** mode.

7. Look for markers on R waves indicating that *sync* mode is operative. If necessary, adjust monitor gain until sync markers occur with each R wave.

8. Select energy dose:
   Initial dose: 0.5-1 J/kg
   Subsequent doses: 2 J/kg

9. Announce "Charging defibrillator," and press *charge* on defibrillator controls or apex paddle.

10. When defibrillator is fully charged, state firm chant, such as "I am going to shock on three." Then count. "All clear!"

11. After confirming all personnel are clear of the patient, press the *shock* button on the defibrillator or press the 2 paddle *discharge* buttons simultaneously. Hold paddles in place until shock is delivered.

12. Check the monitor. If tachycardia persists, increase energy and prepare to cardiovert again.

13. Reset the **sync** mode after each synchronized cardioversion, because most defibrillators default back to unsynchronized mode. This default allows an immediate shock if the cardioversion produces VF.

Note: If VF develops, immediately begin CPR and prepare to deliver an unsynchronized shock (see the Critical Concept box "Manual Defibrillation" in Part 10).

Increase the gain of the ECG lead being monitored or select a different ECG lead.

- Synchronization may take extra time (e.g., if it is necessary to attach separate ECG electrodes or if the operator is unfamiliar with the equipment).

Indications

Synchronized cardioversion is used for

- Hemodynamically unstable patients (poor perfusion, hypotension, or heart failure) with tachyarrhythmias (SVT, atrial flutter, VT) but with palpable pulses
- Elective cardioversion, under the direction of a pediatric cardiologist, for children with hemodynamically stable SVT, atrial flutter, or VT

Energy Dose

In general, cardioversion requires less energy than defibrillation. Start with an energy dose of 0.5 to 1 J/kg for cardioversion of SVT or VT. If the initial dose is ineffective, increase the dose to 2 J/kg. The experienced provider may increase the shock dose more gradually (e.g., 0.5 J/kg, then 1 J/kg, followed by 2 J/kg for subsequent doses). If the rhythm does not convert to sinus rhythm, reevaluate the diagnosis of SVT versus ST.

Medication Therapy

Table 1 reviews common agents used in the management of tachyarrhythmias.

Table 1. Medication Therapy Used in the Pediatric Tachycardia With a Pulse and Adequate Perfusion and Pediatric Tachycardia With a Pulse and Poor Perfusion Algorithms

Drug	Indications/Precautions	Dosage/Administration
Adenosine	**Indications** • Drug of choice for treatment of SVT • Effective for SVT caused by reentry at the AV node (both accessory pathway and AV nodal reentry mechanisms) • May be helpful in distinguishing atrial flutter from SVT • Not effective for treatment of atrial flutter, atrial fibrillation, or tachycardias caused by mechanisms other than reentry through the AV node **Mechanism of Action** • Blocks conduction through the AV node temporarily (for about 10 seconds) **Precautions** • A common cause of adenosine cardioversion "failure" is that the drug is administered too slowly or with inadequate IV flush. • A brief period (10 to 15 seconds) of bradycardia (asystole or third-degree heart block) may ensue after administration of adenosine (Figure 5).	**Dose** • With continuous ECG monitoring, administer 0.1 mg/kg (maximum initial dose 6 mg) as a rapid IV bolus. • If the drug is effective, the rhythm will convert to sinus rhythm within 15 to 30 seconds of administration (Figure 5). • If there is no effect, give 1 dose of 0.2 mg/kg (maximum second dose 12 mg). This dose is more likely to be needed when the drug is administered into a peripheral (rather than central) vein. • Decrease the initial dose for patients receiving carbamazepine or dipyridamole or those with transplanted hearts. **Administration** • Because adenosine has a very short half-life (<10 seconds), administer as rapidly as possible. • The drug is rapidly taken up by vascular endothelial cells and red blood cells and metabolized by an enzyme on the surface of red blood cells (adenosine deaminase). • To enhance delivery to the site of action in the heart, use a rapid flush technique (5 to 10 mL NS). • Adenosine may be given by the IO route.

(continued)

(continued)

Drug	Indications/Precautions	Dosage/Administration
Amiodarone	**Indications** • Effective for the treatment of a wide variety of atrial and ventricular tachyarrhythmias in children • May be considered in the treatment of hemodynamically stable SVT refractory to vagal maneuvers and adenosine • Safe and effective for hemodynamically unstable VT in children **Mechanism of Action** • Inhibits α- and β-adrenergic receptors, producing vasodilation and AV nodal suppression (this slows conduction through the AV node) • Inhibits the outward potassium current so it prolongs the QT interval • Inhibits sodium channels, which slows conduction in the ventricles and prolongs QRS duration **Precautions** • Drug effects may be beneficial in some patients but may also increase the risk for polymorphic VT (torsades de pointes) by prolonging the QT interval. • Rare but significant acute side effects of amiodarone include bradycardia, hypotension, and polymorphic VT. • Use with caution if hepatic failure is present. • Because the pharmacology of amiodarone is complex, and it has slow and incomplete oral absorption, long half-life, and potential for long-term adverse effects, a pediatric cardiologist or similarly experienced provider should direct long-term amiodarone therapy.	**Dose** • For supraventricular and ventricular arrhythmias with poor perfusion, a loading dose of 5 mg/kg infused over 20 to 60 minutes is recommended. (Maximum single dose: 300 mg.) Because this drug can cause hypotension and decrease cardiac contractility, a slower rate of delivery is recommended for treatment of a perfusing rhythm than for cardiac arrest. Providers must weigh the potential for causing hypotension against the need to achieve a rapid drug effect. • Repeat doses of 5 mg/kg may be given up to a maximum of 15 mg/kg per day as needed (should not exceed the maximum recommended adult cumulative daily dose of 2.2 g over 24 hours). **Administration** • Rapid administration of amiodarone may cause vasodilation and hypotension; it may also cause heart block or polymorphic VT. • Monitor blood pressure frequently during administration. • Seek expert consultation when using amiodarone. • Routine use of amiodarone in combination with another agent that prolongs the QT interval (e.g., procainamide) is not recommended.

(continued)

(continued)

Drug	Indications/Precautions	Dosage/Administration
Procainamide	**Indications** • Can be used to treat a wide range of atrial and ventricular arrhythmias in children, including SVT and VT • Can terminate SVT that is resistant to other drugs • May be considered for treatment of hemodynamically stable SVT refractory to vagal maneuvers and adenosine • Effective in the treatment of atrial flutter and atrial fibrillation • May be used to treat or suppress VT **Mechanism of Action** • Blocks sodium channels so it prolongs the effective refractory period of both the atria and ventricles and depresses conduction velocity within the conduction system • By slowing intraventricular conduction, prolongs QT, QRS, and PR intervals **Precautions** • Paradoxically shortens the effective refractory period of the AV node and increases AV nodal conduction; may cause increased heart rate when used to treat ectopic atrial tachycardia and atrial fibrillation • Can cause hypotension in children through its potent vasodilator effect • Reduce dose for patients with poor renal or cardiac function	**Dose** • Infuse a loading dose of 15 mg/kg over 30 to 60 minutes with continuous ECG monitoring and frequent blood pressure monitoring. **Administration** • Procainamide must be given by slow infusion to avoid toxicity from heart block, hypotension, and prolongation of the QT interval (which predisposes to VT or torsades de pointes). • Monitor blood pressure frequently during administration. • Procainamide, like amiodarone, may increase the risk of polymorphic VT (torsades de pointes). • Routine use of procainamide in combination with another agent (e.g., amiodarone) that prolongs the QT interval is not recommended without expert consultation. **Other** • Seek expert consultation when using procainamide. • Despite a long history of use, there are limited data in children comparing the effectiveness of procainamide with other antiarrhythmic agents.
Lidocaine	**Indications** • Alternative agent for treatment of stable VT • Not effective for supraventricular arrhythmias **Mechanism of Action** • Sodium channel blocker that decreases automaticity and suppresses wide-complex ventricular arrhythmias **Precautions** • High plasma concentrations and lidocaine toxicity may develop in patients with persistently low cardiac output and hepatic or renal failure • Contraindicated for bradycardia with wide-complex ventricular escape beats and high-degree heart block	**Dose/Administration** • Loading bolus IV dose of 1 mg/kg • Consider an infusion of 20 to 50 mcg/kg per minute. • If there is a delay of >15 minutes between the bolus dose and the start of an infusion, consider giving a second bolus of 0.5 to 1 mg/kg to reestablish therapeutic concentrations.
Magnesium sulfate	**Indications** • Treatment of torsades de pointes or VT with hypomagnesemia	**Dose** • 25 to 50 mg/kg IV/IO (maximum dose 2 g) given over 10 to 20 minutes (faster for torsades de pointes with cardiac arrest)

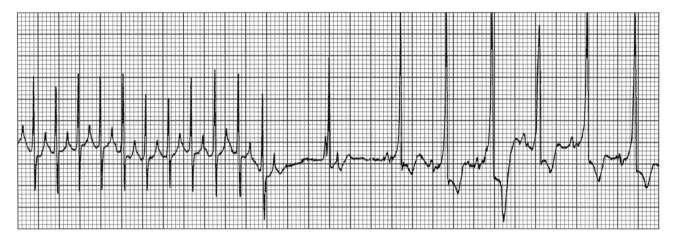

Figure 5. SVT converting to sinus rhythm with administration of adenosine.

Other Interventions

Many other interventions (e.g., digoxin, short-acting β-blockers, overdrive pacing) have been used for treatment of SVT in children but should be reserved for expert consultation.

Verapamil, a calcium channel blocking agent, *should not be used routinely* to treat SVT in infants because refractory hypotension and cardiac arrest have been reported following administration. Use verapamil with caution in children because it may cause hypotension and myocardial depression. If using verapamil in children ≥1 year of age, infuse the drug in a dose of 0.1 mg/kg (up to 5 mg) over at least 2 minutes with continuous ECG monitoring.

Summary of Emergency Interventions

The following specific emergency interventions are used to treat tachyarrhythmias with pulses, based on the width of the observed QRS complex (narrow versus wide):

Intervention	Narrow-Complex Tachyarrhythmia	Wide-Complex Tachyarrhythmia
Vagal maneuvers	Used for SVT	Used for SVT
Synchronized cardioversion	Used for • SVT • Atrial flutter (seek expert consultation)	Used for VT with palpable pulses
Medication therapy	Used for SVT: • Adenosine • Amiodarone (seek expert consultation) • Procainamide (seek expert consultation) • Verapamil for children ≥1 year of age (seek expert consultation) Drugs used for other SVT with a pulse (e.g., atrial flutter): Seek expert consultation	Used for VT with palpable pulses: • Amiodarone (seek expert consultation) • Procainamide (seek expert consultation) • Lidocaine Drug used for torsades de pointes: • Magnesium Drugs used for SVT with abnormal/aberrant intraventricular conduction: • Adenosine • Amiodarone (seek expert consultation) • Procainamide (seek expert consultation)

Pediatric Tachycardia With a Pulse and Adequate Perfusion Algorithm

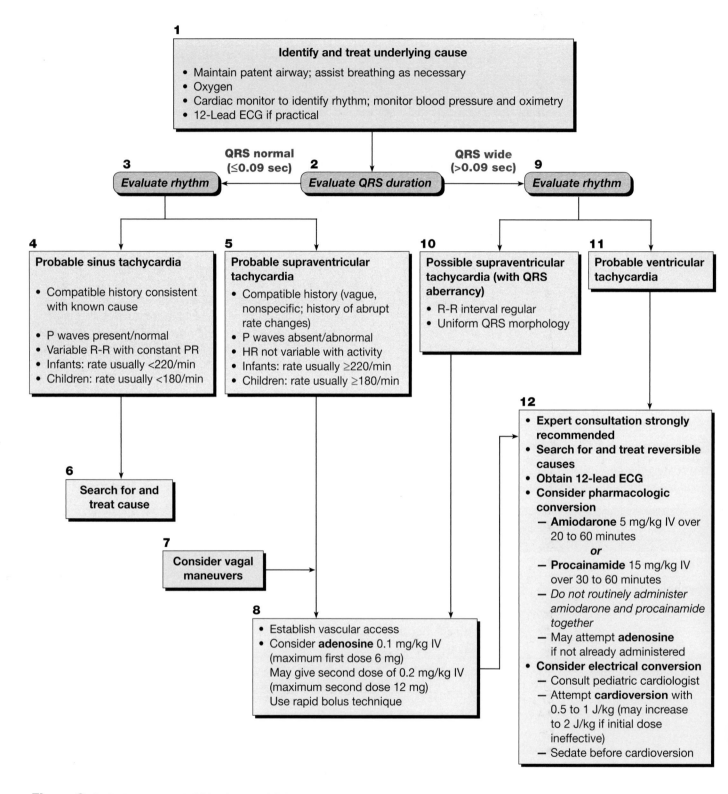

1

Identify and treat underlying cause

- Maintain patent airway; assist breathing as necessary
- Oxygen
- Cardiac monitor to identify rhythm; monitor blood pressure and oximetry
- 12-Lead ECG if practical

QRS normal (≤0.09 sec)

2 *Evaluate QRS duration*

QRS wide (>0.09 sec)

3 *Evaluate rhythm*

9 *Evaluate rhythm*

4 Probable sinus tachycardia

- Compatible history consistent with known cause

- P waves present/normal
- Variable R-R with constant PR
- Infants: rate usually <220/min
- Children: rate usually <180/min

5 Probable supraventricular tachycardia

- Compatible history (vague, nonspecific; history of abrupt rate changes)
- P waves absent/abnormal
- HR not variable with activity
- Infants: rate usually ≥220/min
- Children: rate usually ≥180/min

10 Possible supraventricular tachycardia (with QRS aberrancy)

- R-R interval regular
- Uniform QRS morphology

11 Probable ventricular tachycardia

6 Search for and treat cause

7 Consider vagal maneuvers

8
- Establish vascular access
- Consider **adenosine** 0.1 mg/kg IV (maximum first dose 6 mg) May give second dose of 0.2 mg/kg IV (maximum second dose 12 mg) Use rapid bolus technique

12
- **Expert consultation strongly recommended**
- **Search for and treat reversible causes**
- **Obtain 12-lead ECG**
- **Consider pharmacologic conversion**
  - **Amiodarone** 5 mg/kg IV over 20 to 60 minutes
    or
  - **Procainamide** 15 mg/kg IV over 30 to 60 minutes
  - *Do not routinely administer amiodarone and procainamide together*
  - May attempt **adenosine** if not already administered
- **Consider electrical conversion**
  - Consult pediatric cardiologist
  - Attempt **cardioversion** with 0.5 to 1 J/kg (may increase to 2 J/kg if initial dose ineffective)
  - Sedate before cardioversion

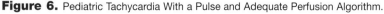

Figure 6. Pediatric Tachycardia With a Pulse and Adequate Perfusion Algorithm.

The Pediatric Tachycardia With a Pulse and Adequate Perfusion Algorithm (Figure 6) outlines the steps for assessment and management of a child presenting with symptomatic tachycardia and adequate perfusion. Box numbers in the text refer to the corresponding boxes in the algorithm.

Initial Management (Box 1)

When systemic perfusion is adequate, you have more time to evaluate the rhythm and the child. Begin the initial management steps, which may include the following:

- Assess and support the airway, oxygenation, and ventilation as needed.
- If O_2 is needed, provide it with a nonrebreathing mask.
- Evaluate the presence and strength of peripheral pulses.
- Attach a continuous ECG monitor/defibrillator and a pulse oximeter.
- Obtain a 12-lead ECG if practical.

Evaluate QRS Duration (Box 2)

Evaluate QRS duration to determine the type of arrhythmia.

QRS Duration	Probable Arrhythmia	Proceed in Algorithm
Normal/narrow (≤0.09 second)	ST or SVT	Boxes 3, 4, 5, 6, 7, 8
Wide (>0.09 second)	Probable VT vs. SVT with aberrant conduction	Boxes 9, 10, 11

Normal QRS: ST or SVT? (Boxes 3-5)

If QRS duration is normal (Box 3), evaluate the rhythm and try *to determine if the rhythm represents ST or SVT.*

Signs and symptoms consistent with ST (Box 4) include

- History is compatible with ST, consistent with a known cause (e.g., the child has fever, dehydration, pain)
- P waves are present and normal
- Heart rate varies with activity or stimulation
- R-R is variable, but PR is constant
- Heart rate is <220/min in an infant or <180/min in a child

Signs and symptoms consistent with SVT (Box 5) include

- History of vague or nonspecific symptoms or palpitations of sudden onset; no history compatible with ST (e.g., no fever, dehydration, or other identifiable cause of ST)
- P waves are absent or abnormal
- Heart rate does not vary with activity or stimulation
- Heart rate is ≥220/min in an infant or ≥180/min in a child

Treatment of ST (Box 6)

Treatment of ST is directed at the cause of ST. Because ST is a symptom, don't attempt to decrease the heart rate by pharmacologic or electrical interventions. Instead, search for and treat the cause. Continuous ECG monitoring will confirm a decrease in heart rate to more normal levels if treatment of the underlying cause is effective.

Treat Cause of SVT (Boxes 7 and 8)

Vagal Maneuvers

Consider vagal maneuvers (Box 7). In the stable patient with SVT, try the following:

- Place a bag with ice water over the upper half of the infant's face (without obstructing the airway).
- Ask an older child to try to blow through an obstructed straw.
- Perform carotid sinus massage in older children.

Monitor and record the ECG continuously before, during, and after attempted vagal maneuvers. If the maneuvers fail, they can be attempted a second time. Do not apply ocular pressure. For more information, see the Critical Concept box "Vagal Maneuvers" in this Part.

Adenosine

For SVT resistant to vagal maneuvers, establish vascular access and administer adenosine (Box 8). Adenosine is the drug of choice for most common forms of SVT caused by a reentrant pathway involving the AV node.

Adenosine	
Route	**Dose**
IV/IO	0.1 mg/kg (maximum first dose 6 mg) If the first dose is ineffective, you may give 1 dose of 0.2 mg/kg (maximum second dose 12 mg).
Use a rapid bolus with a *rapid* flush 2-syringe technique.	

Wide QRS, Possible VT vs. SVT (Boxes 9, 10, and 11)

If QRS duration is wide (>0.09 second), the rhythm is either VT or, less likely, SVT with aberrant intraventricular conduction. In infants and children, treat wide-complex tachycardia as presumed VT unless the child is known to have aberrant conduction.

If the wide QRS-complex tachyarrhythmia has a uniform QRS morphology and regular R-R interval and the child remains hemodynamically stable, consider giving a dose of adenosine (Box 9). If the arrhythmia is VT, adenosine will not be effective but will do no harm. Adenosine is effective in the unusual situation of SVT with aberrancy.

Pharmacologic Conversion vs. Electrical Conversion (Box 12)

If a child with a wide-complex tachycardia is hemodynamically stable, early consultation with a pediatric cardiologist or other provider with appropriate expertise is recommended.

Pharmacologic Conversion

Establish vascular access and consider administering **one** of the following medications:

Medication	Route	Dosage and Administration
Amiodarone	IV/IO	5 mg/kg over 20 to 60 minutes
Procainamide	IV/IO	15 mg/kg over 30 to 60 minutes

Seek expert consultation when giving amiodarone or procainamide. Do not routinely administer amiodarone and procainamide together or with other medications that prolong the QT interval. If these initial efforts do not terminate the rapid rhythm, reevaluate the rhythm.

If not already administered, consider adenosine, because a wide-complex tachycardia could be SVT with aberrant ventricular conduction (Box 12).

Electrical Cardioversion

If SVT or a wide-complex tachycardia does not respond to medication therapy and the child remains hemodynamically stable, it is best to consult a pediatric cardiologist before proceeding with synchronized cardioversion. Base the decision of whether to proceed on the provider's experience. If you proceed with synchronized cardioversion, administer a sedative and analgesic. After the child is sedated, start with an energy dose of 0.5 to 1 J/kg. If the initial dose is ineffective, increase the dose to 2 J/kg. An experienced provider may increase the shock dose more gradually (e.g., 0.5 J/kg, then 1 J/kg, then all remaining shocks at 2 J/kg). *Record and monitor the ECG before, during, and after each cardioversion attempt.* Obtain a 12-lead ECG after cardioversion.

Pediatric Tachycardia With a Pulse and Poor Perfusion Algorithm

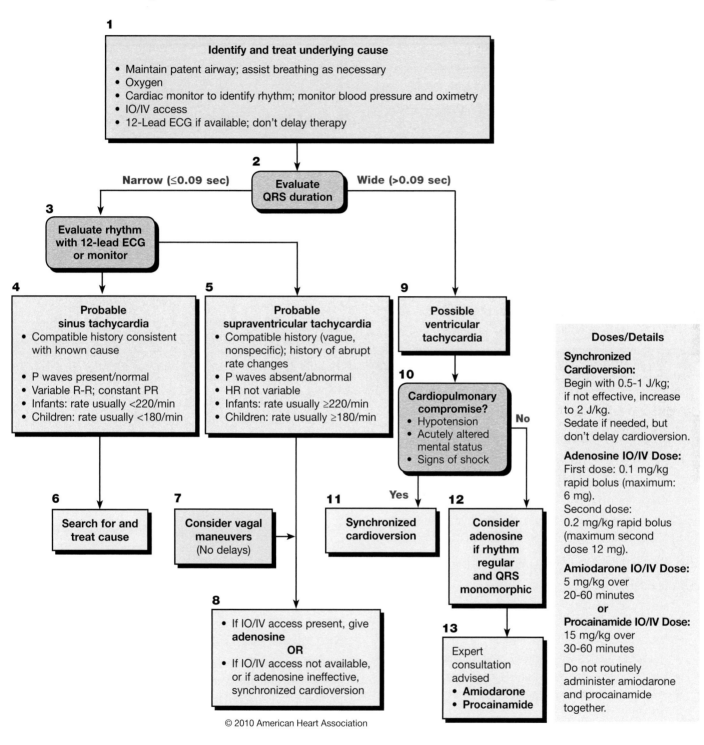

© 2010 American Heart Association

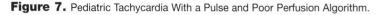

Figure 7. Pediatric Tachycardia With a Pulse and Poor Perfusion Algorithm.

The Pediatric Tachycardia With a Pulse and Poor Perfusion Algorithm (Figure 7) outlines the steps for assessment and management of the child presenting with symptomatic tachycardia and poor perfusion. Box numbers in the text refer to the corresponding boxes in the algorithm.

Initial Management (Box 1)

In a child with tachycardia and palpable pulses but signs of hemodynamic compromise (i.e., poor perfusion, weak pulses), begin initial management steps (Box 1) while attempting to identify and correct the underlying cause. Initial management interventions may include the following:

- Maintain patent airway, assist breathing, and provide O_2 as needed.
- Attach monitors for cardiac rhythm, O_2 saturation, and blood pressure.
- Establish IV/IO access.
- Obtain a 12-lead ECG if available and if it does not delay other care.

Evaluate QRS Duration (Box 2)

Quickly evaluate QRS duration to determine the type of arrhythmia. Although a 12-lead ECG may be useful, initial therapy does not require precise ECG diagnosis of the tachyarrhythmia causing poor perfusion. You can measure QRS width from a rhythm strip.

QRS Duration	Probable Arrhythmia	Proceed in Algorithm
Normal (≤0.09 second)	ST or SVT	Boxes 3, 4, 5, 6, 7, 8
Wide (>0.09 second)	VT	Boxes 9, 10, 11, 12, 13

Normal QRS: ST or SVT? (Boxes 3-5)

If QRS duration is normal, evaluate the rhythm and try *to determine if the rhythm represents ST or SVT* (Box 3).

Signs and symptoms consistent with ST (Box 4) include the following:

- History is compatible with ST or consistent with a known cause (e.g., the child has fever, dehydration, pain).
- P waves are present and normal.
- Heart rate varies with activity or stimulation.
- R-R interval is variable, but PR interval is constant.
- Heart rate is <220/min for an infant or <180/min for a child.

Signs and symptoms consistent with SVT (Box 5) include the following:

- History is compatible with SVT (vague, nonspecific symptoms with abrupt onset of palpitations) and is not consistent with a known cause of ST.
- P waves are absent or abnormal.
- Heart rate does not vary with activity or stimulation.
- Rate changes abruptly.
- Heart rate is ≥220/min in an infant or ≥180/min in a child.

Treat Cause of ST (Box 6)

Treatment of ST is directed at the cause of ST. Because ST is a symptom, do not attempt to decrease the heart rate by pharmacologic or electrical interventions. Instead, search for and treat the cause. Continuous ECG monitoring will confirm a decrease in heart rate to more normal levels if treatment of the underlying cause is effective.

Treatment of SVT (Boxes 7 and 8)

Vagal Maneuvers

Consider vagal maneuvers (Box 7) only while making preparations for pharmacologic or electrical cardioversion. Do not delay definitive treatment to perform vagal maneuvers.

- Place a bag of ice water over the upper half of the infant's face (without obstructing the nose or mouth).
- Have a child try to blow through an obstructed straw.
- Perform carotid sinus massage in older children.

Monitor and record the ECG continuously before, during, and after these attempted vagal maneuvers. Do not apply ocular pressure. For more information, see the Critical Concept box "Vagal Maneuvers" earlier in this Part.

Adenosine

If vascular access (IV/IO) and medications are readily available, administer adenosine (Box 8).

Adenosine	
Route	**Dose**
IV/IO	0.1 mg/kg (maximum first dose 6 mg)
	If the first dose is ineffective, you may give 1 dose of 0.2 mg/kg (maximum second dose 12 mg)
Use a rapid bolus with a *rapid* flush 2-syringe technique.	

Synchronized Cardioversion (Box 8)

If IV/IO access is not readily available or if adenosine is ineffective, attempt synchronized cardioversion. Provide procedural sedation if it will not delay cardioversion. Start with an energy dose of 0.5 to 1 J/kg. If the initial dose is ineffective, increase the dose to 2 J/kg. An experienced provider may increase the shock dose more gradually (e.g., 0.5 J/kg, then 1 J/kg, then 2 J/kg). *Record and monitor the ECG continuously before, during, and immediately after each cardioversion attempt.*

If neither intervention is effective, proceed to Box 13. It is advisable to obtain expert consultation before using amiodarone or procainamide.

Wide QRS, Possible VT (Box 9)

If QRS duration is wide (>0.09 second), treat the rhythm as presumed VT unless the child is known to have aberrant conduction (Box 9).

Treatment of Wide-Complex Tachycardia With Poor Perfusion (Boxes 10-13)

Treat a wide-complex tachycardia with pulses but poor perfusion urgently with synchronized cardioversion, using a starting energy dose of 0.5 to 1 J/kg. Increase the dose to 2 J/kg if the initial dose is ineffective. An experienced provider may increase the shock dose more gradually (e.g., 0.5 J/kg, then 1 J/kg, followed by 2 J/kg). Provide sedation and analgesia before cardioversion, but do not delay cardioversion if the child is hemodynamically unstable.

Because a wide-complex tachycardia could also represent SVT with aberrant intraventricular conduction, consider giving a dose of adenosine first *if it does not delay cardioversion*. Adenosine is not effective but will do no harm if the tachyarrhythmia is VT; adenosine is effective in the unusual situation of SVT with aberrancy.

Refractory Wide-Complex Tachycardia (Box 13)

If a wide-complex tachycardia is refractory to cardioversion, consultation with a pediatric cardiologist is advised before using amiodarone or procainamide.

Consider administration of *one* of the following medications:

Medication	Route	Dosage and Administration
Amiodarone	IV/IO	5 mg/kg over 20 to 60 minutes
Procainamide	IV/IO	15 mg/kg over 30 to 60 minutes

Amiodarone or procainamide can be used for the treatment of wide-complex SVT (unresponsive to adenosine) and VT in children. Both medications must be given by a slow (amiodarone over 20 to 60 minutes, procainamide over 30 to 60 minutes) IV infusion with careful monitoring of blood pressure. Do not routinely administer amiodarone and procainamide together or with other medications that prolong the QT interval.

Suggested Reading List

Benson D Jr, Smith W, Dunnigan A, Sterba R, Gallagher J. Mechanisms of regular wide QRS tachycardia in infants and children. *Am J Cardiol*. 1982;49:1778-1788.

Doniger SJ, Sharieff GQ. Pediatric dysrhythmias. *Pediatr Clin North Am*. 2006;53:85-105, vi.

Gikonyo BM, Dunnigan A, Benson DW Jr. Cardiovascular collapse in infants: association with paroxysmal atrial tachycardia. *Pediatrics*. 1985;76:922-926.

Kugler JD, Danford DA. Management of infants, children, and adolescents with paroxysmal supraventricular tachycardia. *J Pediatr*. 1996;129:324-338.

Manole MD, Saladino RA. Emergency department management of the pediatric patient with supraventricular tachycardia. *Pediatr Emerg Care*. 2007;23:176-185.

Mehta AV, Sanchez GR, Sacks EJ, Casta A, Dunn JM, Donner RM. Ectopic automatic atrial tachycardia in children: clinical characteristics, management and follow-up. *J Am Coll Cardiol*. 1988;11:379-385.

Sanchez J, Christie K, Cumming G. Treatment of ventricular tachycardia in an infant. *Can Med Assoc J*. 1972;107:136-138.

Medications

Burri S, Hug MI, Bauersfeld U. Efficacy and safety of intravenous amiodarone for incessant tachycardias in infants. *Eur J Pediatr*. 2003;162:880-884.

Celiker A, Ceviz N, Ozme S. Effectiveness and safety of intravenous amiodarone in drug-resistant tachyarrhythmias of children. *Acta Paediatr Jpn*. 1998;40:567-572.

Chang PM, Silka MJ, Moromisato DY, Bar-Cohen Y. Amiodarone versus procainamide for the acute treatment of recurrent supraventricular tachycardia in pediatric patients. *Circ Arrhythm Electrophysiol*. 2010;3:134-140.

Dixon J, Foster K, Wyllie J, Wren C. Guidelines and adenosine dosing in supraventricular tachycardia. *Arch Dis Child*. 2005;90:1190-1191.

Drago F, Mazza A, Guccione P, Mafrici A, Di Liso G, Ragonese P. Amiodarone used alone or in combination with propranolol: a very effective therapy for tachyarrhythmias in infants and children. *Pediatr Cardiol*. 1998;19:445-449.

Epstein ML, Kiel EA, Victorica BE. Cardiac decompensation following verapamil therapy in infants with supraventricular tachycardia. *Pediatrics*. 1985;75:737-740.

Figa FH, Gow RM, Hamilton RM, Freedom RM. Clinical efficacy and safety of intravenous amiodarone in infants and children. *Am J Cardiol*. 1994;74:573-577.

Friedman FD. Intraosseous adenosine for the termination of supraventricular tachycardia in an infant. *Ann Emerg Med*. 1996;28:356-358.

Gelband H, Steeg C, Bigger JJ. Use of massive doses of procaineamide in the treatment of ventricular tachycardia in infancy. *Pediatrics*. 1971;48:110-115.

Getschman SJ, Dietrich AM, Franklin WH, Allen HD. Intraosseous adenosine: as effective as peripheral or central venous administration? *Arch Pediatr Adolesc Med*. 1994;148:616-619.

Karlsson E, Sonnhag C. Haemodynamic effects of procainamide and phenytoin at apparent therapeutic plasma levels. *Eur J Clin Pharmacol*. 1976;10:305-310.

Kirk CR, Gibbs JL, Thomas R, Radley-Smith R, Qureshi SA. Cardiovascular collapse after verapamil in supraventricular tachycardia. *Arch Dis Child*. 1987;62:1265-1266.

Kuga K, Yamaguchi I, Sugishita Y. Effect of intravenous amiodarone on electrophysiologic variables and on the modes of termination of atrioventricular reciprocating tachycardia in Wolff-Parkinson-White syndrome. *Jpn Circ J*. 1999;63:189-195.

Laird WP, Snyder CS, Kertesz NJ, Friedman RA, Miller D, Fenrich AL. Use of intravenous amiodarone for postoperative junctional ectopic tachycardia in children. *Pediatr Cardiol*. 2003;24:133-137.

Losek JD, Endom E, Dietrich A, Stewart G, Zempsky W, Smith K. Adenosine and pediatric supraventricular tachycardia in the emergency department: multicenter study and review. *Ann Emerg Med*. 1999;33:185-191.

Luedtke SA, Kuhn RJ, McCaffrey FM. Pharmacologic management of supraventricular tachycardias in children, part 1: Wolff-Parkinson-White and atrioventricular nodal reentry. *Ann Pharmacother*. 1997;31:1227-1243.

Luedtke SA, Kuhn RJ, McCaffrey FM. Pharmacologic management of supraventricular tachycardias in children, part 2: atrial flutter, atrial fibrillation, and junctional and atrial ectopic tachycardia. *Ann Pharmacother*. 1997;31:1347-1359.

Mandapati R, Byrum CJ, Kavey RE, Smith FC, Kveselis DA, Hannan WP, Brandt B III, Gaum WE. Procainamide for rate control of postsurgical junctional tachycardia. *Pediatr Cardiol*. 2000;21:123-128.

Mandel WJ, Laks MM, Obayashi K, Hayakawa H, Daley W. The Wolff-Parkinson-White syndrome: pharmacologic effects of procaine amide. *Am Heart J*. 1975;90:744-754.

Overholt ED, Rheuban KS, Gutgesell HP, Lerman BB, DiMarco JP. Usefulness of adenosine for arrhythmias in infants and children. *Am J Cardiol*. 1988;61:336-340.

Perry JC, Fenrich AL, Hulse JE, Triedman JK, Friedman RA, Lamberti JJ. Pediatric use of intravenous amiodarone: efficacy and safety in critically ill patients from a multicenter protocol. *J Am Coll Cardiol*. 1996;27:1246-1250.

Soult JA, Munoz M, Lopez JD, Romero A, Santos J, Tovaruela A. Efficacy and safety of intravenous amiodarone for short-term treatment of paroxysmal supraventricular tachycardia in children. *Pediatr Cardiol*. 1995;16:16-19.

Part **10**

Recognition and Management
of Cardiac Arrest

Overview

In contrast to adults, cardiac arrest in infants and children does not usually result from a primary cardiac cause (i.e., sudden cardiac arrest). It is typically the end result of progressive respiratory failure or shock. This form of arrest is referred to as a *hypoxic*, *asphyxial*, or a *hypoxic-ischemic arrest*; the term *hypoxic/asphyxial arrest* will be used in this Part. It occurs most often in infants and young children, especially those with underlying disease. Respiratory failure and shock can generally be reversed if identified and treated early. If they progress to cardiac arrest, the outlook is generally poor.

Sudden *cardiac* arrest from ventricular arrhythmia occurs in about 5% to 15% of all pediatric in-hospital and out-of-hospital cardiac arrests. Although a shockable rhythm (i.e., ventricular fibrillation [VF] or pulseless ventricular tachycardia [VT]) is the presenting rhythm in only about 14% of pediatric in-hospital arrests, it is present in up to 27% of such arrests at some point during the resuscitation. For more details see the FYI box below. The incidence of cardiac arrest from VF/pulseless VT increases with age and should be suspected in any patient with a sudden collapse. Increasing evidence suggests that sudden unexpected death in young people is associated with underlying cardiac conditions.

Despite the improved outcome of in-hospital CPR, a majority of children with in-hospital cardiac arrest, and an even larger percentage of children with out-of-hospital cardiac arrest, do not survive or are severely incapacitated. Because outcome from cardiac arrest is so poor, focus should be placed on prevention of cardiac arrest through

- Prevention of disease processes and injuries that can lead to cardiac arrest
- Early recognition and management of respiratory distress, respiratory failure, and shock before they deteriorate to cardiac arrest

Learning Objectives

After completing this Part you should be able to

- Identify the 2 clinical pathways leading to cardiopulmonary failure in children: respiratory failure and shock
- Manage a child as outlined in the Pediatric Cardiac Arrest Algorithm
- Identify the 2 clinical pathways leading to cardiac arrest: hypoxia/asphyxia and sudden cardiac arrest
- List the potential reversible causes of cardiac arrest (H's and T's)
- Recognize the value of family presence during resuscitation
- Describe the impact of family presence on team performance
- Discuss termination of resuscitative efforts and death

Preparation for the Course

During the course you will have the opportunity to practice and be tested on CPR skills. Your performance will also be tested in 2 case scenarios.

Definition of Cardiac Arrest

Cardiac arrest is the cessation of blood circulation resulting from absent or ineffective cardiac mechanical activity. Clinically the child is unresponsive and not breathing or only gasping. There is no detectable pulse. Cerebral hypoxia causes the child to lose consciousness and stop breathing, although agonal gasps may be observed during the first minutes after sudden arrest. When circulation stops, the resulting organ and tissue ischemia can cause cell, organ,

Pathways to Cardiac Arrest

The 2 pathways to cardiac arrest in children are

- Hypoxic/asphyxial
- Sudden cardiac arrest

Hypoxic/Asphyxial Arrest

Hypoxic/asphyxial arrest is the most common cause of cardiac arrest in infants, children, and adolescents. It is the end result of progressive tissue hypoxia and acidosis caused by respiratory failure or shock. Regardless of the initiating event or disease process, the final common pathway preceding cardiac arrest is cardiopulmonary failure (Figure 1).

Sudden Cardiac Arrest

Sudden cardiac arrest (SCA) is less common in children than in adults. It is most often caused by the sudden development of VF or pulseless VT. Predisposing conditions or causes for sudden cardiac arrest may include

- Hypertrophic cardiomyopathy
- Anomalous coronary artery
- Long QT syndrome or other channelopathies
- Myocarditis
- Drug intoxication (e.g., digoxin, ephedra, cocaine)
- Commotio cordis (i.e., sharp blow to the chest)

Primary prevention of some episodes of pediatric cardiac arrest may be possible with cardiovascular screening (e.g., for hypertrophic cardiomyopathy or long QT syndrome) and treatment of predisposing problems (e.g., myocarditis or anomalous coronary artery). Some cases of sudden cardiac arrest in children and young adults are associated with genetic mutations that cause cardiac ion channelopathies. A *channelopathy* is a disorder of the myocyte ion channels that predisposes the heart to arrhythmias. These types of mutations are present in 14% to 20% of sudden cardiac arrest victims in whom no cause of death is found at autopsy. Because these mutations can be genetically inherited, a careful family history to identify sudden and unexplained death (including sudden infant death syndrome [SIDS], drowning, and even a motor vehicle crash) might indicate the presence of a familial channelopathy.

Identify and Intervene Stop Progression to Cardiac Arrest	This course emphasizes the importance of identifying and treating respiratory distress, respiratory failure, and shock before progression to cardiopulmonary failure and cardiac arrest. Early identification and treatment are crucial to saving the lives of seriously ill or injured children.

and patient death if not rapidly reversed.

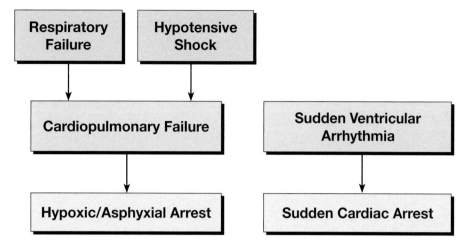

Figure 1. Pathways to different types of cardiac arrest.

Secondary prevention of death from SCA requires prompt and effective resuscitation, including timely defibrillation. Most episodes of SCA in children occur during athletic activity. Prompt treatment of SCA in children will be possible only if coaches, trainers, parents, and the general public are aware that SCA can occur in children. Bystanders must be prepared and willing to activate the emergency response system, provide high-quality CPR, and use an AED as soon as one is available.

Causes of Cardiac Arrest

Causes of cardiac arrest in children vary based on the child's age and underlying health. Causes also vary based on event location (in hospital versus out of hospital).

Most out-of-hospital cardiac arrests in infants and children occur at or near the home. SIDS is a leading cause of death in infants <6 months of age. The frequency of SIDS has decreased with the "Back to Sleep" campaign, which instructs parents to place infants on their backs to sleep. See the Suggested Reading List for a reference on SIDS. Trauma is the predominant cause of death in children 6 months of age through young adulthood. Causes of traumatic cardiac arrest include airway compromise, tension pneumothorax, hemorrhagic shock, and brain injury.

Cardiac arrest in children may be associated with a reversible condition. Review of the H's and T's (see the Identify and Intervene box below) will help you identify reversible causes. The most common immediate causes of pediatric cardiac arrest are respiratory failure and hypotension. Arrhythmia is a less common cause of arrest.

Identify and Intervene *H's and T's*	Cardiac arrest in children may be associated with a reversible condition. If you don't think about reversible causes or complicating factors, you are likely to miss them. Review the following H's and T's to help you identify potentially reversible causes of cardiac arrest or factors that may be complicating resuscitative efforts.

H's	T's
Hypovolemia	**T**ension pneumothorax
Hypoxia	**T**amponade (cardiac)
Hydrogen ion (acidosis)	**T**oxins
Hypoglycemia	**T**hrombosis, pulmonary
Hypo-/Hyperkalemia	**T**hrombosis, coronary
Hypothermia	

Also consider unrecognized trauma as a cause of cardiac arrest, especially in infants and young children.

Figure 2 summarizes common causes of in-hospital and out-of-hospital cardiac arrest, categorized according to respiratory, shock, or sudden cardiac etiologies.

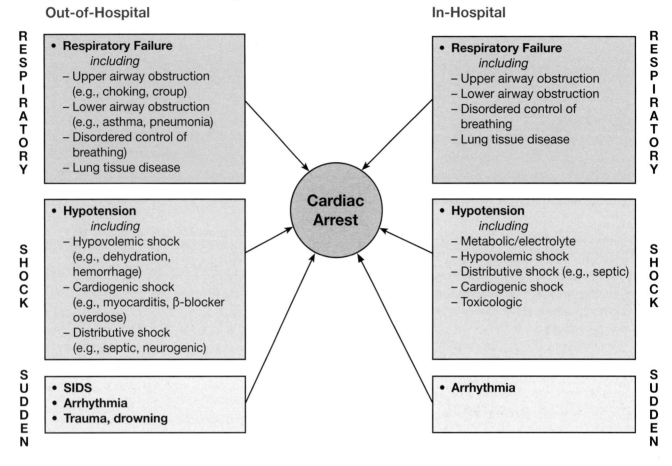

Figure 2. Causes of pediatric cardiac arrest. Based on information from Meert KL, Donaldson A, Nadkarni V, Tieves Kelly S, Schleien Charles L, Brilli RJ, Clark RS, Shaffner DH, Levy F, Statler K, Dalton HJ, van der Jagt EW, Hackbarth R, Pretzlaff R, Hernan L, Dean JM, Moler FW; for the Pediatric Emergency Care Applied Research Network. Multicenter cohort study of in-hospital cardiac arrest. *Pediatr Crit Care Med*. 2009;10:544-553.

Recognition of Cardiopulmonary Failure

Cardiopulmonary failure is defined as a combination of respiratory failure and shock (usually hypotensive shock). It is characterized by inadequate oxygenation, ventilation, and tissue perfusion. Clinically the child appears mottled or cyanotic, is gasping or breathing irregularly, and may be bradycardic. A child in cardiopulmonary failure may be only minutes away from cardiac arrest. Once the child develops cardiopulmonary failure, the process may be difficult to reverse.

If the child is responsive, evaluate by using the primary assessment model. Look for evidence of cardiopulmonary failure, which may include some or all of the following signs:

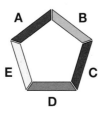

Airway	Possible upper airway obstruction
Breathing	• Bradypnea (i.e., slow respiratory rate) • Irregular, ineffective respirations (decreased and/or asymmetric breath sounds or gasping)
Circulation	• Bradycardia • Delayed capillary refill time (typically >2 seconds) • Weak central pulses • Absent peripheral pulses • Cool extremities • Mottled or cyanotic skin • Hypotension
Disability	Decreased level of consciousness
Exposure	Assess for obvious bleeding/ hemorrhaging, hypo-/hyperthermia

Recognition of Cardiac Arrest

Signs of cardiac arrest are

- Unresponsiveness
- No breathing or only gasping
- No pulse (assess for no more than 10 seconds)

Arrest rhythm may be noted on the cardiac monitor. However, monitoring is not mandatory for recognition of cardiac arrest.

If a child is unresponsive and not breathing (agonal gasps don't count), try to palpate a central pulse (brachial in an infant, carotid or femoral in a child). Because even healthcare providers are unable to reliably detect a pulse, take no more than 10 seconds to try to palpate the pulse. If there is no pulse or you are not sure if a pulse is present, start CPR, beginning with chest compressions.

Arrest Rhythms

Cardiac arrest is associated with one of the following rhythms, also known as *arrest rhythms:*

- Asystole
- Pulseless electrical activity (PEA)
- VF
- Pulseless VT, including torsades de pointes

Asystole and PEA are the most common initial rhythms seen in both in-hospital and out-of-hospital pediatric cardiac arrest, especially in children <12 years of age. Slow wide QRS complex rhythms that immediately precede asystole are often referred to as *agonal rhythms* (Figure 3). VF and pulseless VT are more likely in older children with sudden collapse or in children with underlying cardiovascular conditions.

Asystole

Asystole is cardiac standstill without discernable electrical activity. It is represented by a straight (flat) line on the ECG. Do not rely on the ECG for a diagnosis of cardiac arrest; always confirm it clinically because a "flat line" on the ECG also can be caused by a loose ECG lead.

You can recall potentially reversible causes of asystole by remembering the H's and T's (see the Identify and Intervene box "H's and T's" near the beginning of this Part). Other causes of asystole are drowning and sepsis leading to hypoxia and acidosis.

Pulseless Electrical Activity

PEA is not a specific rhythm. It is a term describing any organized electrical activity (i.e., not VF, VT or asystole) on an ECG or cardiac monitor that is associated with no *palpable* pulses; pulsations may be detected by an arterial waveform or Doppler study, but pulses are not palpable. The rate of electrical activity may be slow (most common), normal, or fast. Very slow PEA may be referred to as *agonal*.

In PEA the ECG may display normal or wide QRS complexes or other abnormalities, including

- Low- or high-amplitude T waves
- Prolonged PR and QT intervals
- AV dissociation, complete heart block, or ventricular complexes without P waves

Reassess the monitored rhythm and note the rate and width of the QRS complexes.

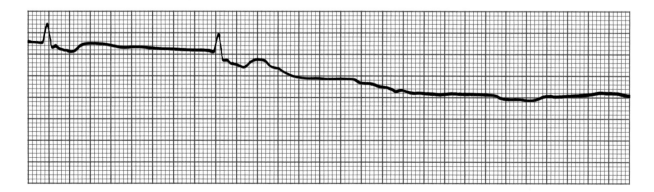

Figure 3. Agonal rhythm (slow ventricular rhythm progressing to asystole).

PEA may be caused by reversible conditions easily recalled by remembering the H's and T's. (See the Identify and Intervene box "H's and T's" near the beginning of this Part.) Unless you can quickly identify and treat the cause of PEA, the rhythm will likely deteriorate to asystole.

Ventricular Fibrillation

When VF is present, the heart has no organized rhythm and no coordinated contractions (Figure 4). Electrical activity is chaotic. The heart quivers and does not pump blood. Therefore, pulses are not palpable. VF may be preceded by a brief period of VT.

Primary VF is uncommon in children. In studies of pediatric cardiac arrest, VF was the initial rhythm in 5% to 15% of both out-of hospital and in-hospital cardiac arrests. Overall prevalence may be higher because VF may occur early during an arrest and quickly deteriorate to asystole. VF has been reported in up to 27% of pediatric in-hospital arrests at some point during the resuscitation.

VF without a previously known underlying cause may occasionally occur in otherwise healthy-appearing teens during sports activities. The cause of VF may be an undiagnosed cardiac abnormality or channelopathy, such as prolonged QT syndrome. Sudden impact to the chest from a collision or moving object may result in commotio cordis, leading to VF. Consider the H's and T's for other potential reversible causes.

Survival and outcome of patients with VF or pulseless VT as the *initial* arrest rhythm are generally better than those of patients presenting with asystole or PEA. Outcome may be improved by prompt recognition and provision of CPR and defibrillation.

Pulseless Ventricular Tachycardia

VT may produce pulses or may be a form of pulseless arrest of ventricular origin. Because the treatment of pulseless VT differs from the treatment of VT with a pulse, pulse assessment is needed to determine appropriate treatment. Almost any cause of VT can present without detectable pulses. Unlike VF, pulseless VT is characterized by organized, wide QRS complexes (Figure 5A). This form of pulseless arrest is usually of brief duration before it deteriorates into VF. See Part 9: "Recognition and Management of Tachycardia" for more information.

Pulseless VT is treated exactly the same as VF. See the Pediatric Cardiac Arrest Algorithm.

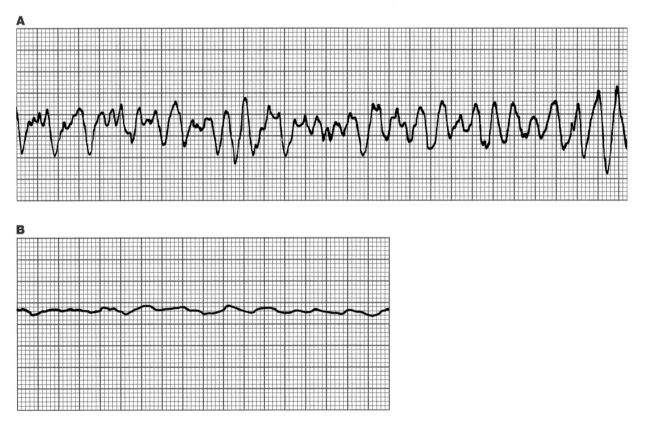

Figure 4. Ventricular fibrillation. **A,** Coarse VF. High-amplitude electrical activity varies in size and shape, representing chaotic ventricular electrical activity with no identifiable P, ORS, or T waves. **B,** Fine VF. Electrical activity is reduced compared with previous (A) rhythm strip.

Torsades de Pointes

Pulseless VT may be monomorphic (ventricular complexes appear uniform) or polymorphic (ventricular complexes do not look alike). Torsades de pointes is a distinctive form of polymorphic VT (Figure 5B). This arrhythmia is seen in conditions distinguished by a prolonged QT interval, including congenital long QT syndrome, drug toxicity, and electrolyte abnormalities (e.g., hypomagnesemia). See Part 9 for more information.

Management of Cardiac Arrest
High-Quality CPR

High-quality CPR is the foundation of basic and advanced life support for the management of cardiac arrest.

The *2010 Guidelines for CPR and ECC* recommended a change in the CPR sequence from A-B-C (Airway-Breathing-Circulation/Compressions) to C-A-B (Compressions-Airway-Breathing). This change will primarily affect a single rescuer

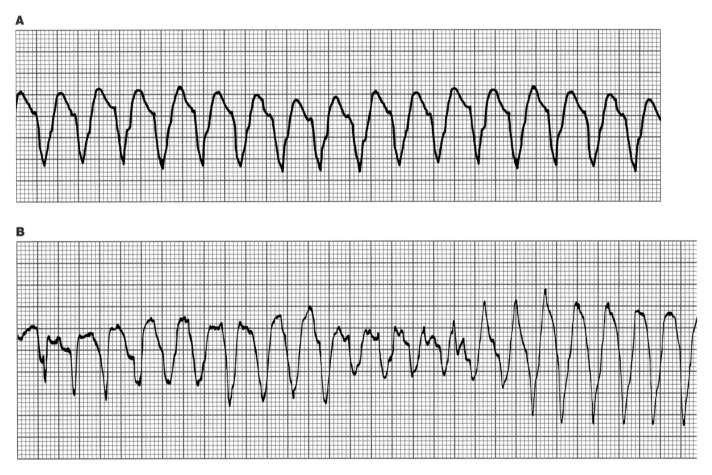

A

B

Figure 5. Ventricular tachycardia. **A,** VT in a child with muscular dystrophy and known cardiomyopathy. The ventricular rhythm is rapid and regular at a rate of 158/min (greater than the minimum 120/min characteristic of VT). The QRS is wide (greater than 0.09 second), and there is no evidence of atrial depolarization. **B,** Torsades de pointes in a child with hypomagnesemia.

Fundamental Fact **High-Quality CPR**	• Push hard—at least one third of anterior-posterior chest diameter, about 4 cm (1.5 inches) in infants and 5 cm (2 inches) in children. • Push fast—at least 100 compressions/min. • Allow complete chest recoil after each compression. • Minimize interruptions in chest compressions. • Avoid excessive ventilation.

who performs actions in sequence. When more rescuers are available, several actions are performed simultaneously rather than in a strict sequence. The change to C-A-B was made for several reasons:

- Only about 30% of victims of sudden death receive any bystander CPR. One of the obstacles to bystander CPR may be the difficulty in opening the airway and giving ventilations. Chest compressions are more easily taught and performed. It is hoped that this change will increase bystander CPR.
- Compressions require no equipment, so CPR can be started immediately without delay.

- The vast majority of cardiac arrest victims are adults with SCA. SCA is best treated with immediate chest compressions and defibrillation.
- Although a combination of chest compressions and ventilations is required for hypoxic/asphyxial arrest (i.e., most pediatric arrests), the C-A-B sequence should delay ventilations by about 18 seconds or less.
- A uniform C-A-B sequence for victims of all ages (excluding newly born infants) should be easy to learn, remember, and perform.

Please review the fundamentals of BLS in Table 1. These recommendations are based on the *2010 Guidelines for CPR and ECC*.

Fundamental Fact **Minimize Interruptions in Chest Compressions**	Chest compressions should be interrupted only briefly (<10 seconds) for ventilation (until an advanced airway is placed), rhythm check, and shock delivery.
FYI **Hands-Only (Compression-Only) CPR**	Hands-Only™ (compression-only) CPR is easier for an untrained rescuer to perform and can be more readily guided by dispatchers over the telephone for adult victims of cardiac arrest. In addition, adult survival rates from cardiac arrest of cardiac etiology are similar with either Hands-Only CPR or CPR with both compressions and rescue breathing. However, for the trained lay rescuer who is able and for all healthcare providers, the recommendation remains for the rescuer to perform both compressions and ventilations. Ventilations are more important during resuscitation from hypoxic/asphyxial arrest than during the first minutes of resuscitation from sudden cardiac arrest. Because hypoxic/asphyxial arrest is the most common cardiac arrest etiology in infants and children, and the combination of compressions and ventilations has been shown to improve survival better than compressions alone for this type of arrest, the combination of compressions and ventilations is still recommended for pediatric resuscitation by all rescuers. However, compressions alone are preferable to no CPR for any victim of cardiac arrest.

Table 1. Summary of Key BLS Components for Adults, Children, and Infants*

Component	Recommendations		
	Adults	**Children**	**Infants**
Recognition	Unresponsive (for all ages)		
	No breathing or no normal breathing (i.e., only gasping)	No breathing or only gasping	
	No pulse palpated within 10 seconds for all ages (HCP only)		
CPR sequence	C-A-B		
Compression rate	At least 100/min		
Compression depth	At least 5 cm (2 inches)	At least ⅓ AP diameter About 5 cm (2 inches)	At least ⅓ AP diameter About 4 cm (1½ inches)
Chest wall recoil	Allow complete recoil between compressions HCPs rotate compressors every 2 minutes		
Compression interruptions	Minimize interruptions in chest compressions Attempt to limit interrruptions to <10 seconds		
Airway	Head tilt–chin lift (HCP suspected trauma: jaw thrust)		
Compression-to-ventilation ratio (until advanced airway placed)	30:2 1 or 2 rescuers	30:2 Single rescuer 15:2 2 HCP rescuers	
Ventilations: when rescuer untrained or trained and not proficient	Compressions only		
Ventilations with advanced airway (HCP)	1 breath every 6-8 seconds (8-10 breaths/min) Asynchronous with chest compressions About 1 second per breath Visible chest rise		
Defibrillation	Attach and use AED as soon as available. Minimize interruptions in chest compressions before and after shock; resume CPR beginning with compressions immediately after each shock.		

Abbreviations: AED, automated external defibrillator; AP, anterior-posterior; CPR, cardiopulmonary resuscitation; HCP, healthcare provider.
*Excluding the newly born.

Monitoring for CPR Quality

During the resuscitation the team leader, as well as team members, should monitor CPR quality. Use good team communication to ensure that chest compressions are the appropriate depth and rate, that the chest fully recoils after each compression, and that ventilations are not excessive. (See the Fundamental Fact box "High-Quality CPR" in this Part.)

Many in-hospital patients, especially if they are in an intensive care unit, have advanced monitoring in place; some have an advanced airway and are receiving mechanical ventilation. Continuous monitoring of the child's end-tidal CO_2 (PETCO$_2$) can provide indirect evidence of the quality of chest compressions (Figure 6). If PETCO$_2$ is <10 to 15 mm Hg, cardiac output during CPR is probably low and not much blood is being delivered to the lungs. Efforts should be made to verify that cardiac compressions are

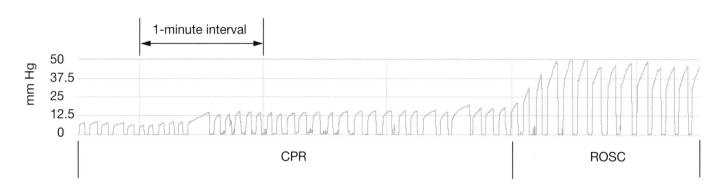

Figure 6. Capnography to monitor effectiveness of resuscitative efforts. This capnography tracing displays the P_{ETCO_2} in mm Hg on the vertical axis over time. This patient is intubated and receiving CPR. Note that the ventilation rate is approximately 8-10 breaths per minute. Chest compressions are given continuously at a rate slightly faster than 100/min but are not visible with this tracing. The initial P_{ETCO_2} is less than 12.5 mm Hg during the first minute, indicating very low blood flow. The P_{ETCO_2} increases to between 12.5 and 25 mm Hg during the second and third minutes, consistent with the increase in blood flow with ongoing resuscitation. Return of spontaneous circulation (ROSC) occurs during the fourth minute. ROSC is recognized by the abrupt increase in the P_{ETCO_2} (visible just after the fourth vertical line) to over 40 mm Hg, which is consistent with a substantial improvement in blood flow.

effective, with a goal of increasing the P_{ETCO_2} to >10 to 15 mm Hg. If the child has an indwelling arterial catheter, use the waveform as feedback to evaluate hand position and chest compression depth. A minor adjustment of hand position or depth of compression can significantly improve the amplitude of the arterial waveform, reflecting better chest compression–induced stroke volume. Verify that ventilation is not excessive. Both the end-tidal CO_2 and arterial waveform may be useful in identification of return of spontaneous circulation (ROSC).

Pediatric Advanced Life Support in Cardiac Arrest

The immediate goal of therapeutic interventions in cardiac arrest is ROSC, the restoration of a spontaneous and perfusing heart rhythm. ROSC has occurred when there is resumption of an organized cardiac electrical rhythm on the monitor plus palpable central pulses. Corresponding clinical evidence of perfusion will also be apparent (e.g., sudden increase in P_{ETCO_2}, measurable blood pressure).

Advanced life support may include the following:

- Rhythm assessment (shockable versus nonshockable)
- Vascular access
- Defibrillation
- Medication therapy
- Advanced airway management

Rhythm Assessment

Identifying the rhythm as shockable or nonshockable determines the applicable pathway of the Pediatric Cardiac Arrest Algorithm. The algorithm outlines the recommended sequence of CPR, shocks, and medication administration for both shockable and nonshockable arrest rhythms. Although the algorithm depicts actions sequentially, many actions (e.g., compressions and medication administration) are typically performed simultaneously when multiple rescuers are present.

Vascular Access

Priorities for drug delivery routes during PALS are

- Intravenous
- Intraosseous
- Endotracheal

When the critically ill child develops cardiac arrest, vascular access may already be established. If vascular access is not present, it should be established immediately. Peripheral IV access is acceptable during resuscitation if it can be placed rapidly, but placement may be difficult in critically ill children. Limit the time you spend trying to obtain IV access in a seriously ill or injured child. If IV access is not already present and you cannot achieve reliable IV access immediately, establish IO access. IO access is useful as the initial vascular access in cases of

---

Fundamental Fact

Factors of a Successful Resuscitation

Remember that the success of any resuscitation is built on a strong base of high-quality CPR, timely shock delivery for any shockable rhythm, and good teamwork.

cardiac arrest. For this reason, in the Pediatric Cardiac Arrest Algorithm and throughout this Part, if drugs can be administered by either intravenous or intraosseous route, the intraosseous route is listed first (i.e., IO/IV). Elsewhere in this manual, drugs that can be given by either route are labeled with the intravenous abbreviation first (i.e., IV/IO).

Intravenous Route

In most cases peripheral IV access is preferred over central venous access for medication and fluid administration during resuscitation. Although a central line is more secure than a peripheral line, central venous access is not needed during most resuscitation attempts, and its placement requires interruptions in chest compressions. Complications of central line placement attempts while performing chest compressions may include vascular lacerations, hematomas, pneumothorax, and bleeding. If a central venous catheter is already in place, it is the preferred route for drug and fluid administration. Central venous administration of medications provides more rapid onset of action and higher peak concentration than peripheral venous delivery.

Establishing a peripheral line does not require interruption of CPR, but drug delivery to the central circulation may be delayed. To improve drug delivery to the central circulation, do the following when administrating drugs into a peripheral IV line:

- Give the drug by bolus injection.
- Give the drug while continuing chest compressions.
- Follow with a 5-mL flush of NS to move the drug from the peripheral to the central circulation.

Intraosseous Route

If IV access is not available, drugs and fluids can be delivered safely and effectively via the IO route. In fact, the IO route is useful as the initial vascular access in cases of cardiac arrest. Important points about IO access are

- IO access can be established in all age groups.
- IO access can often be achieved in 30 to 60 seconds.
- The IO route is preferred over the ET route.

- Any drug or fluid that can be administered IV can be administered IO.

IO cannulation provides access to a noncollapsible marrow venous plexus, which serves as a rapid, safe, and reliable route for administration of resuscitation drugs and fluids. The technique uses a rigid needle, preferably a specially designed IO or bone marrow needle. Although an IO needle with a stylet is preferred to prevent obstruction of the needle with cortical bone during insertion, butterfly needles, standard hypodermic needles, and spinal needles can be inserted successfully and used effectively. See "Resources for Management of Circulatory Emergencies" at the end of Part 7: "Management of Shock" for more information on IO access.

Endotracheal Route

The IV and IO routes are preferable to the ET route for administration of drugs. Lipid-soluble drugs can be given by the ET route. These include lidocaine, epinephrine, atropine, and naloxone (LEAN) and vasopressin. There are limited human studies to provide dosing guidelines for vasopressin, however.

When considering administration of drugs via the ET route during CPR, keep these concepts in mind:

- Drug absorption from the tracheobronchial tree is unpredictable, so drug levels and drug effects will be unpredictable.
- The optimal dose of most drugs given by the ET route is unknown.
  - Drug administration into the trachea results in lower blood levels than the same dose given via IV or IO routes.
  - Animal data suggest that the lower epinephrine concentrations achieved when the drug is delivered by the ET route may produce transient but detrimental β-adrenergic–mediated vasodilation.
- Recommended drug doses administered by the ET route are higher than for the IV/IO route.
  - The recommended ET dose of epinephrine is 10 times the IV/IO dose.
  - The typical ET dose of other drugs is 2 to 3 times the IV/IO dose.

Fundamental Fact **Technique for Administering Medication by ET Route**	If a drug is given by the ET route, administer it as follows: - Instill drug into the ET tube (briefly pause compressions during instillation). - Follow with a minimum of 5 mL NS flush; a smaller volume may be used in neonates. - Provide 5 rapid positive-pressure ventilations after the drug is instilled.

Defibrillation

A defibrillation shock "stuns" the heart by depolarizing a critical mass of the myocardium. If a shock is successful, it terminates VF. This allows the heart's natural pacemaker cells to resume an organized rhythm. The return of an organized rhythm alone, however, does not ensure survival. The organized rhythm must ultimately produce effective cardiac mechanical activity that results in ROSC, defined by the presence of palpable central pulses. If the child's end-tidal CO_2 ($PETCO_2$) or intra-arterial pressure is being monitored, it also can be used to provide an indication of ROSC (Figure 6).

When attempting defibrillation, provide compressions until the defibrillator is charged, deliver 1 shock, and immediately resume CPR, starting with chest compressions. If a shock eliminates VF, continue CPR because most victims have asystole or PEA immediately after shock delivery. Chest compressions are needed to maintain blood flow to the heart (the coronary circulation) and brain until cardiac contractility resumes. There is no evidence that performance of chest compressions in a child with spontaneous cardiac activity is harmful. If VF is not eliminated by a shock, the heart is probably ischemic. Resumption of chest compressions is likely to be of greater value to the child than immediate delivery of a second shock.

In an out-of-hospital or unmonitored setting, do not waste time looking for a shockable rhythm or palpating a pulse immediately after shock delivery; neither is likely to be present. Resume high-quality CPR beginning with chest compressions. This sequence may be modified at a provider's direction in hospital units with invasive arterial monitoring. In in-hospital settings with invasive monitoring in place, return of an arterial waveform or a sudden increase in $PETCO_2$ suggests ROSC. When evidence of ROSC is indicated by monitored parameters, confirm by palpating a central pulse.

For more information about the manual defibrillation procedure, see the Critical Concept box "Manual Defibrillation" later in this Part.

Medication Therapy

The objectives for medication administration during cardiac arrest are to

- Increase coronary and cerebral perfusion pressures and blood flow
- Stimulate spontaneous or more forceful myocardial contractility
- Accelerate heart rate
- Correct and treat the possible cause of cardiac arrest
- Suppress or treat arrhythmias

Medications that may be used during treatment of pediatric cardiac arrest are listed in Table 2.

Table 2. Pediatric Cardiac Arrest Medications

Vasopressors	
Epinephrine	The α-adrenergic–mediated vasoconstriction of *epinephrine* increases aortic diastolic pressure and thus coronary perfusion pressure, a critical determinant of successful resuscitation. Both beneficial and toxic physiologic effects of epinephrine administration during CPR have been shown in animal and human studies. Although epinephrine has been used universally in resuscitation, there is little evidence to show that it improves survival in humans. There is no survival benefit from the routine use of *high-dose IV/IO epinephrine* (0.1 to 0.2 mg/kg or 0.1 to 0.2 mL/kg of 1:1000 solution). High doses may be harmful, particularly in hypoxic/asphyxial arrest. High-dose epinephrine may be considered for special resuscitation circumstances, such as β-blocker overdose.
Vasopressin	There is insufficient evidence to recommend for or against the routine use of *vasopressin* during cardiac arrest in children. Vasopressin given after lack of response to epinephrine may result in ROSC during pediatric cardiac arrest. A large pediatric National Registry of CPR case series, however, suggested that vasopressin therapy is associated with lower ROSC and a trend toward lower 24-hour and discharge survival rates. In a clinical trial in adult patients with asystole, the combination of epinephrine and vasopressin improved ROSC and survival to hospital discharge. This combination, however, did not improve intact neurologic survival when compared with giving epinephrine alone.
Antiarrhythmics	
Amiodarone	*Amiodarone* may be considered for treatment of shock-refractory or recurrent VF/VT. Amiodarone has α-adrenergic and β-adrenergic blocking activity; affects sodium, potassium, and calcium channels; slows AV conduction; prolongs the AV refractory period and QT interval; and slows ventricular conduction (widens the QRS). Studies in adults showed increased rates of survival to hospital admission but not to hospital discharge when amiodarone was compared with placebo or lidocaine for shock-resistant VF. One study in children demonstrated the effectiveness of amiodarone for life-threatening ventricular arrhythmias, but there have been no published studies on the use of amiodarone for pediatric cardiac arrest from VF.
Lidocaine	*Lidocaine* has long been recommended for the treatment of ventricular arrhythmias in infants and children because it decreases automaticity and suppresses ventricular arrhythmias. Data from a study of shock-refractory VT in adults showed that lidocaine was inferior to amiodarone. Lidocaine has been recommended as a second-line drug in shock-refractory VF cardiac arrest when amiodarone is not available. Indications for the use of lidocaine in the treatment of other ventricular arrhythmias are uncertain. There have been no published studies on the use of lidocaine in pediatric VF cardiac arrest.
Magnesium sulfate	*Magnesium sulfate* is used for the treatment of torsades de pointes and for hypomagnesemia. There is insufficient evidence to recommend for or against the routine use of magnesium in pediatric cardiac arrest not associated with these conditions.
Other Agents	
Atropine	*Atropine* is indicated for the treatment of bradycardia, especially if the bradycardia results from excessive vagal tone. There are no published studies suggesting its efficacy for treatment of cardiac arrest in pediatric patients. See Part 8: "Recognition and Management of Bradycardia" for a complete discussion.
Calcium	Routine use of *calcium* in cardiac arrest is not recommended because it does not improve survival and may be harmful. Calcium is indicated for the treatment of documented ionized hypocalcemia and hyperkalemia, particularly in children with hemodynamic compromise. Ionized hypocalcemia is relatively common in critically ill children, particularly during sepsis or after cardiopulmonary bypass. Calcium may also be considered for the treatment of hypermagnesemia or calcium channel blocker overdose.
Sodium bicarbonate	Routine administration of *sodium bicarbonate* in cardiac arrest is not recommended. Sodium bicarbonate is recommended for the treatment of symptomatic patients with hyperkalemia, tricyclic antidepressant overdose, or an overdose of other sodium channel blocking agents.

Advanced Airway Management

In managing the airway and ventilation in pediatric victims of cardiac arrest, consider the following:

- Avoid excessive ventilation during resuscitation.
  - Excessive ventilation can be harmful because it impedes venous return and decreases cardiac output.
  - Increased intrathoracic pressure from positive-pressure ventilation also elevates right atrial pressure and thus reduces coronary perfusion pressure.
  - When ventilating with a mask (in cycles of 15 compressions and 2 breaths), give each breath over 1 second and provide just enough volume to make the chest rise.
  - Excessive tidal volume or pressure during bag-mask ventilation may distend the stomach. Gastric distention impedes ventilation and increases the risk of aspiration.
- Avoid routine use of cricoid pressure if it interferes with intubation or ventilation.
- Use waveform capnography or capnometry to confirm and monitor ET tube placement.
- Colourimetric exhaled CO_2 devices may fail to detect the presence of exhaled CO_2 (i.e., lack of a colour change indicates no CO_2 detected) during cardiac arrest despite correct placement of the ET tube. Use direct laryngoscopy to confirm tube placement if exhaled CO_2 is not detected and there is evidence that the tube is in the trachea (e.g., chest rise and bilateral breath sounds).
- When providing ventilations via an ET tube during CPR, provide 1 breath every 6 to 8 seconds (8 to 10 breaths/min) without pausing chest compressions. Chest compressions are delivered without interruption at a rate of at least 100/min. For more details see

"Insertion of an Advanced Airway During CPR" later in this Part.

An advanced airway (e.g., ET tube) can be placed during CPR. However, in a study of out-of-hospital cardiac arrest when emergency medical services (EMS) transport time was short and providers had limited ongoing experience in pediatric intubation, there was no demonstrated survival advantage of ET intubation over effective bag-mask ventilation. This study does not address ET intubation in the in-hospital setting but suggests that immediate intubation may not be necessary. For more details see Gausche et al, 2000 (full reference in the Suggested Reading List at the end of this Part).

Pediatric Cardiac Arrest Algorithm

The Pediatric Cardiac Arrest Algorithm (Figure 7) outlines assessment and management steps for an infant or child in cardiac arrest who does not respond to BLS interventions. The Pediatric Cardiac Arrest Algorithm is based on expert consensus. It is designed to maximize uninterrupted periods of CPR while enabling efficient delivery of electrical therapy and medications as appropriate. Although the actions are listed sequentially, when several rescuers are involved, some actions will occur simultaneously.

Step numbers in the text below refer to the corresponding steps in the algorithm. The algorithm consists of 2 pathways, depending on the cardiac rhythm as seen on a monitor or interpreted by an AED:

- A shockable rhythm (VF/VT) pathway is displayed on the left side of the algorithm.
- A nonshockable rhythm (asystole/PEA) pathway is displayed on the right side of the algorithm.

Critical Concept

Coordination of Team Members During Resuscitation

Using the Pediatric Cardiac Arrest Algorithm, providers should structure assessments and interventions around 2-minute periods of uninterrupted high-quality CPR. This requires organization so that every member of the team knows his or her responsibilities. When all team members are familiar with the algorithm, they can anticipate and prepare for the next steps, getting equipment ready and drawing up the proper doses of medications. Chest compressors should rotate about every 2 minutes.

Pediatric Cardiac Arrest

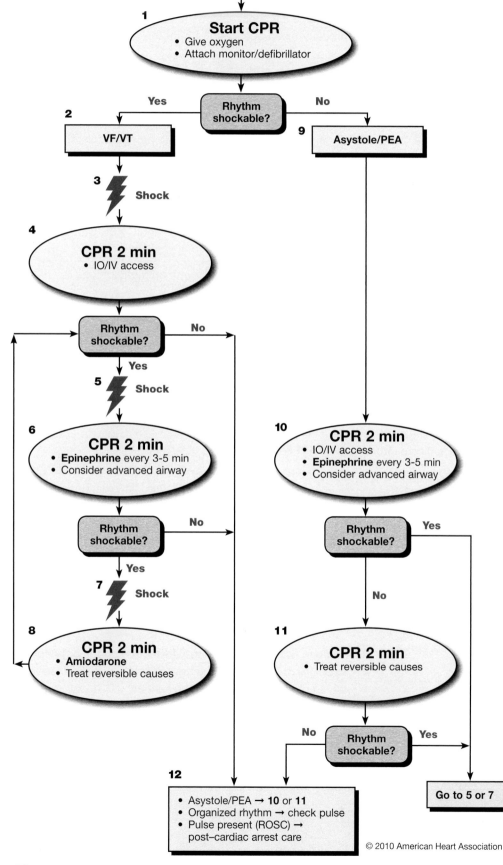

Shout for Help/Activate Emergency Response

1 Start CPR
- Give oxygen
- Attach monitor/defibrillator

Rhythm shockable?

Yes → **2 VF/VT**

No → **9 Asystole/PEA**

3 Shock

4 CPR 2 min
- IO/IV access

Rhythm shockable?

No →

Yes ↓

5 Shock

6 CPR 2 min
- **Epinephrine** every 3-5 min
- Consider advanced airway

Rhythm shockable?

No →

Yes ↓

7 Shock

8 CPR 2 min
- **Amiodarone**
- Treat reversible causes

10 CPR 2 min
- IO/IV access
- **Epinephrine** every 3-5 min
- Consider advanced airway

Rhythm shockable?

Yes →

No ↓

11 CPR 2 min
- Treat reversible causes

Rhythm shockable?

No / Yes

12
- Asystole/PEA → **10** or **11**
- Organized rhythm → check pulse
- Pulse present (ROSC) → post–cardiac arrest care

Go to 5 or 7

© 2010 American Heart Association

Doses/Details

CPR Quality
- Push hard (≥1/3 of anterior-posterior diameter of chest) and fast (at least 100/min) and allow complete chest recoil
- Minimize interruptions in compressions
- Avoid excessive ventilation
- Rotate compressor every 2 minutes
- If no advanced airway, 15:2 compression-ventilation ratio. If advanced airway, 8-10 breaths per minute with continuous chest compressions

Shock Energy for Defibrillation
First shock 2 J/kg, second shock 4 J/kg, subsequent shocks ≥4 J/kg, maximum 10 J/kg or adult dose.

Drug Therapy
- **Epinephrine IO/IV Dose:** 0.01 mg/kg (0.1 mL/kg of 1:10 000 concentration). Repeat every 3-5 minutes. If no IO/IV access, may give endotracheal dose: 0.1 mg/kg (0.1 mL/kg of 1:1000 concentration).
- **Amiodarone IO/IV Dose:** 5 mg/kg bolus during cardiac arrest. May repeat up to 2 times for refractory VF/pulseless VT.

Advanced Airway
- Endotracheal intubation or supraglottic advanced airway
- Waveform capnography or capnometry to confirm and monitor ET tube placement
- Once advanced airway in place give 1 breath every 6-8 seconds (8-10 breaths per minute)

Return of Spontaneous Circulation (ROSC)
- Pulse and blood pressure
- Spontaneous arterial pressure waves with intra-arterial monitoring

Reversible Causes
- **H**ypovolemia
- **H**ypoxia
- **H**ydrogen ion (acidosis)
- **H**ypoglycemia
- **H**ypo-/hyperkalemia
- **H**ypothermia
- **T**ension pneumothorax
- **T**amponade, cardiac
- **T**oxins
- **T**hrombosis, pulmonary
- **T**hrombosis, coronary

Figure 7. Pediatric Cardiac Arrest Algorithm.

Start CPR (Step 1)

As soon as the child is found to be unresponsive with no breathing (or only gasping), shout for help and activate emergency response, send for a defibrillator (manual or AED), check a pulse, and start CPR, beginning with chest compressions. Attach the ECG monitor or AED pads as soon as they are available. Throughout resuscitation, provide high-quality CPR (give chest compressions of adequate rate and depth, allow complete chest recoil after each compression, minimize interruptions in compressions, and avoid excessive ventilation). Use a compression-ventilation ratio of 30:2 for 1 rescuer and 15:2 for 2 rescuers. Administer O_2 with ventilations as soon as it is available.

Once the monitor/defibrillator is attached, check the rhythm. Determine whether the rhythm is shockable (VF/VT) or nonshockable (asystole/PEA). If the rhythm is shockable, follow the left side of the algorithm.

Shockable Rhythm: VF/VT (Step 2)

If the rhythm is shockable, deliver 1 unsynchronized shock (Step 3). Perform CPR while the defibrillator is charging, if possible. The shorter the interval is between the last compression and shock delivery, the higher the potential shock success (elimination of VF) will be. Therefore, try to keep that interval as short as possible, ideally <10 seconds. Immediately after shock delivery, resume high-quality CPR, beginning with chest compressions. In a monitored setting this approach may be modified at the provider's discretion.

If the resuscitation takes place in a critical care setting and the child has intra-arterial monitoring in place, the presence of a waveform with an adequate arterial pressure can be useful in identifying ROSC. In other settings that determination will be made after about 2 minutes of CPR during the next rhythm check. A sharp increase in the exhaled CO_2 pressure (P_{ETCO_2}) can also indicate ROSC.

Defibrillation devices for children are the

- AED (able to distinguish pediatric shockable from nonshockable rhythms and ideally equipped with a pediatric dose attenuator)
- Manual cardioverter/defibrillator (capable of variable shock doses)

Institutions that care for children at risk for arrhythmias and cardiac arrest (e.g., hospitals, emergency departments) ideally should have defibrillators available that are capable of energy adjustment appropriate for children.

AED

AEDs are programmed to evaluate the child's ECG to determine if a shockable rhythm is present, charge to a predetermined dose, and prompt the rescuer to deliver a shock. The AED provides voice and visual prompts to assist the operator. Many, but not all, AED algorithms have been shown to be sensitive and specific for recognizing shockable arrhythmias in children. Many are equipped with pediatric pad-cable systems that attenuate the adult dose to deliver a smaller energy dose appropriate for children. These dose attenuators should be used for children <8 years of age and less than about 25 kg in weight.

Weight/Age	AED Energy Dose
≥25 kg (≥8 years)	• Standard "adult" AED with adult pad-cable system
<25 kg (≥1 year and <8 years)	• AED with attenuated dose if available • AED with adult system if pediatric dose attenuator is not available
<1 year	• Manual defibrillator if available • AED with pediatric dose attenuator if manual defibrillator not available • AED with adult system if neither of the above is available

Manual Defibrillator

The optimal electrical energy dose for pediatric defibrillation is unknown. For manual defibrillation, an initial dose of 2 to 4 J/kg is acceptable, and for ease of teaching a 2 J/kg (biphasic or monophasic waveform) may be considered. If VF or pulseless VT persists at the next rhythm check, deliver a dose of 4 J/kg for the second shock. If VF persists after the second shock, use at least 4 J/kg or higher, not to exceed 10 J/kg or the maximum adult dose. Successful resuscitation using shock doses up to 9 J/kg have been reported in children.

You can use either self-adhesive electrode pads or paddles to deliver shocks with a manual defibrillator. Self-adhesive pads are preferred because they are easy to apply and reduce the risk of current arcing. They also can be used to monitor the heart rhythm. If you use paddles, apply a conducting gel, cream, paste, or an electrode pad between the paddle and the child's chest to reduce transthoracic impedance. Do not use saline-soaked gauze pads, sonographic gels, or alcohol pads. Alcohol pads may pose a fire hazard and cause chest burns.

See the Critical Concept box "Manual Defibrillation" later in this Part for the universal steps for operating a manual defibrillator.

Paddles/Pads

Use the largest paddles or self-adhering electrode pads that will fit on the chest wall without contact between the pads. Recommended paddle sizes are based on the child's weight/age.

Weight/Age	Paddle Size
>10 kg (approximately 1 year or older)	Large "adult" paddles (8 to 13 cm)
<10 kg (<1 year)	Small "infant" paddles (4.5 cm)

Note: The selection of pediatric pads versus adult pads is manufacturer specific. Refer to package instructions to determine the appropriate size.

Place the paddles/electrode pads so that the heart is between them. Place one paddle/electrode pad on the upper right side of the victim's chest below the right clavicle and the other to the left of the left nipple in the anterior axillary line directly over the heart. Allow at least 3 cm between paddles; when pads are used, place them so they don't touch. When using paddles, apply firm pressure to create good contact with the skin.

Modifications may be required in special situations (e.g., if the child has an implanted defibrillator).

Clearing for Defibrillation

To ensure the safety of rescuers during defibrillation, perform a visual check of the child and the resuscitation team just before you deliver a shock. Make sure that high-flow O_2 is not directed across the child's chest. Warn others that you are about to deliver a shock and that everyone must stand clear. State a "warning chant" firmly and in a forceful voice before delivering each shock (this entire sequence should take <5 seconds). See the Critical Concept box "Manual Defibrillation."

Resume CPR, Establish IV/IO Access (Step 4)

Immediately after the shock, resume CPR, beginning with chest compressions. Give about 2 minutes of CPR. (For 2 rescuers this will be about 10 cycles of 15 compressions followed by 2 ventilations.) While CPR is being performed, if vascular access (IO or IV) is not already present, another member of the resuscitation team should establish vascular access in anticipation of the need for medications.

Before the rhythm check the team leader should ensure that the team is prepared to do the following:

- Rotate compressors.
- Calculate appropriate shock dose to administer if VF/pulseless VT persists.
- Prepare drugs for administration if indicated.

Check Rhythm

After 2 minutes of CPR, check the rhythm. *Try to limit interruptions in CPR to <10 seconds for a rhythm check.*

This rhythm check may indicate the following outcomes from the previous shock and CPR:

- Termination of VF/VT to a "nonshockable" rhythm (asystole, PEA, or an organized rhythm with a pulse)
- Persistence of a shockable rhythm (VF/VT)

FYI
Anterior-Posterior Pad Placement

Some defibrillator manufacturers recommend placement of self-adhesive electrode pads in an anterior-posterior position, with one over the victim's heart and the other over the back. Anterior-posterior placement may be necessary in an infant, particularly if only large electrode pads are available.

Place the electrode pads according to the recommendations of the defibrillator manufacturer. These are typically illustrated on the pads themselves.

Termination of VF/VT (i.e., Rhythm Is "Nonshockable") (Step 12)

If the rhythm is nonshockable, check for an "organized" rhythm (i.e., one with regular complexes [Figure 8]). If the rhythm is organized, palpate for a central pulse. If a pulse is present, begin postresuscitation care. If the rhythm is not organized, do not take the time to perform a pulse check; instead, immediately resume CPR (Step 10).

If PEA (an organized rhythm without a palpable pulse) or asystole is present at the rhythm check, resume CPR beginning with compressions and proceed to the right side of the algorithm (Step 10 or 11).

If there is any doubt about the presence of a pulse, immediately resume CPR (Step 10). Chest compressions are unlikely to be harmful to a child with a spontaneous rhythm and weak pulses. *If there is no pulse or you are not sure, resume CPR.*

Critical Concept **Manual Defibrillation (for VF or Pulseless VT)**	*Continue CPR without interruptions during all steps until step 8 in this box. Minimize interval from compressions to shock delivery (do not deliver breaths between compressions and shock delivery).* 1. Turn on defibrillator. 2. Set *lead switch* to *paddles* (or lead I, II, or III if monitor leads are used). 3. Select adhesive pads or paddles. Use the largest pads or paddles that can fit on the patient's chest without touching each other. 4. If using paddles, apply conductive gel or paste. Be sure cables are attached to defibrillator. 5. Position adhesive pads on patient's chest: right anterior chest wall and left axillary positions. If using paddles, apply firm pressure. If patient has an implanted pacemaker, do not position pads/paddles directly over the device. Be sure that oxygen is not directed over patient's chest. 6. Select energy dose: **Initial dose:** 2 J/kg (acceptable range 2-4 J/kg) **Subsequent doses:** 4 J/kg or higher (not to exceed 10 J/kg or standard adult dose) 7. Announce "Charging defibrillator," and press *charge* on defibrillator controls or apex paddle. 8. When defibrillator is fully charged, state firm chant, such as "I am going to shock on three." Then count. "All clear!" (Chest compressions should continue until this announcement.) 9. After confirming all personnel are clear of the patient, press the *shock* button on the defibrillator or press the 2 paddle *discharge* buttons simultaneously. 10. Immediately after shock delivery, resume CPR beginning with compressions for 5 cycles (about 2 minutes), and then recheck rhythm. Interruption of CPR should be brief.
Fundamental Fact **Rhythm and Pulse Checks**	Remember, rhythm and pulse checks should be brief (<10 seconds). Pulse checks are unnecessary unless an organized rhythm (or other evidence of a perfusing rhythm, such as an arterial waveform or an abrupt and sustained increase in $PETCO_2$) is present. In specialized environments (e.g., an intensive care unit) with intra-arterial or other hemodynamic monitoring in place, providers may alter this sequence.

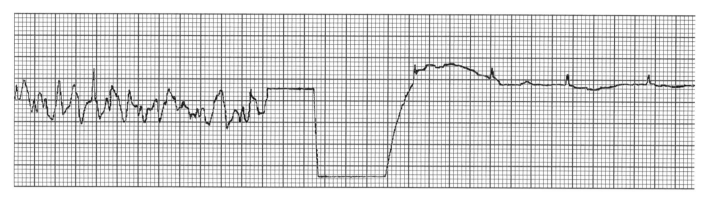

Figure 8. VF converted to organized rhythm after defibrillation (successful shock).

Persistent VF/VT

If the rhythm check reveals a shockable rhythm (i.e., persistent VF/VT), prepare to deliver a second shock with a manual defibrillator (4 J/kg) or AED. Resume chest compressions while the defibrillator is charging. If IV/IO access is established, administer epinephrine while compressions continue. Consider insertion of an advanced airway if one is not in place. Once the defibrillator is charged, "clear" the patient and deliver the shock (Step 5).

Resume CPR with chest compressions immediately after the shock delivery (Step 6). A different compressor should be performing the compressions (i.e., compressors should rotate every 2 minutes). Give about 2 minutes of CPR. (For 2 rescuers, this will be about 10 cycles of 15 compressions followed by 2 ventilations.)

Give Epinephrine (Step 6)

If VF/VT persists despite delivery of 2 shocks and CPR, administer epinephrine as soon as IO/IV access is available while compressions are continuing.

Epinephrine	
Route	**Dose**
IO/IV	0.01 mg/kg (0.1 mL/kg) bolus (1:10 000)
ET	0.1 mg/kg (0.1 mL/kg) bolus (1:1000)
Repeat epinephrine about every 3 to 5 minutes of cardiac arrest. This will generally result in epinephrine delivery after every second (i.e., every other) rhythm check.	

The Pediatric Cardiac Arrest Algorithm and the *2010 Guidelines for CPR and ECC* do not state a specific time for delivery of the first dose of epinephrine. This is because there is no published evidence to guide recommendations for the timing of drug administration. In addition, some patients will have early IO/IV access and hemodynamic monitoring and others will not. Epinephrine administration is not suggested earlier (immediately after the *first* shock) because it might not be necessary if the first shock is successful (i.e., elimination of VF and an organized rhythm may be observed at the rhythm check that follows the first shock and 2 minutes of CPR).

FYI **Timing of Epinephrine Administration**	In a monitored setting a provider may choose to administer epinephrine before or after the second shock. When VF/VT is identified during the rhythm check, the administration of epinephrine can occur during the CPR that precedes (during charging) or immediately follows the shock delivery. Conversely, if, in a monitored setting, an organized rhythm is present during the rhythm check, it is reasonable to check for a pulse to avoid an unnecessary dose of epinephrine because it can produce adverse effects. For example, if the initial VF/VT was related to a cardiomyopathy, myocarditis, or drug toxicity, epinephrine administration immediately after elimination of VF/VT could induce recurrent VF/VT.

Medication Administration During CPR

Ideally, administer IO/IV medications *during compressions* because blood flow generated by compressions helps to circulate the drugs. By consensus the *2010 Guidelines for CPR and ECC* recommend medication administration during compressions immediately *before* (if compressions are performed while the defibrillator is charging) or *after* shock delivery so that the drugs have time to circulate before the next rhythm check (and shock delivery if needed).

Team members responsible for resuscitation drugs should anticipate and prepare the *next* drug dose that might be needed after the next rhythm check. All team members should be familiar with the Pediatric Cardiac Arrest Algorithm and refer to it during the resuscitation to anticipate the next interventions. Drug tables, charts, or other references should be readily available to expedite the calculation of drug doses. Use of a colour-coded length-based resuscitation tape facilitates rapid estimation of appropriate drug doses.

ET administration of resuscitation drugs results in lower blood concentrations than the same dose given intravascularly. Studies also suggest that the lower epinephrine concentration achieved when the drug is delivered by the ET route may produce transient β-adrenergic effects (rather than the α-adrenergic vasoconstrictive effects). The β-adrenergic effects can be detrimental and cause hypotension, lower coronary artery perfusion pressure and flow, and reduce potential for ROSC. Another disadvantage of ET drug delivery is that chest compressions must be interrupted for drug delivery by this route.

Insertion of an Advanced Airway During CPR

The team leader will determine the best time for endotracheal intubation. Because insertion of an advanced airway is likely to require interruption of chest compressions, the team leader must weigh the relative benefits of securing the airway and of minimizing interruptions in compressions. If endotracheal intubation is necessary, careful planning and organization of supplies and personnel will minimize the time that compressions are interrupted. Once the ET tube is inserted, confirm that it is in the correct position.

When an advanced airway is in place during CPR, continuous chest compressions can be provided. See the Critical Concept box "CPR With an Advanced Airway."

Check Rhythm

After 2 minutes of CPR and epinephrine administration, recheck the rhythm. Try to limit interruptions in chest compressions for rhythm checks to <10 seconds. Actions to take based on the rhythm present are listed in the box:

If the Rhythm Check Reveals	Then
Termination of VF/VT	Check for an organized rhythm: • No organized rhythm (asystole/PEA): Go to Step 11. • Organized rhythm: Check pulse. If pulse is present, begin postresuscitation care. If no pulse is present (PEA), go to Step 11.
Persistence of VF/VT	Go to Step 7.

For Persistent VF/VT (Step 7)

Deliver Shock

If VF/VT persists, deliver 1 shock by manual defibrillator (4 J/kg or more, up to 10 J/kg or the maximum adult dose) or AED. Perform chest compressions, if possible, while the defibrillator is charging. When the defibrillator is charged, "clear" the victim and deliver the shock.

Immediately after the shock, resume CPR, beginning with chest compressions. Give about 2 minutes of CPR. (For 2

Critical Concept

CPR With an Advanced Airway

Once an advanced airway (e.g., ET tube) is in place, the CPR sequence changes from "cycles" to *continuous* chest compressions and a regular ventilation rate. One team member compresses the chest at a rate of at least 100/min. Another team member ventilates with 1 breath every 6 to 8 seconds (a rate of about 8 to 10 breaths/min).

Team members performing chest compressions should rotate every 2 minutes to reduce rescuer fatigue and ensure high-quality chest compressions. Limit interruptions of chest compressions to the minimum required for rhythm checks and shock delivery. This sequence may be modified in special settings (e.g., an intensive care unit) with continuous ECG and hemodynamic monitoring in place.

rescuers, this will be about 10 cycles of 15 compressions followed by 2 ventilations.)

Antiarrhythmic Medications (Step 8)

Immediately after resuming chest compressions, administer amiodarone or give lidocaine if amiodarone is not available. If the rhythm check shows torsades de pointes, give magnesium.

Dose antiarrhythmic agents as follows:

Drug	Dose
Amiodarone	5 mg/kg IV/IO bolus (maximum single dose 300 mg); may repeat 5 mg/kg IV/IO bolus up to total dose of 15 mg/kg (2.2 g in adolescents) IV per 24 hours
Lidocaine	1 mg/kg IO/IV
Magnesium	25 to 50 mg/kg IO/IV, maximum dose 2 g

Administer IO/IV drugs during chest compressions.

Summary of the VF/Pulseless VT Sequence

Figure 9 summarizes the recommended sequence of CPR, rhythm checks, shocks, and administration of drugs for VF/pulseless VT based on expert consensus.

Think of the management of pulseless arrest due to VF/VT as provision of nearly continuous CPR. Ideally, CPR is interrupted for only brief periods, for rhythm checks and shock delivery. Drug preparation and administration do not require interruption of CPR and should not delay shock delivery.

Nonshockable Rhythm (Asystole/PEA, Step 9)

If the rhythm is nonshockable, asystole or PEA may be present. The management of this rhythm is outlined in the pathway on the right side of the Pediatric Cardiac Arrest Algorithm (Figure 7). Note that 25% of hospitalized children in the National Registry of CPR developed a shockable rhythm at some point during resuscitation. If VF develops during resuscitation, return to the left side of the Pediatric Cardiac Arrest Algorithm (Step 5 or 7).

Establish Vascular Access (Step 10)

For treatment of asystole or PEA, provide high-quality CPR, deliver epinephrine as appropriate, and try to identify and treat potentially reversible causes of the arrest.

Continue high-quality CPR for about 2 minutes. During this time establish vascular (IO or IV) access and consider endotracheal intubation. As soon as vascular access is established, give a bolus of epinephrine during chest compressions.

Dose epinephrine as follows:

Epinephrine	
Route	**Dose**
IO/IV	0.01 mg/kg (0.1 mL/kg) bolus 1:10 000
ET	0.1 mg/kg (0.1 mL/kg) bolus 1:1000
Repeat epinephrine administration about every 3 to 5 minutes if cardiac arrest persists. This generally results in the administration of epinephrine after every second (i.e., every other) rhythm check.	

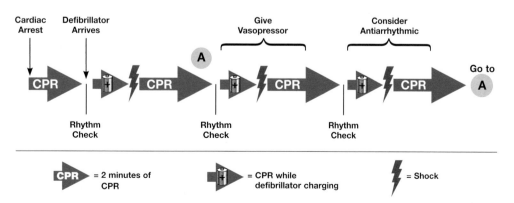

Figure 9. Summary of the VF/pulseless VT cardiac arrest sequence. Prepare next drug before rhythm check. Administer drug during chest compressions, as soon as possible after the rhythm check confirms VF/pulseless VT. Do not delay shock. Continue CPR while drugs are prepared and administered and defibrillator is charging. Ideally, chest compressions should be interrupted only for ventilation (until advanced airway placed), rhythm check, and actual shock delivery.

Check Rhythm

After about 2 minutes of CPR, check the rhythm.

If Rhythm Is	Then
Shockable	Go to Step 7 and proceed through the steps on the left side of the algorithm.
Nonshockable	Go to Step 11.

Nonshockable Rhythm (Step 11)

If the rhythm check reveals a nonshockable rhythm, resume CPR immediately, beginning with chest compressions, and treat potentially reversible causes of cardiac arrest. These can be recalled by remembering the H's and T's mnemonic (see the H's and T's table on this page). After another 2 minutes of CPR, check the rhythm. If it is organized, check for a pulse. If a pulse is present, proceed with postresuscitation care. If a pulse is not palpable or the rhythm is not organized, go to Step 10. If a shockable rhythm is present at any time, go to the left side of the algorithm (Step 5 or 7).

Summary of Asystole/PEA Treatment Sequence

Figure 10 summarizes the recommended sequence of CPR, based on expert consensus, of rhythm checks, shocks, and delivery of drugs for asystole and PEA.

The management of any pulseless arrest includes provision of nearly continuous CPR, interrupted ideally by only brief rhythm checks. Do not interrupt CPR for drug preparation and administration. Administer IO/IV drugs during chest compressions. See the Critical Concept box "CPR With an Advanced Airway" earlier in this Part.

Identifying and Treating Potentially Reversible Causes of Cardiac Arrest

The outcome of pediatric cardiac arrest is generally poor. Rapid recognition, immediate high-quality CPR, and correction of contributing factors and potentially reversible causes offer the best chance for a successful resuscitation. Some cardiac arrests may be associated with a potentially reversible condition. If you can quickly identify the condition and treat it, your resuscitative efforts may be successful.

In a search for potentially reversible causes or contributing factors, do the following:

- Ensure that high-quality CPR is being provided.
- Check that the advanced airway is patent and effective.
- Ensure that ventilations produce visible chest rise without excessive volume or rate.
- Verify that the bag-mask device is connected to a source of high-flow O_2.
- Consider potentially reversible causes by recalling the H's and T's.

H's and T's

Cardiac arrest in children may be associated with a reversible condition.

H's	T's
Hypovolemia	**T**ension pneumothorax
Hypoxia	**T**amponade (cardiac)
Hydrogen ion (acidosis)	**T**oxins
Hyper-/Hypokalemia	**T**hrombosis, pulmonary
Hypoglycemia	**T**hrombosis, coronary
Hypothermia	

Also consider unrecognized trauma as a cause of cardiac arrest, particularly in infants and young children.

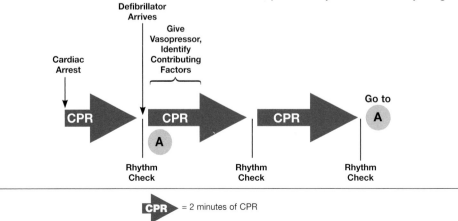

Figure 10. Cardiac arrest treatment sequence: asystole and PEA. If, at any rhythm check, a shockable rhythm is detected, see Figure 9.

Return of Spontaneous Circulation

If resuscitative efforts successfully restore an organized rhythm (or there is other evidence of ROSC, such as an abrupt and sustained increase in $PETCO_2$ or visible pulsations on an arterial waveform), check the child's pulse to determine if a perfusing rhythm is present. If a pulse is present, continue with postresuscitation care.

Pediatric Cardiac Arrest: Special Circumstances

The following special circumstances resulting in pediatric cardiac arrest require specific management:

- Trauma
- Drowning
- Anaphylaxis
- Poisoning
- Congenital heart disease: single ventricle
- Pulmonary hypertension

Cardiac Arrest due to Trauma

Cardiac arrest associated with trauma in children represents a significant subgroup of out-of-hospital pediatric cardiac arrests. Improper resuscitation (including inadequate volume resuscitation) is a major cause of preventable pediatric trauma deaths (for more details see Dykes et al, 1989 [full reference in the Suggested Reading List]). Despite rapid and effective out-of-hospital and trauma centre response, survival of children with out-of-hospital cardiac arrest due to trauma is low. Survival from out-of-hospital pediatric cardiac arrests due to blunt trauma is very low. Factors that may improve outcome from traumatic out-of-hospital cardiac arrest include treatable penetrating injuries and prompt transport (typically ≤10 minutes) to a trauma care facility. For more details see Sasser et al, 2009 (full reference in the Suggested Reading List).

Traumatic cardiac arrest in children has multiple possible causes, including

- Hypoxia secondary to respiratory arrest, airway obstruction, or tracheobronchial injury
- Injury to vital structures (e.g., heart, aorta, pulmonary arteries)
- Severe brain injury with secondary cardiovascular collapse
- Upper cervical spinal cord injury with respiratory arrest, which may be accompanied by spinal shock, progressing to cardiac arrest
- Diminished cardiac output or PEA from tension pneumothorax, cardiac tamponade, or massive hemorrhage

Basic and advanced life support techniques for the pediatric trauma victim in cardiac arrest are fundamentally the same as for the child with nontraumatic cardiac arrest: support of circulation, airway, and breathing. The focus of resuscitation in an out-of-hospital setting is to

- Maintain adequate circulation, airway, and ventilation
- Anticipate airway obstruction by dental fragments, blood, or other debris (use a suction device if necessary)
- Minimize motion of the cervical spine (if indicated)
- Control external bleeding with pressure
- Safely extricate the patient
- Minimize interventions that delay transport to definitive care
- Transport infants and children with multisystem trauma to a trauma centre with pediatric expertise
- Establish IO/IV access and initiate volume resuscitation as needed

The following is a summary of key management principles for traumatic cardiac arrest in children.

Circulation	• Perform high-quality CPR. • Attach a monitor/defibrillator. • Control visible hemorrhage with direct pressure. • Assume that the patient is hypovolemic; establish IO/IV access and replace fluids rapidly. Consider non-crossmatched type O-negative blood for females (and either O-negative or O-positive for males). • Consider pericardiocentesis for possible cardiac tamponade (if suspected). • Consider spinal shock (i.e., loss of sympathetic innervation) resulting in fluid-refractory hypotension and bradycardia. Vasopressor therapy is indicated if spinal shock is suspected.
Airway	• Open and maintain the airway by using a jaw-thrust maneuver. • Restrict cervical spine motion by manual stabilization of the head and neck.

Breathing	• Ventilate with a bag-mask device using 100% O_2; a 2-person bag-mask ventilation technique is preferable to maintain manual stabilization of the head and neck. • If ET intubation is attempted, one rescuer should stabilize the head and neck in a neutral position. • Avoid excessive ventilation. • Consider empiric bilateral needle decompression for tension pneumothorax (if suspected). • Seal any significant open pneumothorax and insert a thoracostomy tube.

Cardiac Arrest due to Drowning

Immediate high-quality CPR is the single most important factor influencing survival in drowning. Chest compressions may be difficult to perform while the victim is still in the water, but you can initiate ventilations immediately. Start chest compressions as soon as you can do so safely, and the child is lying faceup on a firm surface.

No modifications of the standard pediatric BLS sequence are necessary for drowning victims other than consideration of cervical spine injury and the possibility of hypothermia as contributing factors. Rescuers should remove drowning victims from the water by the fastest means available and should begin resuscitation as quickly as possible.

Circulation	• Perform high-quality CPR. • Attach a monitor/defibrillator. • If defibrillation is indicated and the chest is covered with water, quickly wipe the child's chest to minimize electrical arcing between the defibrillation pads or paddles.
Airway	• Open the airway.
Breathing	• Ventilate with a bag-mask device using 100% O_2. • Be prepared to suction the airway because drowning victims often vomit swallowed water; decompress the stomach with a NG/OG tube after the advanced airway is inserted.

If there is reason to suspect a cervical spine injury (e.g., diving injury), restrict spinal motion. Evaluate core body temperature and attempt rewarming if the child is severely hypothermic (core temperature <30°C).

In cardiac arrest associated with hypothermia, it is often difficult to know when to terminate resuscitative efforts. In victims of drowning in icy water, survival is possible after submersion times of as long as 40 minutes and prolonged

duration of CPR (>2 hours). When drowning occurs in ice water, rewarming to a core temperature of at least 30°C is recommended before CPR efforts are abandoned. The heart may be unresponsive to resuscitative efforts until this core temperature is achieved.

Extracorporeal circulation is the most rapid and effective technique for rewarming severely hypothermic cardiac arrest victims after submersion in icy water. Although the patient may be rewarmed with passive techniques or body cavity irrigation in the out-of-hospital or community hospital setting, rapid transfer to a facility that is capable of performing pediatric ECMO or cardiopulmonary bypass is preferred.

Cardiac Arrest due to Anaphylaxis

Near-fatal anaphylaxis produces profound vasodilation, which significantly increases intravascular capacity and produces relative hypovolemia. Anaphylaxis is often accompanied by bronchoconstriction, which compromises oxygenation and further impairs tissue O_2 delivery. If cardiac arrest develops, primary therapy is CPR, bolus fluid administration, and epinephrine. Children with anaphylaxis are often young with healthy hearts and cardiovascular systems. They may respond to rapid correction of vasodilation and low intravascular volume. Effective CPR may maintain sufficient O_2 delivery until the catastrophic effects of the anaphylactic reaction resolve.

If cardiac arrest results from anaphylaxis, management may include the following critical therapies:

Circulation	• Perform effective chest compressions (may maintain sufficient O_2 delivery until the catastrophic effects of the anaphylactic reaction resolve). • Administer large volumes of isotonic crystalloid as quickly as possible by using at least 2 IO catheters or 2 large-bore IVs with pressure bags. • Administer epinephrine in standard doses (0.01 mg/kg IO/IV [0.1 mL/kg of 1:10 000]) or via the ET tube if no vascular access can be obtained (0.1 mg/kg [0.1 mL/kg of 1:1000]). • Titrate epinephrine infusion as needed. • Manage according to the Pediatric Cardiac Arrest Algorithm if the arrest rhythm is asystole or PEA (which is often the case).
Airway	• Open and maintain the airway by using manual maneuvers.

(continued)

(continued)

Breathing	• Perform bag-mask ventilation using 100% O_2. • If ET intubation is performed, be prepared for the possibility of airway edema and the need to use a smaller ET tube than predicted by the child's age or length.

There are sparse data about the value of antihistamines in anaphylactic cardiac arrest, but it is reasonable to assume that administration of antihistamines would result in little harm. Steroids given during cardiac arrest have little effect, but they may have potential value in the management of anaphylaxis. Therefore, administer steroids such as methylprednisolone 1 to 2 mg/kg IV/IO as soon as possible in the postresuscitation period.

Cardiac Arrest Associated With Poisoning

Drug overdose or poisoning may cause cardiac arrest as a result of direct cardiac toxicity or the secondary effects of respiratory depression, peripheral vasodilation, arrhythmias, and hypotension. The myocardium of the poisoning victim is often healthy, but temporary cardiac dysfunction may be present until the effects of the drug or toxin have been reversed or metabolized. This will require a variable amount of time, often several hours, depending on the nature of the toxin, drug, or poison. Because the toxicity may be temporary, prolonged resuscitation efforts and use of advanced support techniques such as extracorporeal life support (ECLS) may result in good long-term survival.

Initiate advanced life support measures according to the Pediatric Cardiac Arrest Algorithm. Pediatric advanced life support treatment for victims of a suspected poisoning should include a search for and treatment of reversible causes. Early consultation with a poison control centre or toxicologist is recommended.

Congenital Heart Disease: Single Ventricle

The prevalence of complex cyanotic congenital heart disease in children is low. Nevertheless, the patient with single ventricle (tricuspid/pulmonary atresia, hypoplastic left heart syndrome, and their variants) represents a large proportion of children who suffer cardiac arrest, particularly in the in-hospital setting. An increasing number of infants and children survive after palliative surgical procedures; these children may require resuscitation postoperatively or during readmission for critical illness.

Single-ventricle physiology is complex and varies with the specific lesion and stage of surgical repair. Therefore, it is important to obtain a history from the caretakers to determine the child's baseline hemodynamic status and arterial O_2 saturation. During cardiac arrest, standard resuscitation care is indicated for all infants with single-ventricle anatomy after stage I (Norwood) palliation or those with a univentricular heart and aortopulmonary shunt to provide pulmonary blood flow. In addition to standard resuscitation, specific measures include the following:

• Heparin administration may be considered for children with aortopulmonary or right ventricular-pulmonary artery shunt if shunt patency is a concern.
• After resuscitation, titrate administered O_2 to achieve an O_2 saturation of approximately 80%.
• End-tidal CO_2 (P_{ETCO_2}) may not be a reliable indicator of CPR quality in a single-ventricle patient because pulmonary blood flow in these patients does not always reflect cardiac output (i.e., it is influenced by additional factors).
• Consider permissive hypoventilation strategies or even negative-pressure ventilation in the prearrest state to improve cardiac output.

FYI **ECLS**	If available, ECLS (e.g., ECMO) may be beneficial for infants and children with acute reversible conditions (e.g., cardiac or respiratory failure due to hypothermia or drug toxicity), especially children with primary cardiac conditions (e.g., after cardiac surgery). It is also used for in-hospital cardiac arrest, provided that high-quality CPR is performed until ECMO is available. ECLS is currently available in a limited number of advanced pediatric centres. Several studies have shown that good outcome can be achieved when extracorporeal circulatory support is established after 30 to 90 minutes of refractory in-hospital arrest with high-quality CPR. For more details see the references under "Extracorporeal Life Support (ECLS)/Extracorporeal Cardiopulmonary Resuscitation (ECPR)" in the Suggested Reading List.

- ECLS or ECMO may be considered for patients in cardiac arrest who have undergone stage I palliation (Norwood) or Fontan-type procedures.

Pulmonary Hypertension

In pulmonary hypertension cardiac output may be impaired by increased resistance to blood flow through the lungs. Standard PALS recommendations should be followed during cardiac arrest. Other measures include the following:

- Correct hypercarbia if present.
- A bolus of isotonic saline may be useful to maintain ventricular preload.
- If the patient was receiving pulmonary vasodilators such as nitric oxide or prostacyclin immediately prior to the arrest, be sure that drug administration continues.
- Consider administration of inhaled nitric oxide or prostacyclin (or IV prostacyclin) to reduce pulmonary vascular resistance.
- ECLS (ECMO) may be useful if instituted early during resuscitation.

Social and Ethical Issues in Resuscitation

Special social and ethical issues during resuscitation of a child in cardiac arrest include

- Family presence during resuscitation
- Termination of resuscitative efforts
- "Do not attempt resuscitation" or "allow natural death" orders

Family Presence During Resuscitation

Studies have shown that most family members would like to be present during the attempted resuscitation of a loved one. Parents or family members may be reluctant to ask if they can be present, but healthcare providers should offer the opportunity whenever possible. Family members may experience less anxiety and depression and more constructive grief behaviors if they are present during resuscitative efforts.

Planning for family-witnessed resuscitation includes the following:

- Discuss the plan in advance with the resuscitation team, if possible.
- Assign one team member to remain with the family to answer questions, clarify information, and offer comfort.
- Provide sufficient space to accommodate all family members who are present.
- Be sensitive to family presence during the resuscitative effort; team members must be mindful of the family members' presence while they communicate with each other.

In the out-of-hospital setting, family members are typically present during the attempted resuscitation of a loved one. Although out-of-hospital providers will be focused on the resuscitative effort, it may comfort family members if providers offer brief explanations and the opportunity for family members to remain with the loved one. Some EMS systems provide a follow-up visit to family members after an unsuccessful resuscitation attempt.

Terminating Resuscitative Efforts

There are no reliable predictors of when to stop resuscitative efforts after a pediatric cardiac arrest (see the next major section, "Predictors of Outcome After Cardiac Arrest"). In the past, children who underwent prolonged resuscitation with absence of ROSC after 2 doses of epinephrine were considered unlikely to survive. However, intact survival after prolonged in-hospital resuscitation with >2 doses of epinephrine has been documented.

The decision to cease resuscitative efforts is influenced by the cause of the arrest, available resources and location of the resuscitation attempt, and the likelihood of any reversible or contributing conditions. Witnessed collapse, bystander CPR, and a short interval from collapse to arrival by professionals improve the chance of successful resuscitation. Prolonged resuscitative efforts should be considered for infants and children with

- Recurring or refractory VF/VT
- Drug toxicity (i.e., to provide time for appropriate toxicologic management or support of the cardiovascular system until the drug effect resolves)
- Primary hypothermic insult (i.e., until appropriate warming measures have been undertaken)

"Do Not Attempt Resuscitation" or "Allow Natural Death" Orders

Scope

The scope of a "do not attempt resuscitation" (DNAR) or an "allow natural death" order should be specific about which interventions are to be withheld. A DNAR/"allow natural death" order does not automatically preclude interventions such as administration of parenteral fluids, nutrition, O_2, analgesia, sedation, antiarrhythmics, or vasopressors unless these are included in the order. For example, some patients may choose to accept defibrillation and chest compressions but not intubation and mechanical ventilation.

Although it is appropriate to offer some interventions and not others based on the patient's or surrogate's preference and the specific potential benefits and burdens of the given intervention, it is never appropriate to write orders to perform a "slow code" designed to give the illusion of attempting effective CPR.

Communication to All Healthcare Providers Involved

Decisions to limit resuscitative efforts must be clearly communicated to all healthcare professionals involved in the patient's care. DNAR/"allow natural death" orders should be reviewed before surgery by the anesthesiologist, attending surgeon, and patient or surrogate to determine their applicability in the operating room and immediate postoperative recovery period.

Predictors of Outcome After Cardiac Arrest

Factors That Influence Outcome

The outcome after cardiac arrest in children may be influenced by

- Interval from collapse to initiation of CPR
- Quality of CPR provided
- Duration of resuscitative efforts
- Underlying conditions
- Other factors

Initiation of prompt CPR is associated with improved outcome. Witnessed events, bystander CPR, and a short interval from collapse to arrival of EMS personnel are important prognostic factors associated with improved outcome in adult cardiac arrest. It seems reasonable to extrapolate these factors to children. A short interval from collapse to initiation of CPR was shown to be a significant prognostic factor in a pediatric study. For more details see Kyriacou et al, 1994 (full reference in the Suggested Reading List at the end of this Part). In out-of-hospital patients who have ROSC before arrival in the emergency department, the chances for long-term survival are improved.

In general, the likelihood of a good outcome declines with the duration of the resuscitative efforts. Six pediatric studies showed that prolonged resuscitation is associated with poor outcome in pediatric cardiac arrest. Although a good outcome is more likely when the duration of CPR is short, successful resuscitations have been documented with longer resuscitative efforts. These include resuscitations in the in-hospital setting when the arrests were witnessed and prompt (presumably high-quality) CPR was provided.

Underlying conditions can significantly influence outcome. Some children with PEA may have reversible causes of arrest that respond to treatment. Children with an initial rhythm of VF/pulseless VT generally have a higher survival rate than children with asystole. This higher survival rate may not be observed in drowning victims with VF/pulseless VT, a rhythm associated with extremely poor prognosis. Similarly, the outcome is worse when VF/pulseless VT develops as a secondary rhythm during the resuscitation of children with in-hospital cardiac arrest. Children with out-of-hospital cardiac arrest caused by blunt trauma rarely survive. For full references see the "Prognostic Indicators" section in the Suggested Reading List at the end of this Part.

Other factors, however, can positively influence outcome despite prolonged resuscitative efforts. Examples include the following:

- Good outcomes for in-hospital pediatric resuscitation in patients with isolated heart disease (usually after surgical intervention) were achieved when ECMO was started after 30 to 90 minutes of high-quality CPR. This demonstrates that 15 to 30 minutes of CPR (as previously taught) does not define the limits of cardiac and cerebral viability.

- Good outcome in an in-hospital witnessed arrest has been reported after 30 to 60 minutes of prompt (and presumably high-quality) CPR.

- Excellent outcome despite prolonged resuscitation has been reported in some children with cardiac arrest caused by environmental hypothermia or drowning in icy water.

Postresuscitation Management

Postresuscitation management begins as soon as ROSC develops. See Part 11: "Postresuscitation Management" for more information.

Suggested Reading List

Cobb LA, Fahrenbruch CE, Walsh TR, Copass MK, Olsufka M, Breskin M, Hallstrom AP. Influence of cardiopulmonary resuscitation prior to defibrillation in patients with out-of-hospital ventricular fibrillation. *JAMA.* 1999;281:1182-1188.

Dykes EH, Spence LJ, Young JG, Bohn DJ, Filler RM, Wesson DE. Preventable pediatric trauma deaths in a metropolitan region. *J Pediatr Surg.* 1989;24:107-110.

Gausche M, Lewis RJ, Stratton SJ, Haynes BE, Gunter CS, Goodrich SM, Poore PD, McCollough MD, Henderson DP, Pratt FD, Seidel JS. Effect of out-of-hospital pediatric endotracheal intubation on survival and neurological outcome: a controlled clinical trial [published correction appears in *JAMA.* 2000;283:3204]. *JAMA.* 2000;283:783-790.

Kyriacou DN, Arcinue EL, Peek C, Kraus JF. Effect of immediate resuscitation on children with submersion injury. *Pediatrics.* 1994;94(pt 1):137-142.

Meert KL, Donaldson A, Nadkarni V, Tieves KS, Schleien CL, Brilli RJ, Clark RS, Shaffner DH, Levy F, Statler K,

Dalton HJ, van der Jagt EW, Hackbarth R, Pretzlaff R, Hernan L, Dean JM, Moler FW. Multicenter cohort study of in-hospital pediatric cardiac arrest. *Pediatr Crit Care Med*. 2009;10:544-553.

Ong ME, Osmond MH, Gerein R, Nesbitt L, Tran ML, Stiell I; OPALS study group. Comparing pre-hospital clinical diagnosis of pediatric out-of-hospital cardiac arrest with etiology by coroner's diagnosis. *Resuscitation*. 2007;72:26-34.

Sasser SM, Hunt RC, Sullivent EE, Wald MM, Mitchko J, Jurkovich GJ, Henry MC, Salomone JP, Wang SC, Galli RL, Cooper A, Brown LH, Sattin RW; National Expert Panel on Field Triage, Centers for Disease Control and Prevention (CDC). Guidelines for field triage of injured patients: recommendations of the National Expert Panel on Field Triage [published correction appears in *MMWR Recomm Rep*. 2009;58:172]. *MMWR Recomm Rep*. 2009;58:1-35.

Smith BT, Rea TD, Eisenberg MS. Ventricular fibrillation in pediatric cardiac arrest. *Acad Emerg Med*. 2006;13:525-529.

Wik L, Hansen TB, Fylling F, Steen T, Vaagenes P, Auestad BH, Steen PA. Delaying defibrillation to give basic cardiopulmonary resuscitation to patients with out-of-hospital ventricular fibrillation: a randomized trial. *JAMA*. 2003;289:1389-1395.

Epidemiology and Outcome

American Heart Association. Get With The Guidelines–Resuscitation (formerly the National Registry of Cardio-pulmonary Resuscitation). www.heart.org/resuscitation. Accessed February 11, 2011.

Atkins DL, Everson-Stewart S, Sears GK, Daya M, Osmond MH, Warden CR, Berg RA. Epidemiology and outcomes from out-of-hospital cardiac arrest in children: the Resuscitation Outcomes Consortium Epistry-Cardiac Arrest. *Circulation*. 2009;119:1484-1491.

Berg MD, Schexnayder SM, Chameides L, Terry M, Donoghue A, Hickey RW, Berg RA, Sutton RM, Hazinski MF; American Heart Association. Part 13: pediatric basic life support: 2010 American Heart Association Guidelines for Cardiopulmonary Resuscitation and Emergency Cardiovascular Care. *Circulation*. 2010;122:S876-S908.

de Mos N, van Litsenburg RR, McCrindle B, Bohn DJ, Parshuram CS. Pediatric in-intensive-care-unit cardiac arrest: incidence, survival, and predictive factors. *Crit Care Med*. 2006;34:1209-1215.

Donoghue AJ, Nadkarni V, Berg RA, Osmond MH, Wells G, Nesbitt L, Stiell IG. Out-of-hospital pediatric cardiac arrest: an epidemiologic review and assessment of current knowledge. *Ann Emerg Med*. 2005;46:512-522.

Gerein RB, Osmond MH, Stiell IG, Nesbitt LP, Burns S. What are the etiology and epidemiology of out-of-hospital pediatric cardiopulmonary arrest in Ontario, Canada? *Acad Emerg Med*. 2006;13:653-658.

Jacobs I, Nadkarni V, Bahr J, Berg RA, Billi JE, Bossaert L, Cassan P, Coovadia A, D'Este K, Finn J, Halperin H, Handley A, Herlitz J, Hickey R, Idris A, Kloeck W, Larkin GL, Mancini ME, Mason P, Mears G, Monsieurs K, Montgomery W, Morley P, Nichol G, Nolan J, Okada K, Perlman J, Shuster M, Steen PA, Sterz F, Tibballs J, Timerman S, Truitt T, Zideman D; International Liaison Committee on Resuscitation. Cardiac arrest and cardiopulmonary resuscitation outcome reports: update and simplification of the Utstein templates for resuscitation registries. A statement for healthcare professionals from a task force of the International Liaison Committee on Resuscitation (American Heart Association, European Resuscitation Council, Australian Resuscitation Council, New Zealand Resuscitation Council, Heart and Stroke Foundation of Canada, InterAmerican Heart Foundation, Resuscitation Council of Southern Africa). *Resuscitation*. 2004;63:233-249.

Meaney PA, Nadkarni VM, Cook EF, Testa M, Helfaer M, Kaye W, Larkin GL, Berg RA. Higher survival rates among younger patients after pediatric intensive care unit cardiac arrests. *Pediatrics*. 2006;118:2424-2433.

Nadkarni VM, Larkin GL, Peberdy MA, Carey SM, Kaye W, Mancini ME, Nichol G, Lane-Truitt T, Potts J, Ornato JP, Berg RA. First documented rhythm and clinical outcome from in-hospital cardiac arrest among children and adults. *JAMA*. 2006;295:50-57.

Reis AG, Nadkarni V, Perondi MB, Grisi S, Berg RA. A prospective investigation into the epidemiology of in-hospital pediatric cardiopulmonary resuscitation using the international Utstein reporting style. *Pediatrics*. 2002;109:200-209.

Rodríguez-Núñez A, López-Herce J, García C, Carrillo A, Domínguez P, Calvo C, Delgado MA; Spanish Study Group for Cardiopulmonary Arrest in Children. Effectiveness and long-term outcome of cardiopulmonary resuscitation in paediatric intensive care units in Spain. *Resuscitation*. 2006;71:301-309.

Samson RA, Nadkarni VM, Meaney PA, Carey SM, Berg MD, Berg RA. Outcomes of in-hospital ventricular fibrillation in children. *N Engl J Med*. 2006;354:2328-2339.

Srinivasan V, Nadkarni VM, Helfaer MA, Carey SM, Berg RA. Childhood obesity and survival after in-hospital pediatric cardiopulmonary resuscitation. *Pediatrics*. 2010;125:e481-e488.

Tibballs J, Kinney S. A prospective study of outcome of in-patient paediatric cardiopulmonary arrest. *Resuscitation*. 2006;71:310-318.

Young KD, Gausche-Hill M, McClung CD, Lewis RJ. A prospective, population-based study of the epidemiology and outcome of out-of-hospital pediatric cardiopulmonary arrest. *Pediatrics*. 2004;114:157-164.

Defibrillation

Berg MD, Banville IL, Chapman FW, Walker RG, Gaballa MA, Hilwig RW, Samson RA, Kern KB, Berg RA. Attenuating the defibrillation dosage decreases postresuscitation myocardial dysfunction in a swine model of pediatric ventricular fibrillation. *Pediatr Crit Care Med*. 2008;9:429-434.

Berg MD, Samson RA, Meyer RJ, Clark LL, Valenzuela TD, Berg RA. Pediatric defibrillation doses often fail to terminate prolonged out-of-hospital ventricular fibrillation in children. *Resuscitation*. 2005;67:63-67.

Meaney PA, Nadkarni VM, Atkins DL, Berg MD, Samson RA, Hazinski MF, Berg RA; American Heart Association National Registry of Cardiopulmonary Resuscitation Investigators. Effect of defibrillation energy dose during in-hospital pediatric cardiac arrest. *Pediatrics*. 2011;127:e16-e23.

Rodríguez-Núñez A, López-Herce J, García C, Domínguez P, Carrillo A, Bellón JM; Spanish Study Group of Cardiopulmonary Arrest in Children. Pediatric defibrillation after cardiac arrest: initial response and outcome. *Crit Care*. 2006;10:R113.

Medications

Duncan JM, Meaney P, Simpson P, Berg RA, Nadkarni V, Schexnayder S; National Registry of CPR Investigators. Vasopressin for in-hospital pediatric arrest: results from the American Heart Association National Registry of Cardiopulmonary Resuscitation. *Pediatr Crit Care Med*. 2009;10:191-195.

Patterson MD, Boenning DA, Klein BL, Fuchs S, Smith KM, Hegenbarth MA, Carlson DW, Krug SE, Harris EM. The use of high-dose epinephrine for patients with out-of-hospital cardiopulmonary arrest refractory to prehospital interventions. *Pediatr Emerg Care*. 2005;21:227-237.

Perondi MB, Reis AG, Paiva EF, Nadkarni VM, Berg RA. A comparison of high-dose and standard-dose epinephrine in children with cardiac arrest. *N Engl J Med*. 2004;350:1722-1730.

Srinivasan V, Morris MC, Helfaer MA, Berg RA, Nadkarni VM. Calcium use during in-hospital pediatric cardiopulmonary resuscitation: a report from the National Registry of Cardiopulmonary Resuscitation. *Pediatrics*. 2008;121:e1144-e1151.

Sudden Cardiac Death

Johnson JN, Tester DJ, Bass NE, Ackerman MJ. Cardiac channel molecular autopsy for sudden unexpected death in epilepsy. *J Child Neurol*. 2010;25:916-921.

Sudden death in the young. Proceedings of the Pediatric and Congenital Electrophysiology Society (PACES) satellite symposium of the Heart Rhythm Society (HRS) meeting in Denver in May 2007. *Pacing Clin Electrophysiol*. 2009;32(suppl 2):S1-S89.

CPR Quality

Abella BS, Alvarado JP, Myklebust H, Edelson DP, Barry A, O'Hearn N, Vanden Hoek TL, Becker LB. Quality of cardiopulmonary resuscitation during in-hospital cardiac arrest. *JAMA*. 2005;293:305-310.

Edelson DP, Abella BS, Kramer-Johansen J, Wik L, Myklebust H, Barry AM, Merchant RM, Hoek TL, Steen PA, Becker LB. Effects of compression depth and pre-shock pauses predict defibrillation failure during cardiac arrest. *Resuscitation*. 2006;71:137-145.

Kitamura T, Iwami T, Kawamura T, Nagao K, Tanaka H, Nadkarni VM, Berg RA, Hiraide A. Conventional and chest-compression-only cardiopulmonary resuscitation by bystanders for children who have out-of-hospital cardiac arrests: a prospective, nationwide, population-based cohort study. *Lancet*. 2010;375:1347-1354.

Maher KO, Berg RA, Lindsey CW, Simsic J, Mahle WT. Depth of sternal compression and intra-arterial blood pressure during CPR in infants following cardiac surgery. *Resuscitation*. 2009;80:662-664.

Morris MC, Nadkarni VM. Pediatric cardiopulmonary-cerebral resuscitation: an overview and future directions. *Crit Care Clin*. 2003;19:337-364.

Sutton RM, Niles D, Nysaether J, Abella BS, Arbogast KB, Nishisaki A, Maltese MR, Donoghue A, Bishnoi R, Helfaer MA, Myklebust H, Nadkarni V. Quantitative analysis of CPR quality during in-hospital resuscitation of older children and adolescents. *Pediatrics*. 2009;124:494-499.

Wik L, Kramer-Johansen J, Myklebust H, Sørebø H, Svensson L, Fellows B, Steen PA. Quality of cardiopulmonary resuscitation during out-of-hospital cardiac arrest. *JAMA*. 2005;293:299-304.

Extracorporeal Life Support (ECLS)/ Extracorporeal Cardiopulmonary Resuscitation (ECPR)

Alsoufi B, Al-Radi OO, Nazer RI, Gruenwald C, Foreman C, Williams WG, Coles JG, Caldarone CA, Bohn DG, Van Arsdell GS. Survival outcomes after rescue extracorporeal cardiopulmonary resuscitation in pediatric patients with refractory cardiac arrest. *J Thorac Cardiovasc Surg*. 2007;134:952-959.e2.

del Nido PJ. Extracorporeal membrane oxygenation for cardiac support in children. *Ann Thorac Surg*. 1996;61:336-339.

Fiser RT, Morris MC. Extracorporeal cardiopulmonary resuscitation in refractory pediatric cardiac arrest. *Pediatr Clin North Am*. 2008;55:929-941.

Lequier L, Joffe AR, Robertson CM, Dinu IA, Wongswadiwat Y, Anton NR, Ross DB, Rebeyka IM; Western Canadian Complex Pediatric Therapies Program Follow-up Group. Two-year survival, mental, and motor outcomes after cardiac extracorporeal life support at less than five years of age. *J Thorac Cardiovasc Surg*. 2008;136:976-983.e3.

Morris MC, Wernovsky G, Nadkarni VM. Survival outcomes after extracorporeal cardiopulmonary resuscitation instituted during active chest compressions following refractory in-hospital pediatric cardiac arrest. *Pediatr Crit Care Med*. 2004;5:440-446.

Prodhan P, Fiser RT, Dyamenahalli U, Gossett J, Imamura M, Jaquiss RD, Bhutta AT. Outcomes after extracorporeal cardiopulmonary resuscitation (ECPR) following refractory pediatric cardiac arrest in the intensive care unit. *Resuscitation*. 2009;80:1124-1129.

Raymond TT, Cunnyngham CB, Thompson MT, Thomas JA, Dalton HJ, Nadkarni VM; American Heart Association National Registry of CPR Investigators. Outcomes among neonates, infants, and children after extracorporeal cardiopulmonary resuscitation for refractory inhospital pediatric cardiac arrest: a report from the National Registry of Cardiopulmonary Resuscitation. *Pediatr Crit Care Med*. 2010;11:362-371.

ETCO$_2$

Aufderheide TP, Sigurdsson G, Pirrallo RG, Yannopoulos D, McKnite S, von Briesen C, Sparks CW, Conrad CJ, Provo TA, Lurie KG. Hyperventilation-induced hypotension during cardiopulmonary resuscitation. *Circulation*. 2004;109:1960-1965.

Falk JL, Rackow EC, Weil MH. End-tidal carbon dioxide concentration during cardiopulmonary resuscitation. *N Engl J Med*. 1988;318:607-611.

Ornato JP, Garnett AR, Glauser FL. Relationship between cardiac output and the end-tidal carbon dioxide tension. *Ann Emerg Med*. 1990;19:1104-1106.

Prognostic Indicators

Hazinski MF, Chahine AA, Holcomb GW III, Morris JA Jr. Outcome of cardiovascular collapse in pediatric blunt trauma. *Ann Emerg Med*. 1994;23:1229-1235.

Nadkarni VM, Larkin GL, Peberdy MA, Carey SM, Kaye W, Mancini ME, Nichol G, Lane-Truitt T, Potts J, Ornato JP, Berg RA. First documented rhythm and clinical outcome from in-hospital cardiac arrest among children and adults. *JAMA*. 2006;295:50-57.

Samson RA, Nadkarni VM, Meaney PA, Carey SM, Berg MD, Berg RA. Outcomes of in-hospital ventricular fibrillation in children. *N Engl J Med*. 2006;354:2328-2339.

SIDS

American Academy of Pediatrics Task Force on Sudden Infant Death Syndrome. The changing concept of sudden infant death syndrome: diagnostic coding shifts, controversies regarding the sleeping environment, and new variables to consider in reducing risk. *Pediatrics*. 2005;116:1245-1255.

Part 11

Postresuscitation Management

Overview

As soon as return of spontaneous circulation (ROSC) develops after cardiac arrest or resuscitation from severe shock or respiratory failure, a systematic approach to assessment and support of the respiratory, cardiovascular, and neurologic systems is critical. In addition, the PALS provider should evaluate and support other body systems (e.g., renal, gastrointestinal) as needed. Although effective resuscitation is a major focus of the PALS Provider Course, ultimate outcome is often determined by the subsequent care the child receives. This includes safe transport to a centre with expertise in caring for seriously ill or injured children.

One objective of optimal postresuscitation management is to avoid common causes of both early and late morbidity and mortality. Early mortality can be caused by hemodynamic instability and respiratory complications. Late morbidity and mortality can result from multiorgan failure or brain injury or both.

For optimal postresuscitation management, identify and treat organ system dysfunction. This includes

- Providing adequate oxygenation and ventilation
- Supporting tissue perfusion and cardiovascular function
- Correcting acid-base and electrolyte imbalances
- Maintaining adequate glucose concentration
- Ensuring adequate analgesia and sedation
- Considering use of therapeutic hypothermia after ROSC following cardiac arrest

The extent of postresuscitation evaluation and management is influenced by the PALS provider's scope of practice and available resources.

Learning Objectives

After completing this Part you should be able to

- List priorities for postresuscitation multisystem evaluation and management
- Differentiate between immediate and subsequent postresuscitation management
- Discuss the importance of effective communication among transferring facilities, among healthcare providers, and with family members
- Summarize how to prepare a child for transfer/transport by using a transport checklist

Preparation for the Course

During the course you will learn about the phases of postresuscitation management. This will include stabilizing cardiopulmonary function, medical management by system, ongoing management of shock, and transport, whether the transport is between hospitals or within a hospital.

Postresuscitation Management

Postresuscitation management consists of 2 general phases to stabilize the child.

The first phase is immediate postresuscitation management. During this phase you will continue to provide advanced life support for immediate life-threatening conditions and focus on the ABCs.

- **Airway and Breathing.** Assess and support oxygenation and ventilation. At this time you will typically use diagnostic tests, such as arterial blood gas analysis and chest x-ray, to further establish the adequacy of oxygenation and ventilation and to confirm endotracheal tube position in the mid trachea.

- **Circulation.** Assess and maintain adequate blood pressure and perfusion. Treat arrhythmias. Diagnostic tests, such as lactate concentration, venous O_2 saturation, and base deficit, provide information on adequacy of tissue perfusion. As you proceed with evaluation, identify and treat any reversible or contributing causes of the arrest or critical illness.

In the second phase of postresuscitation management, provide broader multiorgan supportive care. After the child is stabilized, coordinate transfer or transport to a tertiary care setting as appropriate.

Primary Goals

The primary goals of postresuscitation management are to

- Optimize and stabilize cardiopulmonary function with emphasis on restoring and maintaining vital organ perfusion and function (especially of the brain)
- Prevent secondary organ injury
- Identify and treat the cause of acute illness

- Minimize the risk of deterioration of the child during transport to the next level of care
- Institute measures that may improve long-term, neurologically intact survival

Systematic Approach

Assess the child by using the PALS systematic approach (see Part 2: "Systematic Approach to the Seriously Ill or Injured Child"). In addition to repeated *primary assessments,* your evaluation will often include the secondary assessment as well as diagnostic tests. The *secondary assessment* is a review of patient history and a focused physical examination. *Diagnostic tests* include invasive and noninvasive monitoring and appropriate laboratory and nonlaboratory tests.

This Part discusses evaluation and management of the following systems during the postresuscitation period:

- Respiratory system
- Cardiovascular system
- Neurologic system
- Renal system
- Gastrointestinal system
- Hematologic system

Respiratory System

Management Priorities

Continue to monitor and support the child's airway, oxygenation, and ventilation. Look for clinical signs and objective measurements of adequate oxygenation and ventilation. (See Part 4: "Recognition of Respiratory Distress and Failure" for more information on assessment of the respiratory system.) During resuscitation high-flow O_2, inhaled medications, and ET intubation may be required. In the postresuscitation phase, elective intubation may be appropriate to achieve airway control and support the child during diagnostic studies, such as a CT scan. If the child is being manually ventilated, consider transition to mechanical ventilation.

The goals of respiratory management in the immediate postresuscitation period are as follows:

Goal	Considerations
Maintain adequate oxygenation (generally an O_2 saturation ≥94% but <100%) to reduce the risk of reperfusion injury after cardiac arrest	Once ROSC is achieved, titrate O_2 administration to maintain an O_2 saturation ≥94% but avoid hyperoxia. (An O_2 saturation of 100% can correspond to a Po_2 of approximately 80 to 500 mm Hg.)
	Determining optimal Pao_2 and O_2 saturation requires understanding that O_2 content is an important determinant of tissue O_2 delivery. If the child is anemic, tissue O_2 delivery may be better maintained by achieving a high Pao_2 and O_2 saturation. In comparison, an O_2 saturation ≥94% is typically adequate in a child with a normal hemoglobin concentration and normal O_2 consumption.
Maintain adequate ventilation and acceptable $Paco_2$ levels	The acceptable $Paco_2$ depends on the clinical circumstance. For example, for most patients with neurologic injury, a normal $Paco_2$ is desirable to avoid hypocarbia or hypercarbia. However, in children with asthma and respiratory failure, rapid correction of hypercarbia is not appropriate. Efforts to achieve normocarbia with mechanical ventilation in the child with asthma could result in complications such as pneumothorax.

General Recommendations

General recommendations for assessment and management of the respiratory system may include the following:

Assessment and Management of the Respiratory System	
Assessment	

Monitoring	• Continuously monitor the following parameters (at a minimum):
	  – SpO_2 and heart rate by pulse oximetry (compare pulse oximetry heart rate with ECG and pulse rate to ensure that pulse oximeter readings are accurate)
	  – Heart rate and rhythm
	  – If the patient is intubated, monitor end-tidal CO_2 by capnography if equipment and expertise are available, or intermittently confirm exhaled CO_2 by colourimetric device. Always monitor exhaled CO_2 by either capnography or colourimetric device during intrahospital and interhospital transport to aid in immediate detection of inadvertent extubation.
	• If the child is already intubated, verify tube position, patency, and security.
	• After proper tube position is confirmed, ensure that the tube is well taped and that tube position at the lip or gum is documented.
	
	Providers must use both clinical assessment and confirmatory devices (such as monitoring of exhaled CO_2) to verify proper tube placement immediately after intubation, during transport, and when the child is moved (e.g., from gurney to bed).

Physical examination	• Observe chest rise and auscultate for abnormal or asymmetric breath sounds. • Monitor for evidence of respiratory compromise (e.g., tachypnea, increased work of breathing, agitation, decreased responsiveness, poor air exchange, cyanosis) or inadequate respiratory effort.
Laboratory tests	• Obtain an arterial sample for ABG analysis if possible in children after ROSC or treatment for respiratory failure or severe shock. If the child is mechanically ventilated, obtain the ABG 10 to 15 minutes after establishing initial ventilatory settings; ideally, correlate blood gases with capnographic end-tidal CO_2 concentration to enable noninvasive monitoring of ventilation.
Other tests	• Obtain a chest x-ray to verify correct position of the ET tube (i.e., position in the mid trachea) and to identify pulmonary conditions that may require specific treatment (e.g., pneumothorax, aspiration).
Management	
Oxygenation	• If the child is not intubated, provide supplementary O_2 with a partial or a nonrebreathing mask until you confirm adequate SpO_2. • After ROSC following cardiac arrest, adjust inspired O_2 concentration to achieve an SpO_2 ≥94% but <100% (i.e., 94% to 99%). • If the child has an SpO_2 of <90% while receiving 100% inspired O_2, consider noninvasive ventilatory support or endotracheal intubation with mechanical ventilation and PEEP. • If the child has a cyanotic cardiac lesion, adjust the O_2 saturation goal to the child's baseline SpO_2 and clinical status.
Ventilation	• Assist ventilation as needed, targeting a normal $PaCO_2$ (i.e., 35 to 45 mm Hg) if the child's lung function was previously normal. Remember that normalization of $PaCO_2$ may not be appropriate in all situations. Avoid routine hyperventilation in children with neurologic problems unless there are signs of impending cerebral herniation.

(continued)

(continued)

Respiratory failure	• Intubate the trachea if O_2 administration and other interventions do not achieve adequate oxygenation and ventilation or to maintain a patent airway in the child with decreased level of consciousness. In some patients, CPAP or noninvasive ventilation may be adequate. • Use appropriate ventilator settings (Table 1). • Verify ET tube position, patency, and security; retape if needed before transport. • Assess for a large glottic air leak. Consider reintubation with a cuffed tube or a larger uncuffed tube if the glottic air leak prevents adequate chest rise, oxygenation, or ventilation. Weigh the risk of removing an advanced airway against the benefit of improved tidal volume, oxygenation, and ventilation. • If a cuffed ET tube is in place and is inflated, check the cuff pressure (goal for most tubes is <20 to 25 cm H_2O; follow manufacturer's recommendations) or assess for the presence of a minimal glottic air leak at an inflation pressure of <20 to 25 cm H_2O. • Insert a gastric tube to relieve and help prevent gastric inflation. *Use the "DOPE" mnemonic to troubleshoot acute deterioration in a mechanically ventilated patient. (See the Critical Concept box "Sudden Deterioration in an Intubated Patient" later in this Part.)*
Analgesia and sedation	• Control pain with analgesics (e.g., fentanyl or morphine) and anxiety with sedatives (e.g., lorazepam or midazolam). • Administer sedation and analgesia to all responsive intubated patients. *Use lower doses of sedatives or analgesics if the child is hemodynamically unstable; titrate the dose while stabilizing hemodynamic function. Morphine is more likely than fentanyl to cause hypotension when used in equipotent doses because morphine causes histamine release.*
Neuromuscular blockade	• For the intubated patient with poor oxygenation and ventilation despite adequate sedation and analgesia, assess for acute causes of deterioration by using the DOPE mnemonic. Then consider neuromuscular blocking agents (e.g., vecuronium, pancuronium with sedation). Indications for use of neuromuscular blocking agents include – High peak or mean airway pressure caused by high airway resistance or reduced lung compliance – Patient ventilator asynchrony – Difficult airway *Neuromuscular blockade may reduce the risk of ET tube displacement. Be aware that neuromuscular blockers do not provide sedation or analgesia and will mask seizures. Neuromuscular blockers will also eliminate many signs of agitation that may signal inadequate oxygenation and ventilation. When using neuromuscular blockers, always ensure that the child is adequately sedated by evaluating for signs of stress, such as tachycardia, hypertension, pupil dilation, or tearing.*

Table 1. Initial Ventilator Settings*

O₂	100%, titrate to maintain O₂ saturation ≥94% and <100% (i.e., 94% to 99%)
Tidal volume† (volume ventilation)	6 to 8 mL/kg
Inspiratory time†‡	0.5 to 1 second
Peak inspiratory pressure†‡ (pressure-limited ventilation)	20 to 30 cm H₂O (lowest level that results in adequate chest expansion)
Respiratory rate	Infants: 20 to 30 breaths/min Children: 16 to 20 breaths/min Adolescents: 8 to 12 breaths/min
PEEP	3 to 5 cm H₂O (higher levels may be required in the setting of lung disease to optimize oxygenation)

Abbreviation: PEEP, positive end-expiratory pressure.

*These settings should be adjusted based on clinical assessment, noninvasive monitoring (pulse oximetry and capnography), and arterial blood gas analysis.

†For volume ventilators.

‡For time-cycled, pressure-limited ventilators.

Critical Concept

Sudden Deterioration in an Intubated Patient (DOPE Mnemonic)

Sudden deterioration in an intubated patient may be caused by one of several complications. Use the mnemonic **DOPE** to help remember these:

Displacement of the tube	The tube may be displaced out of the trachea or advanced into the right or left main bronchus.
Obstruction of the tube	Obstruction may be caused by • Secretions, blood, pus, or a foreign body • Kinking of the tube
Pneumothorax	• Simple pneumothorax usually results in a sudden deterioration in oxygenation (reflected by a sudden decrease in SpO₂) and decreased chest expansion and breath sounds on the involved side. • Tension pneumothorax may result in the above plus evidence of hypotension and a decrease in cardiac output. The trachea is usually shifted away from the involved side.
Equipment failure	Equipment may fail for a number of reasons, such as • Disconnection of the O₂ supply from the ventilation system • Leak in the ventilator circuit • Failure of power supply to the ventilator • Malfunction of valves in the bag or circuit

(continued)

(continued)

Evaluating the Patient's Status

If the condition of an intubated patient deteriorates, the first priority is to support oxygenation and ventilation. While attempting this support, rapidly assess the child and attempt to determine and correct the cause of deterioration. If the child is being mechanically ventilated, hand ventilate with a bag while you assess the patient's airway, ventilation, and oxygenation as follows:

- Observe for chest rise and symmetry of chest movement.
- Auscultate over both sides of the anterior chest and at the midaxillary line and over the stomach. Listen carefully over the lateral lung fields for asymmetry in breath sounds or abnormal sounds such as wheezing.
- Check monitors (e.g., pulse oximetry and, if available, capnography).
- Check heart rate.
- Suction the ET tube if you suspect obstruction with secretions.
- Use sedatives or analgesics, with or without neuromuscular blockers, if needed to reduce the child's agitation and control ventilation. Administer these agents only *after* you rule out a correctable cause of the acute distress and are sure that you can provide positive-pressure ventilation.

Your initial assessment will determine the urgency of the required response. If you cannot verify that the ET tube is in the airway, direct visualization of the tube passing through the glottis is advised. If the child's condition is deteriorating and you strongly suspect that the tube is no longer in the trachea, you may need to remove it and ventilate with a bag and mask.

Patient Agitation

Once the ET tube position and patency are confirmed and failure of ventilation equipment and pneumothorax are ruled out, evaluate oxygenation and perfusion. If oxygenation and perfusion are adequate or unchanged, it is possible that agitation, pain, or excessive movement is interfering with adequate ventilation.

If so, try one or more of the following:

- Analgesia (e.g., fentanyl or morphine) to control pain
- Sedation (e.g., lorazepam, midazolam) for anxiety or agitation
- Neuromuscular blocking agents and analgesia or sedation to optimize ventilation and minimize the risk of barotrauma and unintentional tube displacement

Continuous capnography is helpful during mechanical ventilation as an adjunct to clinical assessment. A sudden decrease in exhaled CO_2 can indicate ET tube displacement, while a gradual decrease in exhaled CO_2 may indicate development of ET tube obstruction or decreasing cardiac output. In addition, capnography may help to detect hypoventilation or hyperventilation, and so is particularly useful during transport and diagnostic procedures. A colourimetric detector or capnography should be used during intrahospital and interhospital transport.

Cardiovascular System

Management Priorities

Ischemia resulting from cardiac arrest and subsequent reperfusion can cause circulatory dysfunction that can last for hours after ROSC. Compromised tissue perfusion and oxygenation during shock and respiratory failure can have secondary adverse effects on cardiovascular function. The goals of circulatory management are to maintain adequate blood pressure and cardiac output to restore or maintain tissue oxygenation and delivery of metabolic substrates. Management priorities are to

- Restore and maintain intravascular volume (preload)
- Treat myocardial dysfunction
- Control arrhythmias
- Maintain normal blood pressure and adequate systemic perfusion

- Maintain adequate SpO_2 and PaO_2
- Maintain adequate hemoglobin concentration
- Consider therapies to reduce metabolic demand (e.g., support ventilation and reduce temperature)

This section includes

- General recommendations for advanced evaluation and management of the cardiovascular system
- The PALS Management of Shock After ROSC Algorithm
- Information about administration of maintenance fluids

Review Part 6: "Recognition of Shock" and Part 7: "Management of Shock" for more information about the pathophysiology of shock and the use of medications to maintain cardiac output and tissue perfusion.

General Recommendations

General recommendations for assessment and management of the cardiovascular system may include the following:

Assessment and Management of the Cardiovascular System	
Assessment	

Monitoring	• Monitor the following frequently or continuously:
	  – Heart rate and rhythm by cardiac monitor
	  – Blood pressure and pulse pressure (noninvasively or invasively)
	  – SpO_2 by pulse oximetry
	  – Urine output by urinary catheter
	• In the critical care setting also consider monitoring
	  – Central venous pressure by central venous line
	  – O_2 saturation by central venous cather ($ScvO_2$)
	  – Cardiac function (e.g., echocardiogram) or cardiac output by noninvasive monitoring or pulmonary artery catheter
	
	Noninvasive blood pressure monitoring (i.e., by automated blood pressure devices) is often unreliable in children with poor perfusion or frequent arrhythmias. Blood pressure monitoring with an indwelling arterial line is more reliable in these children, provided the catheter is patent and the transducer is appropriately zeroed and leveled.

Physical examination	• Repeat the physical examination (e.g., evaluate quality of central and peripheral pulses, heart rate, capillary refill, blood pressure, extremity temperature and colour) frequently until the child is stable. • Monitor end-organ function (e.g., neurologic function, renal function, skin perfusion) to detect evidence of worsening circulatory function.

(continued)

(continued)

Laboratory tests	• Arterial or venous blood gas • Hemoglobin and hematocrit • Serum glucose, electrolytes, blood urea nitrogen (BUN), creatinine, calcium • Consider monitoring lactate and central venous O_2 saturation. In addition to pH, note the magnitude of any metabolic acidosis (base deficit). A persistent metabolic (lactic) acidosis suggests inadequate cardiac output and O_2 delivery. Serum electrolytes can help identify an anion gap acidosis. If the child has an elevated anion gap but normal lactate, consider other causes of acidosis, such as toxins or uremia. The difference in O_2 saturation between the arterial and central venous circulations [S(a-v)O_2] provides information about the adequacy of tissue O_2 delivery. Assuming that O_2 consumption remains constant, a high S(a-v)O_2 difference (>35 to 40) suggests low cardiac output with increased O_2 extraction in the tissues (i.e., blood flow and O_2 delivery are decreased, so O_2 extraction must increase). Troponin levels are frequently elevated after cardiac arrest, especially if defibrillation was performed.
Nonlaboratory tests	• Perform a chest x-ray to evaluate ET tube position and heart size and to identify pulmonary edema or other pathology. • Evaluate 12-lead ECG for arrhythmias or evidence of myocardial ischemia. • Consider echocardiography if there is concern about pericardial tamponade or myocardial dysfunction. *Radiographic evaluation of heart size may aid in initial and subsequent assessment of intravascular volume. In the absence of heart disease, a small heart is consistent with hypovolemia. In the absence of a pericardial effusion, a large heart is consistent with volume overload or heart failure.*

Management	
Intravascular volume	• Establish secure vascular access (if possible, 2 catheters, either IV or IO). • Administer fluid boluses (10 to 20 mL/kg of isotonic crystalloid over 5 to 20 minutes) as needed to restore intravascular volume. Smaller boluses of fluid (5 to 10 mL/kg) administered over 10 to 20 minutes may be appropriate in the setting of heart failure. Adjust the fluid administration rate to replace fluid deficits and meet ongoing requirements. Avoid excessive fluid administration in the presence of myocardial dysfunction or respiratory failure. • Consider the need for colloid or blood administration. • Calculate maintenance fluid requirements and administer as appropriate. **Do not use boluses of hypotonic or dextrose-containing fluids for volume resuscitation.** *See "Administration of Maintenance Fluids" later in this Part.*
Blood pressure	• **Treat hypotension aggressively,** titrating volume and vasoactive medications as appropriate. • If hypotension is due to excessive vasodilation (e.g., sepsis), early use of a vasopressor may be indicated. • The use of adrenergic agents during resuscitation may produce elevation in systemic vascular resistance and hypertension. Because the half-life of these agents is relatively short, assess for other causes of hypertension in the postresuscitation phase (e.g., pain, anxiety, seizures). *Treatment of hypotension is crucial to avoid secondary multisystem injury. See the PALS Management of Shock After ROSC Algorithm for more information about management of hypotensive and normotensive shock.*
Tissue oxygenation	• Provide supplementary O_2 in a high concentration to ensure adequate oxygenation. • After ROSC following cardiac arrest, titrate O_2 to maintain SpO_2 94% to 99%. • Support adequate perfusion. • Consider transfusion with packed red blood cells (PRBCs) for patients with low hematocrit and signs of inadequate O_2 delivery.

(continued)

(continued)

Metabolic demand	• Consider ET intubation and assisted ventilation to reduce the work of breathing. • Control pain with analgesia (e.g., morphine, fentanyl). • Control agitation with sedation (e.g., lorazepam, midazolam); rule out hypoxemia, hypercarbia, or poor perfusion as potential causes of agitation. • Control fever with antipyretics. *Caution: Sedatives or analgesics may cause hypotension. Consider expert consultation before elective endotracheal intubation. The use of sedatives or analgesics and initiation of positive-pressure ventilation can precipitate cardiovascular collapse in a child with poor myocardial function.*
Arrhythmias	• Control tachyarrhythmias and bradyarrhythmias with drugs or electrical therapy. • Seek expert consultation for arrhythmia management. *See Part 8: "Recognition and Management of Bradycardia" and Part 9: "Recognition and Management of Tachycardia" for more information.*
Postarrest myocardial dysfunction	• Anticipate postarrest myocardial dysfunction in the first 24 hours after ROSC. • Consider vasoactive agents to improve contractility and/or decrease afterload if blood pressure is adequate. • Correct metabolic abnormalities that can contribute to poor myocardial function (e.g., acidosis, hypocalcemia, hypoglycemia). • Consider positive-pressure ventilation (noninvasive ventilation or via ET tube) to improve left ventricular function. *Myocardial dysfunction is common in children after resuscitation from cardiac arrest. Postarrest myocardial dysfunction can produce hemodynamic instability and secondary organ injury and may precipitate another cardiac arrest.*

PALS Postresuscitation Treatment of Shock

After resuscitation from cardiac arrest or shock, hemodynamic compromise may result from a combination of

- Inadequate intravascular volume
- Decreased cardiac contractility
- Increased systemic vascular resistance (SVR) or pulmonary vascular resistance or very low SVR

Very low SVR most commonly occurs in children with early septic shock. When children with septic shock do not respond to bolus fluid administration (i.e., the shock is fluid refractory), they may have high rather than low SVR and poor myocardial function, similar to cardiogenic shock. Children with cardiogenic shock typically have poor myocardial function and a compensatory increase in systemic and pulmonary vascular resistances in an attempt to maintain an adequate blood pressure. The increased SVR may become detrimental because it increases left ventricular afterload.

Support of Systemic Perfusion

The following parameters can be manipulated to optimize systemic perfusion:

Parameters	Action (When Needed)
Preload	• Bolus fluid administration
Contractility	• Administer inotropes or inodilators. • Correct hypoxia, electrolyte and acid-base imbalances, and hypoglycemia/hypocalcemia. • Treat poisonings (e.g., administer antidotes if available).
Afterload (SVR)	• Administer vasopressors or vasodilators as appropriate.
Heart rate	• Administer chronotropes for bradycardia (e.g., epinephrine). • Administer antiarrhythmics. • Correct hypoxia. • Consider pacing.

See the section "Pathophysiology of Shock" in Part 6 for a discussion of preload, afterload, and contractility.

Overview of Algorithm

The PALS Management of Shock After ROSC Algorithm (Figure 1) outlines evaluation and management steps after cardiac arrest. Box numbers in the text refer to the corresponding boxes in the algorithm.

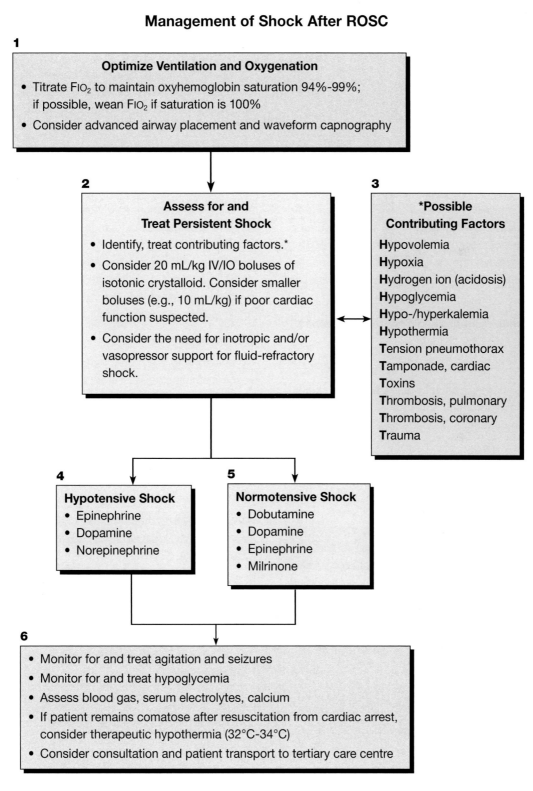

Management of Shock After ROSC

1
Optimize Ventilation and Oxygenation
- Titrate F_{IO_2} to maintain oxyhemoglobin saturation 94%-99%; if possible, wean F_{IO_2} if saturation is 100%
- Consider advanced airway placement and waveform capnography

2
Assess for and Treat Persistent Shock
- Identify, treat contributing factors.*
- Consider 20 mL/kg IV/IO boluses of isotonic crystalloid. Consider smaller boluses (e.g., 10 mL/kg) if poor cardiac function suspected.
- Consider the need for inotropic and/or vasopressor support for fluid-refractory shock.

3
***Possible Contributing Factors**
Hypovolemia
Hypoxia
Hydrogen ion (acidosis)
Hypoglycemia
Hypo-/hyperkalemia
Hypothermia
Tension pneumothorax
Tamponade, cardiac
Toxins
Thrombosis, pulmonary
Thrombosis, coronary
Trauma

4
Hypotensive Shock
- Epinephrine
- Dopamine
- Norepinephrine

5
Normotensive Shock
- Dobutamine
- Dopamine
- Epinephrine
- Milrinone

6
- Monitor for and treat agitation and seizures
- Monitor for and treat hypoglycemia
- Assess blood gas, serum electrolytes, calcium
- If patient remains comatose after resuscitation from cardiac arrest, consider therapeutic hypothermia (32°C-34°C)
- Consider consultation and patient transport to tertiary care centre

Figure 1. PALS Management of Shock After ROSC Algorithm.

Optimize Oxygenation and Ventilation (Box 1)

An important component of supporting cardiovascular function is achieving adequate oxygenation and ventilation. Titrate FIO_2 to maintain an O_2 saturation 94% to 99%; wean O_2 concentration if saturation is 100%. Consider placement of an advanced airway and use waveform capnography if not yet established.

Postarrest Shock and Fluid Therapy (Box 2)

The first intervention for signs of shock is administration of a bolus of 10 to 20 mL/kg of isotonic crystalloid. If you suspect postarrest myocardial dysfunction, consider administering a smaller fluid bolus (5 to 10 mL/kg) over 10 to 20 minutes, and then reassess. *If the child demonstrates signs of poor cardiac function (e.g., large liver, pulmonary edema, jugular venous distention, large heart on chest x-ray), carefully evaluate the need for fluid administration. Excessive fluid administration can worsen cardiopulmonary function.*

Reassess the child frequently to determine response to therapy.

Possible Contributing Factors (Box 3)

Consider factors that may contribute to postarrest shock, including metabolic derangements and conditions such as hypovolemia and cardiac tamponade (H's and T's).

Hypotensive Shock (Box 4)

If the child remains hypotensive after bolus fluid administration, consider infusion of one or a combination of the following drugs.

Medication	Route	Dose and Administration
Epinephrine	IV/IO	0.1 to 1 mcg/kg per minute
and/or		
Dopamine	IV/IO	Begin at approximately 10 to 20 mcg/kg per minute
and/or		
Norepinephrine	IV/IO	0.1 to 2 mcg/kg per minute

Ensure that preload is adequate; base your choice of drug on the most likely cause of hypotension (inadequate heart rate, poor contractility, excessive vasodilation, or a combination of factors). If the heart rate is abnormally low, catecholamine administration may increase the heart rate and cardiac output. However, when catecholamines markedly increase heart rate they increase myocardial O_2 demand.

Epinephrine

Epinephrine is a potent vasoactive agent that can either lower or increase SVR depending on the infusion dose. Low-dose infusions generally produce β-adrenergic action (potent chronotropy, inotropy, and vasodilation); higher doses generally produce α-adrenergic effects (vasoconstriction). Because there is great interpatient variability, titrate the drug to the desired clinical effect. Epinephrine may be preferable to dopamine in children (especially infants) with marked circulatory instability and hypotensive shock.

Dopamine

Titrate the dopamine infusion to treat shock associated with poor contractility and/or low SVR that is unresponsive to fluid administration. At doses >5 mcg/kg per minute, dopamine stimulates cardiac β-adrenergic receptors, but this effect may not be as significant in infants and in patients with chronic congestive heart failure. Doses of 10 to 20 mcg/kg per minute increase SVR due to the α-adrenergic effect. Infusion rates >20 mcg/kg per minute may result in excessive vasoconstriction.

Norepinephrine

Norepinephrine is a potent inotropic and peripheral vasoconstricting agent. Titrate the infusion to treat shock with low SVR (septic, anaphylactic, spinal) that is unresponsive to bolus fluid administration.

Normotensive Shock (Box 5)

If the child is normotensive but remains poorly perfused after bolus fluid administration, consider administration of one or a combination of the following drugs:

Medication	Route	Dose and Administration
Dobutamine	IV/IO	2 to 20 mcg/kg per minute
and/or		
Dopamine	IV/IO	2 to 20 mcg/kg per minute
and/or		
Low-dose epinephrine	IV/IO	0.1 to 0.3 mcg/kg per minute
and/or		
Milrinone	IV/IO	Load with 50 mcg/kg over 10 to 60 minutes. Loading doses may cause hypotension. Infusion: 0.25 to 0.75 mcg/kg per minute.

Dobutamine

Dobutamine has a selective effect on β_1-adrenergic and β_2-adrenergic receptors and has intrinsic α-adrenergic blocking activity. It increases myocardial contractility and usually decreases systemic vascular resistance. Titrate an infusion to improve cardiac output.

Dopamine

See "Dopamine" in the discussion of Box 4.

Low-Dose Epinephrine

See "Epinephrine" in the discussion of Box 4.

Milrinone

Milrinone is an inodilators that augment cardiac output with little effect on heart rate and myocardial O_2 demand. Use an inodilator for treatment of myocardial dysfunction with increased systemic or pulmonary vascular resistance. You may need to administer additional fluids because the vasodilatory effects will expand the vascular space.

Compared with drugs like dopamine and norepinephrine, inodilators have a long half-life. In addition, whenever the infusion rate is changed, there will be a long delay in reaching a new steady-state hemodynamic effect (4.5 hours with milrinone). In case of toxicity, the adverse effects may persist for several hours after you stop the infusion.

Other Postarrest Considerations (Box 6)

Multiple organ systems are affected after ROSC. Treat agitation and seizures with appropriate medications. Correct metabolic derangements, noting that treatment of metabolic acidosis is best accomplished by treating the underlying cause of the acidosis (i.e., restore perfusion in shock). Consider postarrest therapeutic hypothermia for children who remain comatose. Arrange for transfer to an appropriate pediatric critical care unit.

Administration of Maintenance Fluids

Maintenance Fluid Composition

Consider administration of maintenance fluids once intravascular volume has been restored and fluid deficits have been replaced. When you calculate the maintenance fluid requirements and plan for fluid administration, be sure to include the fluid administered with vasoactive drug infusions.

In the first hours after resuscitation the appropriate composition of maintenance IV fluids is an isotonic crystalloid (0.9% NaCl or lactated Ringer's), with or without dextrose, based on the child's condition and age. Avoid hypotonic fluids in critically ill children in the postresuscitation phase.

Specific components may be added to maintenance fluids based on the clinical condition:

- Dextrose should generally be included in maintenance fluids for infants and for children who are hypoglycemic or at risk for hypoglycemia.
- Potassium chloride (KCl) 10 to 20 mEq/L is typically added for children with adequate renal function and documented urine output once periodic monitoring of potassium is available. Do not add KCl to maintenance fluid in children with hyperkalemia, renal failure, muscle injury, or severe acidosis.

• Fluid Rate Calculation by 4-2-1 Method

The 4-2-1 method is a practical approach to estimating hourly maintenance fluid requirements in children (Table 2).

An alternative calculation of maintenance hourly fluid rate for patients weighing >20 kg is weight in kilograms + 40 mL/h.

Once you have calculated the estimated maintenance fluid requirements, adjust the actual rate of fluid administration to the child's clinical condition (e.g., pulse, blood pressure, systemic perfusion, urine output) and level of hydration.

Table 2. Estimation of Maintenance Fluid Requirements

Weight (kg)	Estimated Hourly Fluid Requirements	Sample Calculation
<10	4 mL/kg per hour	8-kg infant: 4 mL/kg per hour × 8 kg = 32 mL/h
10 to 20	40 mL/h + 2 mL/kg per hour for each kilogram between 10 and 20 kg	15-kg child: 40 mL/h + 2 mL/kg per hour × 5 kg = 50 mL/h
>20	60 mL/h + 1 mL/kg per hour for each kilogram above 20 kg	30-kg child: 60 mL/h + 1 mL/kg per hour × 10 kg = 70 mL/h

Neurologic System
Management Priorities

The goals of neurologic management during the postresuscitation period are to preserve brain function and prevent secondary neuronal injury. Management priorities are to

- Maintain adequate brain perfusion
- Maintain normoglycemia
- Control temperature
- Treat increased intracranial pressure (ICP)
- Treat seizures aggressively; search for and treat cause

General Recommendations

General recommendations for assessment and management of the neurologic system include the following:

Assessment and Management of the Neurologic System	
Assessment	
Monitoring	• Monitor temperature. • Monitor heart rate and systemic blood pressure. *In children with poor peripheral perfusion, reliable monitoring of core temperature requires invasive devices (rectal, bladder, esophageal thermometer).*
Physical examination	• Perform frequent, brief neurologic assessments (e.g., Glasgow Coma Scale, pupil responses, gag reflex, corneal reflexes, oculocephalic reflexes). • Identify signs of impending cerebral herniation. • Identify seizure activity, both convulsive and nonconvulsive. • Identify abnormal neurologic findings, including abnormal movements (posturing/myoclonus/hyperreflexia). *Signs of impending cerebral herniation include unequal or dilated unresponsive pupils, posturing, hypertension, bradycardia, respiratory irregularities or apnea, and reduced response to stimulation. A sudden increase in ICP (if monitoring is in place) is often observed. Other causes of central nervous system dysfunction are hypoxic-ischemic brain injury, hypoglycemia, convulsive or nonconvulsive seizures, toxins/drugs, electrolyte abnormalities, hypothermia, traumatic brain injury, stroke or intracranial hemorrhage, and central nervous system infection.* *See the section "Disability" in Part 2 for more information on neurologic assessment.*
Laboratory tests	• Evaluate point-of-care glucose; repeat measurement after treatment of hyperglycemia or hypoglycemia. • Obtain serum electrolytes, point-of-care glucose, and ionized calcium concentration if seizure activity is present; measure anticonvulsant concentrations if the child was receiving these agents. • Consider toxicologic studies if poisoning or overdose is suspected. • Consider cerebral spinal fluid studies if central nervous system infection is suspected, but defer a lumbar puncture if the patient's cardiopulmonary status has not been stabilized.
Nonlaboratory tests	• Consider CT scan if central nervous system dysfunction or neurologic deterioration is present. • Consider an electroencephalogram (EEG) if nonconvulsive status epilepticus is suspected or seizures are a concern in the presence of neuromuscular blockade.
Management	
Brain perfusion	• Optimize brain perfusion by supporting cardiac output and arterial O_2 content. • Avoid hyperventilation unless there are signs of impending cerebral herniation. *Support cardiac output by optimizing heart rate, preload, afterload, and contractility. See the section "Support of Systemic Perfusion" earlier in this Part for more information.*

(continued)

(continued)

Blood glucose	• Treat hypoglycemia. • Monitor glucose concentration. In general, try to avoid causing or worsening hyperglycemia. • In the critical care setting, consider treating persistent hyperglycemia; careful monitoring is needed to prevent hypoglycemia. *Although hyperglycemia is associated with poor outcome in critically ill children, the role of active treatment of hyperglycemia in critically ill children remains uncertain. In most animal studies, hyperglycemia at the time of cerebral ischemia produces a worse outcome, but the effect of hyperglycemia occurring after ROSC is less clear.*
Temperature control	Avoid hyperthermia and consider therapeutic hypothermia. **Hyperthermia** • Avoid hyperthermia; adjust environmental temperature as needed. • Treat elevated temperatures aggressively with antipyretics and cooling devices or procedures. *Fever adversely influences recovery from ischemic brain injury and is associated with poor outcome after resuscitation from cardiac arrest. Metabolic O_2 demand increases by 10% to 13% for each degree Celsius elevation of temperature above normal. Increased metabolic demand may worsen neurologic injury. Furthermore, fever increases the release of inflammatory mediators, cytotoxic enzymes, and neurotransmitters, which increase brain injury.* **Hypothermia** • Do not actively rewarm a hypothermic post–cardiac arrest patient (i.e., with temperature between 32°C and 37°C) after ROSC unless hypothermia is contributing to hemodynamic instability. • Consider initiating therapeutic hypothermia in normothermic patients who remain comatose after resuscitation from cardiac arrest. During cooling, treatment or prevention of shivering is often required. • Monitor for and treat complications of hypothermia. *In adults, cooling to a core temperature of 32°C to 34°C for 12 to 24 hours or longer after resuscitation from a cardiac arrest improved neurologically intact survival after sudden witnessed VF arrest. Hypothermia was also beneficial for newborns with moderate perinatal hypoxic-ischemic encephalopathy. Complications of therapeutic hypothermia include diminished cardiac output, arrhythmia, infection, pancreatitis, coagulopathy, thrombocytopenia, hypophosphatemia, and hypomagnesemia.*
Increased ICP	• Elevate head of bed to 30° if blood pressure is adequate. • Keep head in midline. • Ventilate to maintain normocapnia. • If signs of impending cerebral herniation develop, short periods of hyperventilation may be performed as a temporizing measure. • Consider mannitol or hypertonic saline for acute herniation syndrome. • For children with neurosurgical conditions (e.g., traumatic brain injury, intracranial hemorrhage), obtain expert consultation regarding indications for monitoring of ICP and/or neurosurgical intervention. *Prolonged hyperventilation is not effective to treat increased ICP, and excessive hyperventilation may worsen neurologic outcome. Hypocarbia results in cerebral vasoconstriction, reducing cerebral blood flow. Hyperventilation also reduces venous return and cardiac output, contributing to cerebral ischemia.*
Seizures	• Treat seizures aggressively. Therapeutic options include a benzodiazepine (e.g., lorazepam, midazolam), fosphenytoin/phenytoin, levetiracetam or a barbiturate (e.g., phenobarbital). Monitor blood pressure carefully if phenytoin or phenobarbital is used, because these drugs may cause hypotension. • Search for a correctable metabolic cause, such as hypoglycemia, hyponatremia, or hypocalcemia. • Consider toxins or metabolic disease as the etiology. • Consult a neurologist if available.

Renal System

Management Priorities

If renal dysfunction develops following resuscitation, the goals of therapy are to minimize secondary renal injury and maintain fluid and electrolyte balance. Management priorities for support of the renal system are to

- Optimize renal perfusion and function
- Correct acid-base imbalance

General Recommendations

General recommendations for assessment and management of the renal system may include the following:

Assessment and Management of the Renal System	
Assessment	
Monitoring	• Monitor for adequate urine output (>1 mL/kg per hour in infants and children or >30 mL per hour in adolescents) by urinary catheter. • Monitor for inappropriately high urine output. Causes of excessive urine output include glucosuria, diabetes insipidus, and osmotic and nonosmotic diuretics. *Insert a urinary catheter to accurately measure urine output. Consider using a urinary catheter with a temperature probe to enable continuous monitoring of core temperature.*
Physical examination	• Examine the abdomen for a distended bladder. In addition, assess for a diffusely distended and tight abdomen, which may impair renal perfusion (abdominal compartment syndrome). • Examine for evidence of hypovolemia and circulatory dysfunction resulting in oliguria. • Ensure that the urinary catheter is patent. *Common causes of oliguria are prerenal conditions (e.g., hypovolemia or inadequate systemic perfusion), intrinsic renal disease (including hypoxic-ischemic injury), and urinary tract obstruction.*

Laboratory tests	• Assess renal function
	  – BUN/creatinine
	  – Serum electrolytes, especially potassium and bicarbonate
	• Obtain urinalysis if indicated by history or examination.
	• Assess metabolic state
	  – ABG (acid-base)
	  – Serum glucose
	  – Anion gap
	  – Lactate concentration
	
	Urine glucose testing is important when evaluating urine output; glucosuria can be caused by a stress response after resuscitation and may cause increased urine output.

Management	
Renal function	• Augment renal perfusion by restoring intravascular volume and supporting systemic perfusion with vasoactive drugs if needed. • Consider treating children with volume overload/CHF and normal blood pressure with a trial of loop diuretics (e.g., furosemide). • Avoid nephrotoxic medications if possible; if renal function is impaired, adjust dose and timing of medications excreted by the kidneys. • If renal function is poor or the child is oliguric, do not routinely add potassium to IV fluids until serum potassium level is measured. • The oliguric patient may have intrinsic renal failure; if so, it may be necessary to restrict fluids once intravascular volume is adequate. *Bolus fluid administration augments preload in volume-depleted patients. Vasoactive drugs may improve renal perfusion by improving cardiac output and renal blood flow.*

(continued)

(continued)

Acid-base balance	• Correct lactic acidosis by improving tissue perfusion (i.e., with fluid administration and, if necessary, vasoactive agents).
	• Consider correcting non–anion gap metabolic acidosis with sodium bicarbonate, particularly if the history or signs suggest bicarbonate loss.
	• Sodium bicarbonate is not indicated for treatment of hyperchloremic metabolic acidosis (e.g., associated with normal saline boluses used for resuscitation).

Gastrointestinal System

Management Priorities

One major goal of gastrointestinal management during postresuscitation care is to restore and maintain gastrointestinal function, including liver and pancreatic function. Another major goal is to minimize the risk of aspiration of gastric contents into the airway. Management priorities are to

- Support systemic perfusion
- Relieve gastric distention
- Correct electrolyte abnormalities (e.g., hypomagnesemia or hypokalemia) that may be contributing to ileus
- Support hepatic function

General Recommendations

General recommendations for assessment and management of the gastrointestinal system may include the following:

Assessment and Management of the Gastrointestinal System	
Assessment	
Monitoring	• Monitor type and quantity of gastric (NG/OG) tube drainage.
Physical examination	• Perform a careful abdominal examination with attention to bowel sounds, abdominal girth, and abdominal tightness. *Critically ill or injured children may have delayed gastric emptying.* *A tensely distended or painful abdomen that is difficult to compress should raise concern about a possible intra-abdominal catastrophe such as a perforated bowel or bleeding. Additional studies (e.g., abdominal ultrasound or CT scan) and early surgical consultation may be indicated.*

Laboratory tests	Obtain laboratory tests of liver and pancreatic function based on the child's condition and etiology of the arrest. Assess for evidence of bowel ischemia.
	
	• Evaluate liver function
	  – Transaminases (alanine aminotransferase [ALT]/aspartate aminotransferase [AST])
	  – Biliary function (bilirubin, alkaline phosphatase)
	  – Glucose
	  – Ammonia (if concerned about liver failure)
	  – Coagulation studies (PT, activated partial thromboplastin time [aPTT], international normalized ratio [INR])
	• Evaluate for pancreatic injury
	  – Amylase/lipase
	• Evaluate for evidence of bowel ischemia
	• Evaluate acid-base balance (assess for anion-gap metabolic acidosis, rising serum lactate)

Nonlaboratory tests	• Consider ultrasound to evaluate liver, gall bladder, pancreas, and bladder and to assess for intra-abdominal fluid. • Consider abdominal CT scan, particularly when evaluating abdominal trauma.
Management	
Gastric distention	• Insert OG or NG tube and aspirate stomach air and contents. Ideally, use a sump tube rather than a single-lumen feeding tube to decompress the stomach.
Ileus	• Insert OG or NG tube and continuously suction gastric contents. • Assess, restore, and maintain electrolyte and fluid balance.
Hepatic failure	• Infuse glucose at a rate to maintain normal glucose concentration. High infusion rate may be needed. • When bleeding is present, correct clotting factor deficiency by using fresh frozen plasma, cryoprecipitate, and/or activated factor VII as needed.

Hematologic System

Management Priorities

The goals of hematologic management during the postresuscitation period are to optimize blood O_2-carrying capacity and coagulation function.

General Recommendations

General recommendations for assessment and management of the hematologic system may include the following:

Assessment and Management of the Hematologic System	
Assessment	
Physical examination	• Identify external or internal hemorrhage. • Assess skin and mucous membranes for pallor, petechiae, or bruising.
Laboratory tests	• Hemoglobin and hematocrit • Platelet count • Prothrombin time (PT), activated partial thromboplastin time (aPTT), international normalized ratio (INR), fibrinogen, D-dimer and fibrin split products
Management	

Blood component therapy	• If hemorrhagic shock is refractory to isotonic crystalloid (2 or 3 boluses of 20 mL/kg), transfuse with 10 mL/kg PRBCs.
	
	 Type-specific blood is generally available within 5 minutes and is preferred over transfusion with O-negative blood when time precludes complete crossmatching. Complications of massive transfusion (greater than the equivalent of patient's blood volume) include hypothermia, hyperkalemia, hypokalemia, hypocalcemia, and coagulopathy from dilution of platelets and clotting factors. Massive transfusion scenarios require the use of PRBCs, fresh frozen plasma, and platelets. Seek expert consultation.
	
	 • Correct thrombocytopenia
	   – If the platelet count is <50 000 to 100 000/mm³ (consult hospital protocol) and active bleeding is present, transfuse with platelets. Transfusion at higher platelet counts may be indicated if intracranial hemorrhage is present.
	   – If the platelet count is <20 000/mm³ and the child is not bleeding, consider platelet transfusion.
	   – In general, 1 unit of random donor platelets per 5 kg of body weight will increase the platelet count by 50 000/mm³.
	
	 Platelets should be ABO and Rh compatible; platelet crossmatching is not necessary.
	
	 • Administer fresh frozen plasma (10 to 15 mL/kg) if coagulation tests are abnormal and the child is actively bleeding or is at high risk for bleeding.
	 • Consider administration of vitamin K for elevated PT. The elevated PT may be associated with depletion of vitamin K–dependent clotting factors.
	 • Ensure that serum ionized calcium is normal because it is a cofactor in clotting and can decrease with administration of blood products.
	
	 Fresh frozen plasma contains all clotting factors but no platelets. Be aware that fresh frozen plasma uses citrate as an anticoagulant; rapid infusions of fresh frozen plasma may acutely lower plasma ionized calcium concentration, causing vasodilation and reduced cardiac contractility.

Postresuscitation Transport

The PALS principles of postresuscitation—evaluation, monitoring, intervention, stabilization, communication, and documentation—apply to the transport of the pediatric patient. These apply whether transport is interhospital or intrahospital.

Important considerations of transport include coordination with the receiving facility, advance preparation, and infectious disease considerations. In addition, communicating among providers and facilities, as well as with the family, is critical. Finally, decisions must be made regarding the best mode of transport and the composition of the transport team.

Coordination With Receiving Facility

Coordinate transport and transfer with receiving providers at the tertiary care centre to ensure that the child is delivered safely in stable or improved condition. Both referring and receiving facilities should have well-defined protocols for specific clinical situations. Protocols, contracts, and agreements should be established *before* a seriously ill or injured child requires transport. Federal regulations, known as *EMTALA* (Emergency Medical Treatment and Active Labor Act), apply to the interfacility transfer of patients with emergency medical conditions in the United States. EMTALA delineates responsibilities of the referring physician and hospital, including provision of stabilizing care to the best of the institution's ability; identification of an accepting hospital and physician; and use of qualified personnel and appropriate equipment to prevent patient deterioration during transfer.

Advance Preparation for Transport

Advance preparation by the referring facility for interhospital transport may include the following:

- List of pediatric tertiary care facilities and telephone numbers
- List of nearest alternative hospital (even in another state) if there is only 1 pediatric tertiary care centre in the area
- List of pediatric critical care transport systems and telephone numbers
- If transport is to be performed by personnel from the referring facility, maintain a list of pediatric equipment and supplies to supplement standard EMS equipment. Ideally pediatric transport packs, containing equipment of the correct size and medication doses for the particular emergency situation, should be prepared in advance. Provide transport-specific training for staff who may not be familiar with the mobile environment and equipment.

- Evaluate transport vehicle equipment periodically to ensure that
  - The entire range of pediatric equipment sizes (i.e., for all ages and sizes) is included
  - Lost or missing equipment is immediately replaced
- Use administrative protocols and a transport checklist to ensure that all appropriate interventions are provided and appropriate documents are sent with the patient.

Infectious Disease Considerations

If the child is suspected of having a communicable disease, obtain appropriate cultures (if not already obtained), but do not delay antibiotic therapy if the child is critically ill. Early (within 1 hour of medical contact) antibiotic administration is critical when sepsis or meningitis is suspected. Transport personnel should take appropriate precautions (e.g., gloves, masks) to avoid disease transmission.

Immediate Preparation Before Transport

Immediately before transport consider the following:

- Obtain consent to transport
- Prepare the child for transport
- Anticipate requirements of the transport team

Obtain Consent to Transport

If the transport team is not based in the referring or receiving hospital, the referring hospital must assist in the efficient transfer of the child. Obtain written consent to transport from the child's legal guardian if possible. Many transport teams request that the parents remain at the referring hospital to give consent directly to the team.

Prepare the Child for Transport

Because it is challenging to perform advanced airway management in a transport vehicle, consider insertion of an advanced airway (e.g., an ET tube) before transport. Verify placement with clinical assessment and a confirmation device (e.g., exhaled CO_2 detector). If radiology services are readily available or if there is uncertainty about the ET tube position, check depth of insertion with a chest x-ray. Tape intravascular lines and the advanced airway securely in place. Provide sedation as needed. Vascular catheters and ET tubes may become dislodged during transport if not adequately secured for a moving environment. Before transporting a trauma patient, stabilize the cervical spine (if indicated) and any fractured bones.

Anticipate Requirements of the Transport Team

For more efficient transfer, anticipate the requirements of the transport team. Make copies of the child's chart and x-rays before the team arrives. If blood products may be required during transport, prepare a supply in advance to accompany the child. Anticipate the need for vasoactive drug support and prepare infusions.

Communication Between Referring and Receiving Healthcare Providers

Good communication is important before patient transfer. The initial call to transfer a patient should be from the provider who is responsible for the child's care (referring provider) to the provider who will be accepting responsibility for the child's care (receiving provider). This is an opportunity for the receiving provider to make recommendations for patient stabilization before arrival of the transport team. For more details see Seidel and Knapp, 2000 (full reference in the "Transport" section in the Suggested Reading List at the end of this Part). Use of trained communication specialists can facilitate logistical aspects of the transport and decrease mobilization time.

Other important components of this discussion and follow-up documentation may include the following:

- Consult the child's chart at the time of the call and give specific details about estimated weight, vital signs, fluids and medications administered, and timing of events.
- In a crisis give a brief history of the illness or injury, interventions, and the child's current clinical status to facilitate decisions about treatment and method of transport.
- Document the names of the receiving physician and hospital.
- Document the advice provided by the receiving physician; the transport team may need additional specific information to select the proper equipment for transport.
- Discuss any potential need for infection precautions so arrangements can be made at the receiving hospital.

Communication Among Facilities and With Other Healthcare Providers

Successful communication among receiving and referring facilities, as well as with other healthcare providers, is essential for successful transport. Important communications may include the following:

- Nurses from the receiving and referring facilities should respectively request and provide updates on the child's status.
- When the transport team arrives, the referring physician should personally provide a current report about the child directly to the transport team.
- If the receiving hospital's transport team is not involved in the transport, the referring physician should telephone the receiving physician immediately before the child's departure and report the child's most recent vital signs, current clinical status, and estimated time of arrival at the receiving hospital.
- Include copies of all records, laboratory results, and x-rays with the child. Note any laboratory results that are pending at the time of transport. Include the laboratory phone number with the child's record so the receiving physician can obtain the results.

Communication With the Family

Communication with the family is an essential part of postresuscitation care and transport care. Update the family about all interventions and diagnostic tests. Answer questions, clarify information, and offer comfort.

Posttransport Documentation and Follow-up

Posttransport follow-up provides important feedback that can improve the performance of the transport team and referring hospital. Providing information to the transport team and referring hospital may require written consent from the child's parent or guardian. Patient information should be provided in accordance with local policies and practice.

Critical Concept **If Child's Condition Changes**	The referring physician should notify the receiving facility if the child's condition changes significantly at any time before arrival of the transport team.

Who	Action
Receiving physician	Contact the referring physician after the transport is complete to provide feedback about management and give an update on the child's status. Address any transport issues.
Receiving hospital	Provide personnel at the referring hospital with follow-up information about the child's condition, including the ultimate outcome.
Referring physician	Communicate any laboratory results that become available after the child was transported to the receiving hospital. If the receiving hospital does not provide communication about the child's condition and ultimate outcome, contact the medical director of the transport system. Express any concerns about transport. Such a discussion can often clarify misunderstandings, such as the necessity for interventions or timing of transport.

Mode of Transport and Transport Team Composition

The mode of transport and composition of the transport team should be determined by the anticipated level of care required by the patient and applicable logistical issues. Once the child has been stabilized, providers must determine the most appropriate method of transfer to a tertiary care facility and the appropriate personnel to care for the child during transport. Interhospital transport can be provided by

- Ground transportation by ambulance (e.g., local EMS ambulance, advanced life support unit, or critical care transport vehicle)
- Helicopter
- Fixed-wing aircraft

Ground Transportation by Ambulance

Ambulances, whether operated by local EMS providers or a critical care transport team from the receiving hospital, provide readily available ground transportation. Transportation by ambulance is relatively inexpensive and spacious (compared with most transport aircraft). Ambulances are operable in most weather conditions and can stop easily if a procedure must be performed. One disadvantage of ground ambulance transport is increased transport time over long distances. Another disadvantage is the risk of traffic-related delays.

Helicopter

Barring weather delays, rotor-wing transport is faster than ground transport for longer-distance transports, allowing rapid transfer of care from the referring hospital to the receiving hospital without concern for traffic delays. Children with time-sensitive conditions, such as a surgical emergency (e.g., epidural hematoma), are most likely to benefit from use of a helicopter transport. Disadvantages include difficulty in monitoring or evaluating the child and the challenge of performing emergency procedures during transport. Other disadvantages are lack of pressurization, extreme variability of temperatures, inability to fly in all weather conditions, increased safety concerns, and high cost.

Fixed-Wing Aircraft

Fixed-wing aircraft are primarily used for long-distance transport or when it is necessary to reach a remote area, such as an island. These aircraft are pressurized and land at controlled sites. It is easier to monitor the child and perform interventions in a fixed-wing aircraft than in a helicopter. The disadvantages are longer mobilization times (usually offset by speed of flight) and the need to transfer the child from hospital to ambulance to aircraft with a reverse transfer sequence on landing.

Transport Team

Transport team members should have specific training and experience in pediatric evaluation, stabilization, and resuscitation. Members of the transport team may be

- Local EMS personnel
- Medical and nursing personnel from the referring hospital
- Critical care transport teams
- Specialized pediatric critical care transport teams

Local EMS teams rarely have the training, experience, or equipment for long-distance transport of a critically ill or injured child after resuscitation. The use of local EMS personnel may also deprive the community of service in the event of other local emergencies.

Medical and nursing personnel from the referring hospital can be rapidly mobilized. But their involvement on the transport team may deprive their facility of necessary personnel unless they are specifically scheduled for transport. Personnel with limited experience in pediatric prehospital and critical care will find patient management especially difficult in a moving vehicle with limited or unfamiliar equipment (e.g., portable monitors). Anticipated care during transfer should not exceed the level that the transport team is capable of providing.

Critical Concept

Pediatric Critical Care Transport Teams

It is often best to wait for the arrival of a team experienced in pediatric critical care to transport a critically ill or injured child even if this is not the fastest method of transfer. This type of transport team can initiate pediatric critical care interventions at the referring hospital and maintain that level of care during transport. An exception to this rule is the child who requires immediate surgical intervention (e.g., a craniotomy for epidural hematoma) at the tertiary care centre.

Critical care transport teams who transport patients of all ages may have variable training, experience, and equipment for optimum care of a critically ill or injured child. Evaluate the ability of transport teams to care for critically ill or injured children before this type of care is needed.

Pediatric critical care transport teams provide optimum services for critically ill children and often provide continuity of care from the referring to the receiving hospital. Unfortunately such teams are not available in all areas, and they may not have access to all types of transport vehicles. Use the most qualified team that is available within an acceptable time interval based on the child's condition.

Transport Triage

No specific criteria are available to reliably determine the need for a pediatric critical care transport team. The following are broad criteria:

- Children who are expected to require admission to the pediatric intensive care unit at the receiving hospital are likely to benefit from that level of care and monitoring during transport.
- Children with respiratory, cardiovascular, or neurologic conditions who have significant potential for deterioration during transport.
- Children who have recently experienced a life-threatening event (even if they are stable at the time of transport) because the event may recur; examples are neonates and infants with a history of apnea and any child who has required aggressive stabilization (e.g., after seizure with apnea or after resuscitation from severe shock).

Summary: Transport Checklist

Transport Checklist	
Coordination with receiving facility	
☐	Identify pediatric tertiary care centre and receiving providers. Phone number:
Advance preparation for transport	
☐	Identify nearest alternative hospital if there is only 1 pediatric tertiary care centre in the area. Phone number:
☐	Locate administrative protocol for interhospital patient transport.
Mode of transport	
☐	Determine appropriate mode of transport for patient and weather condition (ground ambulance, helicopter, fixed-wing aircraft).
Infectious disease considerations	
☐	Practice universal precautions.
☐	Obtain appropriate cultures if the patient is suspected of having an infectious disease.
☐	Administer antibiotics if sepsis or meningitis is suspected.
☐	Consider the need for infection precautions (i.e., respiratory or contact).
Preparation immediately before transport	
☐	Obtain consent to transport.
☐	Prepare the patient for transport.
☐	Anticipate requirements of the transport team (medications, fluids, blood products).
Communication between physicians	
☐	Identify and document the name of the receiving physician:
☐	Communicate appropriate patient details with the receiving physician.
Communication between facilities and with other healthcare providers	
☐	Notify the receiving facility if the patient's condition changes significantly at any time before arrival of the transport team.
☐	Nurses from the referring facility should provide a report and updates as needed on the patient's status.
☐	The referring physician should provide a current report about the patient directly to the transport team.
☐	If the receiving hospital's transport team is not involved in transport, the referring physician should contact the receiving physician immediately before departure to provide the most current information about the patient and estimated time of arrival.
☐	Send copies of all records, laboratory results, and x-rays with the patient.
☐	Note laboratory results pending at the time of transport and include the laboratory phone number with the patient's record so that the receiving physician can obtain the results.
Communication with family	
☐	Communicate the results of all interventions and diagnostic studies to the family. Answer questions, clarify information, and offer comfort.
Posttransport documentation and follow-up	
☐	Contact the medical director of the transport system if no follow-up information is received from the receiving facility about the patient's condition and outcome.

Suggested Reading List

Bembea MM, Nadkarni VM, Diener-West M, Venugopal V, Carey SM, Berg RA, Hunt EA. Temperature patterns in the early postresuscitation period after pediatric inhospital cardiac arrest. *Pediatr Crit Care Med*. 2010;11:723-730.

Brierley J, Carcillo JA, Choong K, Cornell T, Decaen A, Deymann A, Doctor A, Davis A, Duff J, Dugas MA, Duncan A, Evans B, Feldman J, Felmet K, Fisher G, Frankel L, Jeffries H, Greenwald B, Gutierrez J, Hall M, Han YY, Hanson J, Hazelzet J, Hernan L, Kiff J, Kissoon N, Kon A, Irazuzta J, Lin J, Lorts A, Mariscalco M, Mehta R, Nadel S, Nguyen T, Nicholson C, Peters M, Okhuysen-Cawley R, Poulton T, Relves M, Rodriguez A, Rozenfeld R, Schnitzler E, Shanley T, Kache S, Skippen P, Torres A, von Dessauer B, Weingarten J, Yeh T, Zaritsky A, Stojadinovic B, Zimmerman J, Zuckerberg A. Clinical practice parameters for hemodynamic support of pediatric and neonatal septic shock: 2007 update from the American College of Critical Care Medicine. *Crit Care Med*. 2009;37:666-688.

Checchia PA, Sehra R, Moynihan J, Daher N, Tang W, Weil MH. Myocardial injury in children following resuscitation after cardiac arrest. *Resuscitation*. 2003;57:131-137.

Kilgannon JH, Jones AE, Shapiro NI, Angelos MG, Milcarek N, Hunter K, Parrillo JE, Trzeciak S; Emergency Medicine Shock Research Network (EmShockNet) Investigators. Association between arterial hyperoxia following resuscitation from cardiac arrest and in-hospital mortality. *JAMA*. 2010;303:2165-2171.

Kleinman ME, Chameides L, Schexnayder SM, Samson RA, Hazinski MF, Atkins DL, Berg MD, de Caen AR, Fink EL, Freid EB, Hickey RW, Marino BS, Nadkarni VM, Proctor LT, Qureshi FA, Sartorelli K, Topjian A, van der Jagt EW, Zaritsky AL. Part 14: pediatric advanced life support: 2010 American Heart Association Guidelines for Cardiopulmonary Resuscitation and Emergency Cardiovascular Care. *Circulation*. 2010;122:S876-S908.

Kleinman ME, Srinivasan V. Postresuscitation care. *Pediatr Clin North Am*. 2008;55:943-967, xixx.

Manole MD, Kochanek PM, Fink EL, Clark RS. Postcardiac arrest syndrome: focus on the brain. *Curr Opin Pediatr*. 2009;21:745-750.

Neumar RW, Nolan JP, Adrie C, Aibiki M, Berg RA, Bottiger BW, Callaway C, Clark RS, Geocadin RG, Jauch EC, Kern KB, Laurent I, Longstreth WT Jr, Merchant RM, Morley P, Morrison LJ, Nadkarni V, Peberdy MA, Rivers EP, Rodriguez-Nunez A, Sellke FW, Spaulding C, Sunde K, Vanden Hoek T. Post-cardiac arrest syndrome: epidemiology, pathophysiology, treatment, and prognostication.

A consensus statement from the International Liaison Committee on Resuscitation (American Heart Association, Australian and New Zealand Council on Resuscitation, European Resuscitation Council, Heart and Stroke Foundation of Canada, InterAmerican Heart Foundation, Resuscitation Council of Asia, and the Resuscitation Council of Southern Africa); the American Heart Association Emergency Cardiovascular Care Committee; the Council on Cardiovascular Surgery and Anesthesia; the Council on Cardiopulmonary, Perioperative, and Critical Care; the Council on Clinical Cardiology; the Stroke Council. *Circulation*. 2008;118:2452-2483.

Tømte O, Andersen GO, Jacobsen D, Drægni T, Auestad B, Sunde K. Strong and weak aspects of an established post-resuscitation treatment protocol—a five-year observational study [published online ahead of print May 14, 2011]. *Resuscitation*. doi:10.1016/j.resuscitation.2011.05.003.

van den Berghe G, Wouters P, Weekers F, Verwaest C, Bruyninckx F, Schetz M, Vlasselaers D, Ferdinande P, Lauwers P, Bouillon R. Intensive insulin therapy in the critically ill patients. *N Engl J Med*. 2001;345:1359-1367.

Therapeutic Hypothermia

Doherty DR, Parshuram CS, Gaboury I, Hoskote A, Lacroix J, Tucci M, Joffe A, Choong K, Farrell R, Bohn DJ, Hutchison JS. Hypothermia therapy after pediatric cardiac arrest. *Circulation*. 2009;119:1492-1500.

Fink EL, Clark RS, Kochanek PM, Bell MJ, Watson RS. A tertiary care center's experience with therapeutic hypothermia after pediatric cardiac arrest. *Pediatr Crit Care Med*. 2010;11:66-74.

Hickey RW, Kochanek PM, Ferimer H, Graham SH, Safar P. Hypothermia and hyperthermia in children after resuscitation from cardiac arrest. *Pediatrics*. 2000;106(pt 1):118-122.

Hypothermia after Cardiac Arrest Study Group. Mild therapeutic hypothermia to improve the neurologic outcome after cardiac arrest. *N Engl J Med*. 2002;346:549-556.

Kochanek PM, Fink EL, Bell MJ, Bayir H, Clark RS. Therapeutic hypothermia: applications in pediatric cardiac arrest. *J Neurotrauma*. 2009;26:421-427.

Therapeutic Hypothermia to Improve Survival After Cardiac Arrest in Pediatric Patients—THAPCA-IH [In Hospital] Trial. National Institutes of Health clinical trials website. http://clinicaltrials.gov/ct2/show/NCT00880087. Updated January 28, 2011. Accessed June 20, 2011.

Transport

Orr RA, Felmet KA, Han Y, McCloskey KA, Dragotta MA, Bills DM, Kuch BA, Watson RS. Pediatric specialized transport teams are associated with improved outcomes. *Pediatrics*. 2009;124:40-48.

Seidel JS, Knapp JF. *Childhood Emergencies in the Office, Hospital, and Community.* Elk Grove Village, IL: American Academy of Pediatrics; 2000.

Warren J, Fromm RE Jr, Orr RA, Rotello LC, Horst HM. Guidelines for the inter- and intrahospital transport of critically ill patients. *Crit Care Med*. 2004;32:256-262.

Woodward G, ed. *Guidelines for Air and Ground Transport of Neonatal and Pediatric Patients.* 3rd ed. Elk Grove Village, IL: American Academy of Pediatrics Section on Transport Medicine; 2006.

Part 12

Pharmacology

Overview

This Part contains information on drugs referenced in the *PALS Provider Manual.*

The scientific basis for the pharmacologic treatment of seriously ill or injured infants and children is dynamic. Advances in management options and drug therapies occur rapidly. Readers are advised to check for changes in recommended doses, indications, and contraindications in the following sources: *Highlights of Emergency Cardiovascular Care*, which is available at **heartandstroke. ca/CPRguidelines**; the *2010 Handbook of Emergency Cardiovascular Care for Healthcare Providers*; and the package insert product information sheet for each drug and medical device.

This Part contains selected pharmacology information. The focus of this information is the pharmacology of these agents when used for the treatment of seriously ill or injured children. The contents of this Part should not be considered complete information on the pharmacology of these drugs.

Preparation for the Course

During the course you will be expected to be familiar with all of the drugs used in the PALS recommendations for pediatric resuscitation and postresuscitation care. During the course you should be familiar with the indications and doses of adenosine, amiodarone, atropine, epinephrine, and O_2.

Pharmacology

Adenosine

Classification: Antiarrhythmic

Indications: SVT

Available Forms: Injection: 3 mg/mL

Dose and Administration:

SVT		
IV/IO	First dose	0.1 mg/kg *rapid* push (maximum dose 6 mg)
	Second dose	0.2 mg/kg *rapid* push (maximum dose 12 mg)

Actions:

- Stimulates adenosine receptors in heart and vascular smooth muscle
  - Transiently blocks conduction through AV node
  - Interrupts reentry pathways through AV node
  - Allows return of normal sinus rhythm in patients with SVT, including SVT associated with Wolff-Parkinson-White syndrome
- Depresses sinus node automaticity

Pharmacokinetics:

Absorption	(Not applicable with IV/IO route of administration)
Distribution	Erythrocytes, vascular endothelium
Metabolism	Erythrocytes, endothelium rapidly take up and metabolize adenosine
Excretion	Inactive metabolites in urine
Half-life	≤10 seconds

Pharmacodynamics:

IV/IO

- Onset—Rapid if given by rapid bolus
- Peak—Unknown
- Duration—Usually <1 minute

Monitoring: Monitor blood pressure frequently and ECG continuously.

Adverse Effects:

CNS	Light-headedness, dizziness, arm tingling, numbness, apprehension, blurred vision, headache
EENT	Metallic taste, throat tightness
RESP	Dyspnea, hyperventilation, bronchospasm
CV	Hypotension, transient bradycardia or asystole, atrial tachyarrhythmias, angina, palpitations
GI	Nausea
SKIN	Facial and systemic flushing, sweating

Special Considerations:

- If possible, record multiple-lead rhythm strip during administration.
- Administer via central venous access if present; otherwise by IV/IO at most proximal injection site.
- Push adenosine rapidly IV/IO followed immediately by NS flush (5 to 10 mL).
- Theophylline is an adenosine receptor antagonist and reduces adenosine effectiveness.
- Limited adult data suggest the need to reduce dose in patients taking carbamazepine or dipyridamole and in patients with transplanted hearts.

Albumin

Classification: Blood product derivative (plasma volume expander)

Indications:

- Shock
- Trauma
- Burns

Available Forms: Injection: 5% (5 g/100 mL), 25% (25 g/100 mL)

Dose and Administration:

Shock, Trauma, Burns	
IV/IO	0.5 to 1 g/kg by *rapid* infusion (10 to 20 mL/kg of 5% solution)

Actions:

- Expands intravascular volume through colloid oncotic effect. As a large molecule, albumin is more likely to remain in the intravascular space for a longer time than crystalloid. Oncotic effect may help expand the intravascular space by pulling water and sodium from the extravascular compartment.
- Augments preload and thus cardiac output.

Pharmacokinetics:

Absorption	(Not applicable with IV/IO route of administration)
Distribution	Initially intravascular space, then throughout extracellular space at a rate determined by capillary permeability
Metabolism	Liver
Excretion	Unknown
Half-life	Variable (affected by clinical setting); usually <24 hours

Pharmacodynamics:

IV/IO

- Onset—15 to 30 minutes
- Peak—Unknown
- Duration—Unknown

Monitoring: Monitor cardiopulmonary function and systemic perfusion.

Adverse Effects:

RESP	Pulmonary edema (if fluid overloaded), increased respiratory rate, bronchospasm (rare allergic reaction)
CV	Fluid overload (can produce hypertension), hypotension, tachycardia
SKIN	Rash, urticaria, flushing
MISC	Fever, hypocalcemia

Precautions:

- Monitor for signs of pulmonary edema.
- Albumin binds calcium, so rapid infusions may decrease ionized calcium concentration, leading to hypotension.
- Albumin also binds many drugs, such as phenytoin, which may reduce free drug concentration and therapeutic effect.

Special Considerations:

- Blood product—transfusion-like reactions rarely occur.
- For IV administration, use within 4 hours of opening vial.
- 5% albumin is generally used undiluted; 25% albumin may be given undiluted or diluted in NS.

Alprostadil (Prostaglandin E$_1$ [PGE$_1$])

Classification: Vasodilator, prostaglandin

Indications: To maintain patency of ductus arteriosus for ductal-dependent congenital heart disease, such as

- Cyanotic defects (e.g., transposition of great vessels, tricuspid atresia, tetralogy of Fallot)
- Left heart or ascending aortic obstructive lesions (e.g., hypoplastic left heart syndrome, critical aortic stenosis, coarctation of aorta, interrupted aortic arch)

Available Forms: Injection: 500 mcg/mL

Dose and Administration:

Ductal-Dependent Congenital Heart Disease (All Forms)		
IV/IO	Initial	0.05 to 0.1 mcg/kg per minute infusion
	Maintenance	0.01 to 0.05 mcg/kg per minute infusion, titrated to response

Actions:

- Acts through PGE$_1$ receptors to cause vasodilation of all arteries and arterioles (including ductus arteriosus)
- Inhibits platelet aggregation
- Stimulates uterine and intestinal smooth muscle

Pharmacokinetics:

Absorption	(Not applicable with IV/IO route of administration)
Distribution	Wide
Metabolism	Endothelium in the lung (90% metabolized in 1 pass)
Excretion	Urine
Half-life	5 to 10 minutes

Pharmacodynamics:

IV/IO

- Onset—Within seconds
- Peak—<1 hour for cyanotic defects; several hours for acyanotic defects

Monitoring: Monitor SpO$_2$, respiratory rate, blood pressure, ECG, and temperature continuously.

Adverse Effects:

CNS	Seizures, jitteriness
RESP	Apnea (common), bronchospasm
CV	Vasodilation (common), hypotension, bradycardia, tachycardia, cardiac arrest
GI	Gastric outlet obstruction, diarrhea
GU	Renal failure
MS	Cortical proliferation of long bones (after prolonged treatment, seen as periosteal new bone formation on x-ray)
SKIN	Flushing, edema, urticaria
ENDO	Hypoglycemia
HEME	Disseminated intravascular coagulation, leukocytosis, hemorrhage, thrombocytopenia
ELECT	Hypocalcemia
MISC	Fever (common)

Precautions:

- Adverse effects are dose related.
- Extravasation may cause tissue sloughing and necrosis.

Special Considerations:

- Drug may also be given via umbilical arterial catheter positioned near ductus arteriosus.
- PGE$_1$ should be refrigerated until administered.

Amiodarone

Classification: Antiarrhythmic (Class III)

Indications:

- SVT
- VT (with pulses)
- VF/pulseless VT

Available Forms: Injection: 50 mg/mL

Dose and Administration:

SVT, VT (With Pulses)	
IV/IO	5 mg/kg *load* over 20 to 60 minutes (maximum dose 300 mg), may give up to 3 doses to maximum daily dose of 15 mg/kg (2.2 g in adolescents)

Pulseless Arrest (VF/Pulseless VT)	
IV/IO	5 mg/kg rapid *bolus* (maximum dose 300 mg), repeat to maximum daily dose of 15 mg/kg (2.2 g in adolescents)

Actions:

- Prolongs action potential duration and effective refractory period
- Slows sinus rate
- Prolongs PR and QT intervals
- Noncompetitively inhibits α-adrenergic and β-adrenergic receptors

Pharmacokinetics:

Absorption	(Not applicable with IV/IO route of administration)
Distribution	Wide
Metabolism	Liver
Excretion	Bile/feces, urine (minimal)
Half-life	15 to 50 days (oral doses have very long half-life)

Pharmacodynamics:

IV/IO

- Onset—Within minutes
- Peak—2 to 3 days to 1 to 3 weeks
- Duration—2 weeks to months after drug is discontinued

Monitoring: Monitor blood pressure frequently and ECG continuously.

Adverse Effects:

CNS	Headache, dizziness, involuntary movement, tremors, peripheral neuropathy, malaise, fatigue, ataxia, paresthesias, syncope
RESP	Pulmonary fibrosis, pulmonary inflammation, ARDS (*Note:* Gasping was reported in neonates as a complication of the benzyl alcohol preservative in non–water-soluble form of the drug; water-soluble product is not associated with this problem)
CV	Hypotension (related to infusion rate), bradycardia, CHF, prolonged QT interval, torsades de pointes
GI	Nausea, vomiting, diarrhea, abdominal pain
SKIN	Rash, photosensitivity, blue-gray skin discolouration, alopecia, ecchymosis, toxic epidermal necrolysis, flushing
ENDO	Hyperthyroidism, hypothyroidism (chronic use)
HEME	Coagulation abnormalities

Precautions:

- Before using in a patient with a perfusing rhythm, expert consultation is strongly recommended.
- Administration in combination with procainamide (or other agents that prolong QT interval) is not recommended without expert consultation.
- Use with caution in patients with hepatic failure.
- Amiodarone inhibits cytochrome P-450 system (a family of enzymes that are involved in drug metabolism) and therefore can increase concentration and risk of toxicity of multiple drugs.

Contraindications: Sinus node dysfunction, second- or third-degree AV block

Special Considerations: Because amiodarone has a long half-life and potential drug interactions, consultation with a cardiologist is recommended before it is used outside the cardiac arrest setting.

Atropine

Classification: Anticholinergic

Indications:

- Symptomatic bradycardia caused by vagal stimulation or primary AV block
- Toxins/overdose (e.g., organophosphate, carbamate)
- Rapid sequence intubation (RSI) (i.e., age <1 year, age 1 to 5 years receiving succinylcholine, age >5 years receiving second dose of succinylcholine)

Available Forms: Injection: 0.05, 0.1, 0.4, 1 mg/mL

Dose and Administration:

Symptomatic Bradycardia	
IV/IO	0.02 mg/kg (minimum dose 0.1 mg, maximum single dose 0.5 mg). May repeat dose once (maximum total dose for child 1 mg; maximum total dose for adolescent 3 mg). Larger doses may be needed for treatment of organophosphate poisoning.
ET	0.04 to 0.06 mg/kg

Toxins/Overdose (e.g., Organophosphate, Carbamate)		
IV/IO	<12 years	0.02 to 0.05 mg/kg initially, then repeated every 20 to 30 minutes until muscarinic symptoms reverse
	>12 years	2 mg initially, then 1 to 2 mg every 20 to 30 minutes until muscarinic symptoms reverse

RSI	
IV/IO	0.01 to 0.02 mg/kg (minimum dose 0.1 mg, maximum dose 0.5 mg)
IM	0.02 mg/kg

Action:

- Blocks acetylcholine and other muscarinic agonists at parasympathetic neuroeffector sites
- Increases heart rate and cardiac output by blocking vagal stimulation
- Reduces saliva production and increases saliva viscosity
- Causes mydriasis

Pharmacokinetics:

Absorption	(Not applicable with IV/IO route of administration)
Distribution	Crosses blood-brain barrier
Metabolism	Liver
Excretion	Urine, unchanged (70% to 90%)
Half-life	2 to 3 hours (6.9 ± 3 hours if age <2 years)

Pharmacodynamics:

IV/IO

- Onset—2 to 4 minutes
- Peak—2 to 4 minutes
- Duration—2 to 6 hours

Monitoring: Monitor ECG, SpO$_2$, and blood pressure continuously.

Adverse Effects:

CNS	Headache, dizziness, involuntary movement, confusion, psychosis, anxiety, coma, flushing, drowsiness, weakness
EENT	Blurred vision, photophobia, glaucoma, eye pain, pupil dilation, nasal congestion, dry mouth, altered taste
CV	Tachycardia, hypotension, paradoxical bradycardia, angina, premature ventricular contractions, hypertension
GI	Nausea, vomiting, abdominal pain, constipation, paralytic ileus, abdominal distention
GU	Urinary retention, dysuria
SKIN	Rash, urticaria, contact dermatitis, dry skin, flushing, decreased sweating

(continued)

Atropine (continued)

Precautions:

- Doses <0.1 mg may cause paradoxical bradycardia.
- Document clearly if used for patients with head injury because atropine causes the pupils to dilate.

Contraindications: Angle closure glaucoma, tachyarrhythmias, thyrotoxicosis

Special Considerations:

- Blocks bradycardic response to hypoxia. Monitor SpO_2 with pulse oximetry.
- Administer if bradycardia present before intubation.
- Consider for prevention of excessive secretions associated with ketamine administration.
- Consider for prevention of succinylcholine-induced bradycardia in infants and young children.

Calcium Chloride

Classification: Electrolyte

Indications:

- Hypocalcemia
- Hyperkalemia
- Consider for treatment of hypermagnesemia
- Consider for treatment of calcium channel blocker overdose

Available Forms: Injection: 100 mg/mL (10%)

Dose and Administration:

Hypocalcemia, Hyperkalemia, Hypermagnesemia, Calcium Channel Blocker Overdose	
IV/IO	• For cardiac arrest: 20 mg/kg (0.2 mL/kg) IV/IO bolus into a central venous line if available; may repeat if documented or suspected clinical indications persist. • In a nonarrest situation: Infuse over 30 to 60 minutes into a central line if available.

Actions:

- For maintenance of nervous, muscular, and skeletal function; enzyme reactions; cardiac contractility; and coagulation.
- Affects secretory activity of endocrine and exocrine glands.

Pharmacokinetics:

Absorption	(Not applicable with IV/IO route of administration)
Distribution	Extracellular
Metabolism	Liver, bone uptake
Excretion	Feces (80%), urine (20%)
Half-life	Unknown

Pharmacodynamics:

IV/IO

- Onset—Immediate
- Peak—Rapid
- Duration—Variable

Monitoring: Monitor ECG continuously and blood pressure frequently.

Adverse Effects:

CV	Hypotension, bradycardia, asystole, shortened QT interval, heart block, cardiac arrest
SKIN	Sclerosis of peripheral veins, venous thrombosis, burn/necrosis from extravasation
ELECT	Hypercalcemia

Precautions:

- Do not use routinely during cardiac arrest (may contribute to cellular injury).
- Avoid rapid administration except during cardiac arrest.

Contraindications: Hypercalcemia, digitalis toxicity

Special Considerations:

- A 20 mg/kg dose of calcium chloride 10% (0.2 mL/kg) IV or IO provides 5.4 mg/kg of elemental calcium. If only calcium gluconate is available, the equivalent dose is 0.6 mL/kg of a 10% solution (60 mg/kg).
- Central venous administration is preferred if available.
- When infusing calcium and sodium bicarbonate, flush the tubing with NS before and after infusion of each drug to avoid formation of an insoluble precipitate in the catheter lumen.

Dexamethasone

Classification: Corticosteroid

Indications:

- Croup
- Asthma

Available Forms:

- Injection: 4, 10 mg/mL
- Elixir: 0.5 mg/5 mL
- Oral solution: 0.1, 1 mg/mL

Dose and Administration:

Croup	
PO/IM/IV	0.6 mg/kg × 1 dose (maximum dose 16 mg)

Asthma	
PO/IM/IV	0.6 mg/kg every 24 hours (maximum dose 16 mg)

Actions:

- Widespread effects on inflammatory response
- Increases expression of β-adrenergic receptors to improve catecholamine responsiveness

Pharmacokinetics:

Absorption	Rapid absorption through oral and IM routes (not applicable with IV route of administration)
Distribution	Wide distribution; acts at intracellular receptor
Metabolism	Liver
Excretion	Urine, bile/feces
Half-life	3 to 4½ hours for clearance; pharmacologic effect is much longer

Pharmacodynamics:

	PO	IM
Onset	1 hour	<1 hour
Peak	1 to 2 hours	8 hours
Duration	2½ days	6 days

Adverse Effects:

CNS	Depression, headache, irritability, insomnia, euphoria, seizures, psychosis, hallucinations, weakness
EENT	Fungal infections, increased intraocular pressure, blurred vision
CV	Hypertension, thrombophlebitis, embolism, tachycardia, edema
GI	Diarrhea, nausea, abdominal distention, pancreatitis, gastrointestinal bleeding
MS	Fractures, osteoporosis
SKIN	Flushing, sweating, acne, poor wound healing, ecchymosis, petechiae, hirsutism
ENDO	Hypothalamic-pituitary-adrenal axis suppression, hyperglycemia, sodium and fluid retention
HEME	Hemorrhage, thrombocytopenia
ELECT	Hypokalemia

Dextrose (Glucose)

Classification: Carbohydrate

Indications: Hypoglycemia (documented or strongly suspected)

Available Forms: Injection: $D_{10}W$ (0.1 g/mL), $D_{25}W$ (0.25 g/mL), $D_{50}W$ (0.5 g/mL)

Dose and Administration:

Hypoglycemia	
IV/IO	0.5 to 1 g/kg
Concentration	**Dose**
$D_{50}W$	1 to 2 mL/kg
$D_{25}W$	2 to 4 mL/kg
$D_{10}W$	5 to 10 mL/kg

Action: Increases blood glucose providing substrate for metabolism.

Monitoring: Use point-of-care glucose test to confirm suspicion of hypoglycemia and monitor response to therapy.

Adverse Effects:

SKIN	Sclerosis of veins (with hypertonic glucose concentrations)
ENDO	Hyperglycemia, hyperosmolarity

Precautions: Do not administer routinely during resuscitation unless hypoglycemia is documented.

Special Considerations:

- Follow bolus of glucose with continuous infusion if continued therapy indicated.
- Maximum recommended concentration for bolus administration is $D_{25}W$ (can be prepared by mixing $D_{50}W$ 1:1 with sterile water or NS).
- Maximum concentration for newborn administration is $D_{12.5}W$ (0.125 g/mL).

Diphenhydramine

Classification: Antihistamine

Indications: Anaphylaxis (after administration of epinephrine)

Available Forms: Injection: 10, 50 mg/mL

Dose and Administration:

Anaphylactic Shock	
IV/IO/IM	1 to 2 mg/kg every 4 to 6 hours (maximum dose 50 mg)

Actions:

- Competes with histamine for H_1-receptor sites
- Decreases allergic response by blocking histamine

Pharmacokinetics:

Absorption	(Not applicable with IV/IO route of administration)
Distribution	Wide
Metabolism	Liver (95%)
Excretion	Urine
Half-life	2 to 8 hours

Pharmacodynamics:

	IM	IV/IO
Onset	30 minutes	Immediate
Peak	1 to 4 hours	Unknown
Duration	4 to 8 hours	4 to 8 hours

Monitoring: Monitor SpO_2 continuously and blood pressure frequently.

Adverse Effects:

CNS	Dizziness, drowsiness, poor coordination, fatigue, anxiety, euphoria, confusion, paresthesia, neuritis, seizures, dystonic reaction, hallucinations, sedation (can cause paradoxical excitation in children)
EENT	Blurred vision, pupil dilation, tinnitus, nasal stuffiness, dry nose/mouth/throat
CV	Hypotension, palpitations, tachycardia
RESP	Chest tightness
GI	Nausea, vomiting, diarrhea
GU	Urinary retention, dysuria, frequency
SKIN	Photosensitivity, rash
HEME	Thrombocytopenia, agranulocytosis, hemolytic anemia
MISC	Anaphylaxis

Precautions: Drug may exacerbate angle closure glaucoma, hyperthyroidism, peptic ulcer, and urinary tract obstruction.

Dobutamine

Classification: Selective β_1-adrenergic agent

Indications: Ventricular dysfunction

Available Forms:

- Injection: 12.5 mg/mL
- Premixed dilutions: 1 mg/mL, 2 mg/mL, 4 mg/mL

Dose and Administration:

Congestive Heart Failure, Cardiogenic Shock	
IV/IO	2 to 20 mcg/kg per minute infusion (titrate to desired response)

Actions:

- Stimulates β_1-receptors (predominant effect)
  - Increases heart rate (sinoatrial node effect)
  - Increases myocardial contractility, automaticity, and conduction velocity (ventricular effect)
- Stimulates β_2-receptors, producing increased heart rate and vasodilation
- Because dobutamine has intrinsic α-adrenergic blocking effects, it increases risk of hypotension in patients with shock complicated by excessive vasodilation (e.g., septic shock)

Pharmacokinetics:

Absorption	(Not applicable with IV/IO route of administration)
Distribution	Extracellular fluid
Metabolism	Liver, kidney
Excretion	Urine
Half-life	2 minutes

Pharmacodynamics:

IV/IO

- Onset—1 to 2 minutes
- Peak—10 minutes
- Duration—<10 minutes when infusion stopped

Monitoring: Monitor ECG continuously and blood pressure frequently.

Adverse Effects:

CNS	Anxiety, headache, dizziness
CV	Hypotension, hypertension, palpitations, tachyarrhythmias, premature ventricular contractions, angina
GI	Nausea, vomiting, mucositis
HEME	Thrombocytopenia

Precautions:

- Do not mix with sodium bicarbonate.
- May produce or exacerbate hypotension.
- May produce tachyarrhythmias.

Special Considerations:

- May be given via peripheral IV.
- Drug is inactivated in alkaline solutions.

Dopamine

Classification: Catecholamine, vasopressor, inotrope

Indications:

- Ventricular dysfunction, including cardiogenic shock
- Distributive shock

Available Forms:

- Injection: 40, 80, 160 mg/mL
- Prediluted in D_5W: 0.8, 1.6, 3.2 mg/mL

Dose and Administration:

Cardiogenic Shock, Distributive Shock	
IV/IO	2 to 20 mcg/kg per minute infusion (titrate to desired response)

Actions:

- Stimulates α-adrenergic receptors (>15 mcg/kg per minute)
  - Increases SVR via constriction of arterioles
- Stimulates $β_1$-adrenergic receptors (5 to 15 mcg/kg per minute)
  - Increases heart rate (sinoatrial node effect)
  - Increases myocardial contractility, automaticity, and conduction velocity (ventricular effect)
- Stimulates $β_2$-adrenergic receptors (5 to 15 mcg/kg per minute)
  - Increases heart rate
  - Decreases SVR

Pharmacokinetics:

Absorption	(Not applicable with IV/IO route of administration)
Distribution	Extracellular space
Metabolism	Liver, kidney, plasma
Excretion	Urine
Half-life	2 minutes

Pharmacodynamics:

IV/IO

- Onset—1 to 2 minutes
- Peak—10 minutes
- Duration—<10 minutes after infusion is stopped

Monitoring: Monitor ECG continuously and blood pressure frequently.

Adverse Effects:

CNS	Headache
RESP	Dyspnea
CV	Palpitations, premature ventricular contractions, SVT, VT, hypertension, peripheral vasoconstriction
GI	Nausea, vomiting, diarrhea
GU	Acute renal failure
SKIN	Local necrosis (with infiltration), gangrene

Precautions:

- High infusion rates (>20 mcg/kg per minute) produce peripheral, renal, and splanchnic vasoconstriction and ischemia; if infusion dose >20 mcg/kg per minute is required, consider addition of alternative adrenergic agent (e.g., epinephrine/norepinephrine).
- Do not mix with sodium bicarbonate.
- Tissue ischemia and necrosis may result if IV infiltration occurs. Infiltration with phentolamine may reduce local toxic effect of dopamine.

Special Considerations:

- Central venous administration is preferred.
- Inactivated in alkaline solutions.

Epinephrine

Classification: Catecholamine, vasopressor, inotrope

Indications:

- Anaphylaxis
- Asthma (when more selective β_2-agonists are not available)
- Bradycardia (symptomatic)
- Croup (nebulized)
- Cardiac arrest
- Shock
- Toxins/overdose (e.g., β-adrenergic blocker, calcium channel blocker)

Available Forms:

- Injection: **1:1000*** aqueous (1 mg/mL), 1:10 000 aqueous (0.1 mg/mL)
  Note: *On this page 1:1000 dilution is bold to differentiate this dilution from the standard 1:10 000 dilution.
- IM autoinjector: 0.15 mg, 0.3 mg
- Racemic solution: 2.25%

Dose and Administration:

Anaphylaxis	
IM	• 0.01 mg/kg (0.01 mL/kg of **1:1000**) every 15 minutes PRN (maximum dose 0.3 mg) *or* • IM autoinjector 0.3 mg (for patient weighing ≥30 kg) or IM junior autoinjector 0.15 mg (for patient weighing 10 to 30 kg)
IV/IO	• 0.01 mg/kg (0.1 mL/kg of 1:10 000) every 3 to 5 minutes (maximum dose 1 mg) if hypotension is present • If hypotension persists despite fluid administration and bolus injection, consider continuous infusion of 0.1 to 1 mcg/kg per minute

Asthma	
Subcutaneous	0.01 mg/kg (0.01 mL/kg of **1:1000**) every 15 minutes (maximum dose 0.3 mg)

Bradycardia (Symptomatic)	
IV/IO	0.01 mg/kg (0.1 mL/kg of 1:10 000) every 3 to 5 minutes (maximum dose 1 mg)

Croup	
Nebulizer	• 0.25 mL racemic solution (2.25%) mixed in 3 mL NS by inhaled nebulizer for moderate to severe illness (i.e., stridor at rest) in infants or young children; up to 0.5 mL mixed in 3 mL NS for older children *or* • 0.5 mL/kg of **1:1000** epinephrine, maximum of 5 mL, dilute in 3 mL NS; this dose is approximately equal to 0.25 mL of racemic solution

Cardiac Arrest	
IO/IV	0.01 mg/kg (0.1 mL/kg of 1:10 000) every 3 to 5 minutes (maximum dose 1 mg)
ET tube	0.1 mg/kg (0.1 mL/kg of **1:1000**) endotracheally every 3 to 5 minutes

Shock	
IV/IO infusion	0.1 to 1 mcg/kg per minute infusion (consider higher doses if needed)

Toxins/Overdose (e.g., β-Adrenergic Blocker, Calcium Channel Blocker)	
IV/IO	0.01 mg/kg (0.1 mL/kg of 1:10 000) (maximum dose 1 mg); if no response, consider higher doses up to 0.1 mg/kg (0.1 mL/kg of **1:1000**)
IV/IO infusion	0.1 to 1 mcg/kg per minute infusion (consider higher doses if hypotension refractory to this dose)

(continued)

Epinephrine (continued)

Actions:

- α-Adrenergic receptor stimulation is dose and age dependent.
- Stimulates β_1-adrenergic receptors
  - Increases heart rate, myocardial contractility, automaticity, and conduction velocity
- Stimulates β_2-adrenergic receptors (predominance at lower doses will be patient specific)
  - Increases heart rate
  - Causes bronchodilation
  - Causes dilation of arterioles (decreases diastolic blood pressure)

Pharmacokinetics:

Absorption	IM absorption is affected by perfusion (not applicable with IV/IO route of administration)
Distribution	Unknown
Metabolism	Liver, kidney, endothelium
Excretion	Unknown
Half-life	2 to 4 minutes

Pharmacodynamics:

	IM	**IV/IO**	**Inhalation**
Onset	5 to 10 minutes	Immediate	1 minute
Peak	Unknown	Within 1 minute	Unknown

Monitoring: Monitor ECG and SpO_2 continuously and blood pressure frequently.

Adverse Effects:

CNS	Tremors, anxiety, insomnia, headache, dizziness, weakness, drowsiness, confusion, hallucinations, intracranial hemorrhage (from severe hypertension)
RESP	Dyspnea
CV	Arrhythmias (especially tachyarrhythmias, e.g., SVT and VT), palpitations, tachycardia, hypertension, ST-segment elevation, postresuscitation myocardial dysfunction
GI	Nausea, vomiting
GU	Renal vascular ischemia
ENDO	Hyperglycemia, postresuscitation hyperadrenergic state
ELECT	Hypokalemia (β_2-adrenergic stimulation causes intracellular potassium shift)
MISC	Gluconeogenesis response increases serum lactate independent of any change in organ perfusion, making interpretation of serum lactate as a marker of ischemia more difficult

Precautions:

- High doses produce vasoconstriction and may compromise organ perfusion.
- Low doses may increase cardiac output with redirection of blood flow to skeletal muscles, producing decreased renal and splanchnic blood flow.
- Myocardial O_2 requirements are increased (as the result of increased heart rate, myocardial contractility, and, with higher doses, increased SVR).
- Tissue ischemia and necrosis may result if IV infiltration occurs. Infiltration with phentolamine may reduce local toxic effect of epinephrine.
- Central venous access is preferred for administration.
- Catecholamines are inactivated in alkaline solutions.
- Observe at least 2 hours after croup treatment for "rebound" (i.e., recurrence of stridor).

Contraindications: Cocaine-induced VT

Special Considerations: When given IM in anaphylaxis, best absorption occurs from injection in thigh rather than deltoid muscle. Subcutaneous administration is not recommended for treatment of anaphylaxis because absorption is delayed.

Etomidate

Classification: Ultrashort-acting nonbarbiturate, nonbenzodiazepine sedative-hypnotic agent with no analgesic properties

Indications:

- Sedation for rapid sequence intubation (RSI)
- Sedative of choice for patients with hypotension, cardiovascular disease, and multiple trauma. Agent of choice for intubation of patients with head injuries.

Available Forms: Injection: 2 mg/mL

Dose and Administration:

RSI	0.2 to 0.4 mg/kg IV/IO (maximum 20 mg) infused over 30 to 60 seconds produces rapid sedation that lasts 10 to 15 minutes

Actions:

- Ultrashort-acting nonbarbiturate, nonbenzodiazepine sedative-hypnotic agent
- No analgesic properties
- Decreases intracranial pressure, cerebral blood flow, and cerebral basal metabolic rate

Pharmacokinetics:

Absorption	(Not applicable with IV/IO route of administration)
Excretion	Hepatic and plasma esterases
Half-life	2.6 hours

Pharmacodynamics:

IV/IO

- Onset—30 to 60 seconds
- Peak—1 minute
- Duration—10 to 15 minutes

Monitoring: Monitor SpO$_2$, respiratory function, and blood pressure frequently.

Adverse Effects:

RESP	Hypoventilation or hyperventilation
CV	Hypotension or hypertension, tachycardia
GI	Nausea, vomiting on emergence from anesthesia, myoclonic activity (coughing, hiccups)
ENDO	Adrenal suppression
MISC	Myoclonus, uncontrolled eye movements, pain at injection site

Precautions:

- May suppress cortisol production after a single dose. Consider administration of stress dose hydrocortisone (2 mg/kg; maximum dose 100 mg).
- Avoid routine use in septic shock.
- May also cause myoclonic activity (coughing, hiccups) and may exacerbate focal seizure disorders.
- Relative contraindications include known adrenal insufficiency or history of focal seizure disorder.
- Contains propylene glycol.

Special Considerations:

- Produces rapid sedation with minimal cardiovascular or respiratory depression.
- Because the drug may cause possible adrenal suppression, should not be used to maintain sedation after intubation.
- Use of benzodiazepines or opioids may decrease myoclonus.

Furosemide

Classification: Loop diuretic

Indications:

- Pulmonary edema
- Fluid overload

Available Forms: Injection: 10 mg/mL

Dose and Administration:

Pulmonary Edema, Fluid Overload	
IV/IM	1 mg/kg (typical maximum dose 20 mg for patient not chronically on loop diuretics)

Actions:

- Acts on ascending limb of loop of Henle, inhibiting reabsorption of sodium and chloride, causing excretion of sodium, chloride, calcium, magnesium, and water; increased potassium excretion occurs in distal tubule in exchange for sodium
- Increases excretion of potassium in distal tubule as indirect effect

Pharmacokinetics:

Absorption	IM absorption not documented (not applicable with IV/IO route of administration)
Distribution	Unknown
Metabolism	Liver (30% to 40%); most excreted unchanged in urine
Excretion	Urine, feces
Half-life	½ to 1 hour

Pharmacodynamics:

	PO	IM	IV
Onset	½ to 1 hour	½ hour	5 minutes
Peak	1 to 2 hours	Unknown	½ hour
Duration	6 to 8 hours	4 to 8 hours	2 hours

Monitoring:

- Monitor blood pressure frequently.
- Monitor serum creatinine, BUN, and electrolytes, especially potassium.

Adverse Effects:

CNS	Headache, fatigue, weakness, vertigo, paresthesias
EENT	Hearing loss, tinnitus, blurred vision, dry mouth, oral irritation
CV	Orthostatic hypotension, angina, ECG changes (from electrolyte abnormalities), circulatory collapse
GI	Nausea, vomiting, diarrhea, abdominal cramps, gastric irritation, pancreatitis
GU	Polyuria, renal failure, glycosuria
MS	Muscle cramps, stiffness
SKIN	Pruritus, purpura, Stevens-Johnson syndrome, sweating, photosensitivity, urticaria
ENDO	Hyperglycemia
HEME	Thrombocytopenia, agranulocytosis, leukopenia, anemia, neutropenia
ELECT	Hypokalemia, hypochloremia, hypomagnesemia, hyperuricemia, hypocalcemia, hyponatremia
MISC	Metabolic alkalosis

Special Considerations: Hypokalemia may be significant and requires close monitoring and replacement therapy.

Hydrocortisone

Classification: Corticosteroid

Indications: Adrenal insufficiency (may be associated with septic shock)

Available Forms: Sodium succinate injectable in 100, 250, 500, 1000 mg/vial

Dose and Administration:

Adrenal Insufficiency	
IV/IO	2 mg/kg bolus (maximum dose 100 mg)

Actions:

- Widespread effects on inflammatory response
- Increases expression of β-adrenergic receptors to improve catecholamine responsiveness

Pharmacokinetics:

Absorption	(Not applicable with IV/IO route of administration)
Distribution	Widely distributed; acts at intracellular receptor
Metabolism	Liver (extensive)
Excretion	Urine
Half-life	3 to 5 hours

Pharmacodynamics:

IV/IO

- Onset—Rapid
- Peak—Unknown
- Duration—8 to 24 hours

Adverse Effects:

CNS	Depression, headache, mood changes
EENT	Fungal infections, increased intraocular pressure, blurred vision
CV	Hypertension
GI	Diarrhea, nausea, abdominal distention, peptic ulcer
MS	Fractures, osteoporosis, weakness
SKIN	Flushing, sweating, thrombophlebitis, edema, acne, poor wound healing, ecchymosis, petechiae, pruritus
ENDO	Hyperglycemia, suppression of hypothalamic-pituitary axis
MISC	Increased risk of infection

Ipratropium Bromide

Classification: Anticholinergic, bronchodilator

Indications: Asthma

Available Forms:

- Nebulized solution: 0.02% (500 mcg/2.5 mL)
- MDI: 17 mcg/puff

Dose and Administration:

Asthma	
Nebulizer	250 to 500 mcg (inhaled) every 20 minutes × 3 doses

Actions:

- Blocks action of acetylcholine at parasympathetic sites in bronchial smooth muscle, resulting in bronchodilation
- Inhibits secretions from serous and seromucous glands lining the nasal mucosa

Pharmacokinetics:

Absorption	Minimal
Distribution	Does not cross blood-brain barrier
Metabolism	Liver (minimal)
Excretion	Unknown
Half-life	2 hours

Pharmacodynamics:

Inhalation

- Onset—1 to 15 minutes
- Peak—1 to 2 hours
- Duration—3 to 6 hours

Monitoring: Monitor SpO_2 continuously.

Adverse Effects:

CNS	Anxiety, dizziness, headache, nervousness
EENT	Dry mouth, blurred vision (pupil dilation)
RESP	Cough, worsening bronchospasm
CV	Palpitations
GI	Nausea, vomiting, abdominal cramps
SKIN	Rash

Special Considerations:

- Ipratropium is not absorbed into the bloodstream; its cardiovascular side effects are minimal.
- Nebulized ipratropium may cause pupil dilation if the nebulized solution enters the eyes.

Lidocaine

Classification: Antiarrhythmic (Class IB)

Indications:

- VF/pulseless VT
- Wide-complex tachycardia (with pulses)
- Rapid sequence intubation (RSI): Administer before laryngoscopy to blunt increase in intracranial pressure (ICP)

Available Forms:

- Injection: 0.5%, 1%, 2%
- Premixed injection in D_5W: 0.4% (4 mg/mL), 0.8% (8 mg/mL)

Dose and Administration:

VF/Pulseless VT, Wide-Complex Tachycardia (With Pulses)		
IV/IO	Initial	1 mg/kg loading bolus; repeat bolus dose if infusion initiated more than 15 minutes after initial bolus
	Maintenance	20 to 50 mcg/kg per minute infusion (to follow bolus therapy)
ET	2 to 3 mg/kg	
RSI		
IV/IO	1 to 2 mg/kg	

Actions:

- Increases electrical stimulation threshold of ventricle and His-Purkinje system (stabilizing cardiac membrane and decreasing automaticity)
- Reduces ICP through inhibition of sodium channels in neurons, which reduces metabolic activity

Pharmacokinetics:

Absorption	(Not applicable with IV/IO administration)
Distribution	Erythrocytes, vascular endothelium
Metabolism	Liver, active metabolites
Excretion	Urine
Half-life	Biphasic (8 minutes, 1 to 3 hours)

Pharmacodynamics:

IV/IO

- Onset—1 to 2 minutes
- Peak—Unknown
- Duration—10 to 20 minutes because of rapid redistribution; terminal elimination 1½ to 2 hours

Monitoring: Monitor ECG continuously and blood pressure frequently.

Adverse Effects:

CNS	Seizures (high concentrations), headache, dizziness, involuntary movement, confusion, tremor, drowsiness, euphoria
EENT	Tinnitus, blurred vision
CV	Hypotension, myocardial depression, bradycardia, heart block, arrhythmias, cardiac arrest
RESP	Dyspnea, respiratory depression or arrest
GI	Nausea, vomiting
SKIN	Rash, urticaria, edema, swelling, phlebitis at IV site

Precautions: High plasma concentration may cause myocardial and circulatory depression and CNS complications (seizures).

Contraindication: Wide-complex ventricular escape beats associated with bradycardia.

Special Considerations:

- Reduce infusion dose if severe CHF or low cardiac output is compromising hepatic and renal blood flow.
- Drug may decrease ICP response during laryngoscopy.
- Drug attenuates intraocular pressure response during laryngoscopy.

Magnesium Sulfate

Classification: Electrolyte, bronchodilator

Indications:

- Asthma (refractory status asthmaticus)
- Torsades de pointes
- Hypomagnesemia

Available Forms:

- Injection: 500 mg/mL (4.06 mEq/mL)
- Premixed in D_5W: 10 mg/mL (0.08 mEq/mL), 20 mg/mL (0.16 mEq/mL)
- Premixed in sterile water for injection: 40 mg/mL (0.65 mEq/mL)

Dose and Administration:

Asthma (Refractory Status Asthmaticus), Torsades de Pointes, Hypomagnesemia	
IV/IO	• Status asthmaticus: 25 to 50 mg/kg by slow infusion (15 to 30 minutes) (maximum dose 2 g) • Pulseless VT with torsades: 25 to 50 mg/kg bolus (maximum dose 2 g) • VT with pulses associated with torsades or hypomagnesemia: 25 to 50 mg/kg over 10 to 20 minutes (maximum dose 2 g)

Actions:

- Smooth muscle relaxation
- Antiarrhythmic

Pharmacokinetics:

Absorption	(Not applicable with IV/IO route of administration)
Distribution	Wide
Metabolism	Taken up by cells and bone
Excretion	Urine
Half-life	Unknown

Pharmacodynamics:

IV/IO

- Onset—Immediate
- Peak—Depends on duration of infusion
- Duration—30 minutes

Monitoring: Monitor ECG and SpO_2 continuously and blood pressure frequently.

Adverse Effects (Most Are Related to Hypermagnesemia):

CNS	Confusion, sedation, depressed reflexes, flaccid paralysis, weakness
RESP	Respiratory depression
CV	Hypotension, bradycardia, heart block, cardiac arrest (may develop with rapid administration)
GI	Nausea, vomiting
MS	Cramps
SKIN	Flushing, sweating
ELECT	Hypermagnesemia

Precautions: Rapid bolus may cause severe hypotension and bradycardia.

Contraindication: Renal failure

Special Considerations: Have calcium chloride (or calcium gluconate) available if needed to reverse magnesium toxicity.

Methylprednisolone

Classification: Corticosteroid

Indications:

- Asthma (status asthmaticus)
- Anaphylactic shock

Available Forms: Injection: 40, 125, 500, 1000, 2000 mg

Dose and Administration: (For IV use sodium succinate salt)

Asthma (Status Asthmaticus), Anaphylactic Shock		
IV/IO/IM	Load	2 mg/kg (maximum 60 mg)
IV	Maintenance	0.5 mg/kg every 6 hours or 1 mg/kg every 12 hours up to 120 mg/day

Actions:

- Widespread effects on inflammatory response
- Increases expression of β-adrenergic receptors to improve catecholamine responsiveness

Pharmacokinetics:

Absorption	(Not applicable with IV/IO route of administration)
Distribution	Wide distribution; binds to intracellular steroid receptor
Metabolism	Liver (extensive)
Excretion	Urine
Half-life	3 to 5 hours for clearance; duration of effect is longer

Pharmacodynamics:

IV/IO

- Onset—Rapid
- Peak—Unknown
- Duration—1 to 2 days

Adverse Effects:

CNS	Depression, headache, mood changes, weakness
CV	Hypertension
GI	Hemorrhage, diarrhea, nausea, abdominal distention, pancreatitis, peptic ulcer
MS	Fractures, osteoporosis, arthralgia
ENDO	Hyperglycemia
HEME	Transient leukocytosis
MISC	Anaphylaxis (rare)

Milrinone

Classification: Phosphodiesterase inhibitor, inodilator

Indications: Myocardial dysfunction with increased systemic vascular resistance (SVR)/pulmonary vascular resistance (PVR) (e.g., cardiogenic shock with high SVR, post–cardiac surgery CHF)

Available Forms:

- Injection: 1 mg/mL
- Premixed injection in D_5W: 200 mcg/mL

Dose and Administration:

Myocardial Dysfunction and Increased SVR/PVR	
IV/IO	• Loading dose of 50 mcg/kg IV/IO over 10 to 60 minutes (give over longer period if patient is unstable) • Maintenance dose (continuous IV infusion): 0.25 to 0.75 mcg/kg per minute

Actions:

- Increases myocardial contractility
- Reduces preload and afterload through relaxation of vascular smooth muscle

Pharmacokinetics:

Absorption	(Not applicable with IV/IO route of administration)
Distribution	Unknown
Metabolism	Liver (12%)
Excretion	Urine, unchanged (83%), metabolites (12%)
Half-life	Mean 2.4 hours

Pharmacodynamics:

IV/IO

- Onset—2 to 5 minutes
- Peak—10 minutes
- Duration—Variable (1½ to 5 hours)

Monitoring:

- Monitor ECG continuously and blood pressure frequently.
- Monitor platelet count.

Adverse Effects:

CNS	Headache, tremor
CV	Hypotension, ventricular arrhythmias, angina
GI	Nausea, vomiting, abdominal pain, hepatotoxicity, jaundice
HEME	Thrombocytopenia
ELECT	Hypokalemia

Precautions:

- Hypovolemia may worsen hypotensive effects.
- May accumulate in renal failure and in patients with low cardiac output.
- Avoid in patients with ventricular outflow tract obstruction.

Special Considerations: Use of a longer infusion time to administer loading dose reduces the risk of hypotension.

Naloxone

Classification: Opioid receptor antagonist

Indications: Narcotic (opiate) reversal

Available Forms: Injection: 0.4, 1 mg/mL

Dose and Administration:

Narcotic (Opiate) Reversal

Note: Total reversal is indicated for narcotic toxicity secondary to overdose; significantly smaller doses are required for patients with respiratory depression associated with therapeutic narcotic use.

- Total reversal: 0.1 mg/kg IV/IO/IM/subcutaneous bolus every 2 minutes (maximum dose 2 mg)
- Total reversal not required: 1 to 5 mcg/kg IV/IO/IM/subcutaneous (titrate to response)
- Continuous IV/IO infusion: 0.002 to 0.16 mg/kg per hour (2 to 160 mcg/kg per hour)

Action: Competes with opiates at opioid receptor sites (reversing opioid effects)

Pharmacokinetics:

Absorption	Rapid absorption after IM, subcutaneous administration (not applicable with IV/IO route of administration)
Distribution	Rapid
Metabolism	Liver
Excretion	Urine
Half-life	1 hour (up to 3 hours in neonates)

Pharmacodynamics:

IV/IO

- Onset—1 to 2 minutes
- Peak—Unknown
- Duration—20 to 60 minutes (variable and dose dependent)

Monitoring: Monitor ECG and SpO_2 continuously and blood pressure frequently.

Adverse Effects:

CNS	Seizures, drowsiness, nervousness
RESP	Hyperpnea, pulmonary edema
CV	VF/VT, tachycardia, hypertension, asystole (especially if total reversal dose administered)
GI	Nausea, vomiting

Precautions:

- Repeat dosing is often required because half-life of naloxone is often shorter than half-life of opioid being reversed.
- Administration to newborns of addicted mothers may precipitate seizures or other withdrawal symptoms.
- In overdose patients, establish effective assisted ventilation before administration of naloxone to avoid excessive sympathetic nervous system stimulation.
- Consider administration of nonopioid analgesics for treatment of pain.

Special Considerations: Drug exerts some analgesic effects.

Nitroglycerin

Classification: Vasodilator, antihypertensive

Indications:

- Congestive heart failure
- Cardiogenic shock

Available Forms:

- Injection: 5 mg/mL
- Prediluted injection in D_5W: 100 mcg/mL, 200 mcg/mL, 400 mcg/mL

Dose and Administration:

Congestive Heart Failure, Cardiogenic Shock	
IV/IO	• Initiate at 0.25 to 0.5 mcg/kg per minute infusion; titrate by 1 mcg/kg per minute every 15 to 20 minutes as tolerated. Typical dose range is 1 to 5 mcg/kg per minute (maximum dose 10 mcg/kg per minute).
	• In adolescents, start with 5 to 10 mcg per minute (*note:* this dose is **not** per kilogram per minute) and increase to maximum of 200 mcg *per minute.*

Action: Releases nitric oxide, which stimulates cyclic guanosine monophosphate (cGMP) production; cGMP is an intracellular messenger that results in vascular smooth muscle relaxation. Action is greatest in venous system and pulmonary vascular bed with relatively less effect on systemic vascular resistance.

Pharmacokinetics:

Absorption	(Not applicable with IV/IO route of administration)
Distribution	Unknown
Metabolism	Liver (extensive); no active metabolites
Excretion	Urine
Half-life	1 to 4 minutes

Pharmacodynamics:

IV/IO

- Onset—1 to 2 minutes
- Peak—Unknown
- Duration—3 to 5 minutes

Monitoring: Monitor ECG continuously and blood pressure frequently.

Adverse Effects:

CNS	Headache, dizziness
RESP	Hypoxemia (due to increased V/Q mismatch)
CV	Postural hypotension, tachycardia, cardiac arrest, syncope, paradoxical bradycardia
SKIN	Flushing, pallor, sweating

Precautions: May cause hypotension, especially in hypovolemic patients

Nitroprusside (Sodium Nitroprusside)

Classification: Vasodilator, antihypertensive

Indications:

- Cardiogenic shock (characterized by high SVR)
- Hypertension (severe)

Available Forms: Injection: 25 mg/mL

Dose and Administration:

Cardiogenic Shock (High SVR), Hypertension (Severe)	
IV/IO	0.3 to 1 mcg/kg per minute initial dose; then titrate to desired response up to 8 mcg/kg per minute

Action: Relaxes tone in all vascular beds (arteriolar and venous) through release of nitric oxide. This vasodilation reduces cardiac filling pressures and right and left ventricular afterload.

Pharmacokinetics:

Absorption	(Not applicable with IV/IO route of administration)
Distribution	Extracellular fluid
Metabolism	Endothelial cells and RBCs (to cyanide), then liver (to thiocyanate)
Excretion	Urine (thiocyanate)
Half-life	3 to 7 days (thiocyanate)

Pharmacodynamics:

IV/IO

- Onset—1 to 2 minutes
- Peak—Rapid
- Duration—1 to 10 minutes after stopping infusion

Monitoring:

- Monitor ECG continuously and blood pressure frequently.
- Thiocyanate (should be <50 mg/L) and cyanide (toxic is >2 mcg/mL) levels in patients receiving prolonged infusion, particularly if rate is >2 mcg/kg per minute or in patients with renal dysfunction.

Adverse Effects:

CNS	Seizures (thiocyanate toxicity), dizziness, headache, agitation, decreased reflexes, restlessness
CV	Hypotension, bradycardia, tachycardia
GI	Nausea/vomiting/abdominal cramps (thiocyanate toxicity)
ENDO	Hypothyroidism
MISC	Cyanide and thiocyanate toxicity

Precautions:

- Hypovolemia may worsen hypotensive effect.
- Cyanide and thiocyanate toxicity may result if administered at high rates, for >48 hours, or to patients with decreased hepatic or renal function (drug is metabolized by endothelial cells to cyanide, then metabolized in the liver to thiocyanate, and excreted by the kidneys).

Special Considerations:

- Use special administration tubing or wrap drug reservoir in aluminum foil or another opaque material to protect it from deterioration with exposure to light.
- Use solution immediately after preparation.
- Freshly prepared solution may have a very faint brownish tint without change in drug potency.
- May react with a variety of substances to form highly coloured reaction products.

Norepinephrine

Classification: Inotrope, vasopressor, catecholamine

Indications: Hypotensive shock (i.e., associated with low SVR unresponsive to bolus fluid administration)

Available Forms: Injection: 1 mg/mL

Dose and Administration:

Hypotensive Shock	
IV/IO	0.1 to 2 mcg/kg per minute infusion (titrate to desired change in blood pressure and systemic perfusion)

Actions:

- Activates α-adrenergic receptors (increased smooth muscle tone)
- Activates myocardial β_1-adrenergic receptors (increased contractility and heart rate); the heart rate effect is blunted by baroreceptor stimulation that results from the vasoconstrictive effects

Pharmacokinetics:

Absorption	(Not applicable with IV/IO route of administration)
Distribution	Extracellular space
Metabolism	Liver, kidney, sympathetic nerves
Excretion	Urine
Half-life	2 to 4 minutes

Pharmacodynamics:

IV/IO

- Onset—<30 seconds
- Peak—5 to 10 minutes
- Duration—≤10 minutes after stopping infusion

Monitoring: Monitor ECG continuously and blood pressure frequently.

Adverse Effects:

CNS	Headache, anxiety
RESP	Respiratory distress
CV	Hypertension, tachycardia, bradycardia, arrhythmias
GU	Renal failure
SKIN	Local necrosis (infiltration)

Precautions:

- May produce hypertension, organ ischemia, or arrhythmias.
- Tissue infiltration may produce severe ischemia and necrosis. Infiltration with phentolamine may reduce local toxic effect of norepinephrine.
- Do not mix with sodium bicarbonate.

Special Considerations:

- Ideally should be administered via a central venous catheter.
- Drug is inactivated in alkaline solutions.

Oxygen

Classification: Element, gas

Indications:

- Hypoxia/hypoxemia
- Respiratory distress/respiratory failure
- Shock
- Trauma
- Cardiopulmonary failure
- Cardiac arrest

Available Forms: Flow rates and delivery device affect inspired oxygen concentration.

Dose and Administration:

- Administer 100% O_2 initially via high-flow O_2 delivery system; titrate to response.
- After return of spontaneous circulation (ROSC) following cardiac arrest, maintain oxyhemoglobin saturation 94% to 99% (94% or higher, but below 100%) to minimize risk of oxidative/reperfusion injury.

Actions:

- Increases arterial O_2 saturation
- Increases arterial O_2 content
- May improve tissue O_2 delivery if cardiac output is adequate
- Pulmonary vasodilator

Monitoring: Monitor SpO_2 continuously.

Adverse Effects:

CNS	Headache (high-flow rates)
EENT	Dry mucous membranes (high-flow rates)
RESP	Airway obstruction (due to drying of secretions)
GI	Gastric distention (high-flow rates)

Precautions: Insufficient flow rates delivered via O_2 mask, O_2 hood, and O_2 tent may cause CO_2 retention.

Special Considerations: In children with cyanotic heart defects with single-ventricle physiology (e.g., following surgical palliation before correction of hypoplastic left heart syndrome), use O_2 with caution. In these children the balance of systemic versus pulmonary blood flow can be substantially altered by the effects of O_2 administration on pulmonary vascular resistance (PVR). Seek expert advice, if available, before use.

Procainamide

Classification: Antiarrhythmic (Class IA)

- SVT
- Atrial flutter
- VT (with pulses)

Available Forms: Injection: 100, 500 mg/mL

Dose and Administration:

SVT, Atrial Flutter, VT (With Pulses)	
IV/IO	15 mg/kg load over 30 to 60 minutes

Actions:

- Depresses excitability of cardiac muscle to electrical stimulation
- Slows conduction in atrium, bundle of His, and ventricle
- Increases refractory period

Pharmacokinetics:

Absorption	(Not applicable with IV/IO route of administration)
Distribution	Rapid
Metabolism	Liver to active metabolite, *N*-acetyl procainamide (NAPA)
Excretion	Urine, unchanged (50% to 70%)
Half-life	2.5 to 4.5 hours (procainamide); approximately 6 to 8 hours (NAPA)

Pharmacodynamics:

IV/IO

- Onset—Rapid
- Peak—15 to 60 minutes
- Duration—3 to 6 hours

Monitoring: Monitor ECG continuously with focus on QT interval, and monitor blood pressure frequently.

Adverse Effects:

CNS	Headache, dizziness, confusion, psychosis, restlessness, irritability, weakness
CV	Hypotension, negative inotropic effects, prolonged QT interval, torsades de pointes, heart block, cardiac arrest
GI	Nausea, vomiting, diarrhea, hepatomegaly
SKIN	Rash, urticaria, edema, swelling, pruritus, flushing
HEME	Systemic lupus erythematosus syndrome, agranulocytosis, thrombocytopenia, neutropenia, hemolytic anemia

Precautions:

- Before using for a hemodynamically stable patient, expert consultation is strongly recommended.
- Administration in combination with amiodarone (or other agents that prolong QT interval) is not recommended without expert consultation.
- Risk of hypotension and negative inotropic effects increases with rapid administration.
- Reduce dose for patients with poor renal or cardiac function.

Special Considerations: Monitor procainamide and NAPA concentrations.

Salbutamol

Classification: Bronchodilator, β_2-adrenergic agent

Indications:

- Asthma
- Anaphylaxis (bronchospasm)
- Hyperkalemia

Available Forms:

- Nebulized solution: 0.5% (5 mg/mL)
- Prediluted nebulized solution: 0.63 mg/3 mL NS, 1.25 mg/3 mL NS, 2.5 mg/3 mL NS (0.083%)
- Metered-dose inhaler (MDI): 90 mcg/puff

Dose and Administration:

Asthma, Anaphylaxis (Mild to Moderate), Hyperkalemia		
MDI	4 to 8 puffs (inhalation) every 20 minutes PRN with spacer	
Nebulizer	Weight <20 kg	2.5 mg/dose (inhalation) every 20 minutes PRN
	Weight >20 kg	5 mg/dose (inhalation) every 20 minutes PRN
Asthma, Anaphylaxis (Severe)		
Continuous nebulizer	0.5 mg/kg per hour continuous inhalation (maximum dose 20 mg/h)	
MDI (recommended if intubated)	4 to 8 puffs (inhalation) via ET tube every 20 minutes PRN or with spacer if not intubated	

Action: Stimulates β_2-adrenergic receptors, causing bronchodilation, tachycardia, vasodilation, movement of potassium from extracellular to intracellular space (serum potassium concentration will decrease)

Pharmacokinetics:

Absorption	Well absorbed
Distribution	Unknown
Metabolism	Liver (extensive), tissues
Excretion	Urine
Half-life	3 to 8 hours

Pharmacodynamics:

Inhalation

- Onset—5 to 15 minutes
- Peak—1 to 1½ hours
- Duration—4 to 6 hours

Monitoring:

- Monitor SpO_2, blood pressure, breath sounds, and ECG continuously.
- Consider checking serum potassium concentration, especially if low before administration or if high doses of salbutamol used.

Adverse Effects:

CNS	Tremors, anxiety, insomnia, headache, dizziness, hallucinations
EENT	Dry nose and throat, irritation of nose and throat, bad taste
RESP	Wheezing, dyspnea, bronchospasm, cough (rare)
CV	Palpitations, tachycardia, systolic hypertension with wide pulse pressure, angina, hypotension, tachyarrhythmias
GI	Heartburn, nausea, vomiting, diarrhea
SKIN	Flushing, sweating, angioedema

Contraindications: Tachyarrhythmias, severe cardiac disease, or hypersensitivity to salbutamol or adrenergic amines

Special Considerations:

- May be combined in the same nebulizer with ipratropium bromide
- Increased risk of tachyarrhythmias when combined with theophylline or simultaneous use of other adrenergic agents (e.g., terbutaline, dopamine)

Sodium Bicarbonate

Classification: Alkalinizing agent, electrolyte

Indications:

- Metabolic acidosis (severe)
- Hyperkalemia
- Sodium channel blocker overdose (e.g., tricyclic antidepressant)

Available Forms:

- Injection: 4% (0.48 mEq/mL), 4.2% (0.5 mEq/mL), 7.5% (0.89 mEq/mL), 8.4% (1 mEq/mL)
- Injection (premixed): 5% (0.6 mEq/mL)

Dose and Administration:

Metabolic Acidosis (Severe), Hyperkalemia	
IV/IO	1 mEq/kg *slow* bolus; maximum dose 50 mEq
Sodium Channel Blocker Overdose (e.g., Tricyclic Antidepressant)	
IV/IO	1 to 2 mEq/kg bolus, repeat until serum pH is >7.45 (7.50 to 7.55 for severe poisoning); follow with infusion of 150 mEq $NaHCO_3$/L solution, titrated to maintain alkalosis

Action: Increases plasma bicarbonate, which buffers H^+ ion (reversing metabolic acidosis), forming CO_2; elimination of CO_2 via the respiratory tract increases pH

Pharmacokinetics:

Absorption	(Not applicable with IV/IO route of administration)
Distribution	Wide (extracellular fluid)
Metabolism	Combines with protons; taken up by cells
Excretion	Urine, exhalation as CO_2
Half-life	Unknown

Pharmacodynamics:

IV/IO

- Onset—Rapid
- Peak—Rapid
- Duration—Unknown

Monitoring:

- Monitor SpO_2 and ECG continuously.
- Monitor ABG.

Adverse Effects:

CNS	Irritability, headache, confusion, stimulation, tremors, hyperreflexia, tetany, seizures, weakness
RESP	Respiratory depression, apnea
CV	Arrhythmia, hypotension, cardiac arrest
GI	Abdominal distention, paralytic ileus
GU	Renal calculi
SKIN	Cyanosis, edema, sclerosis/necrosis (infiltration), vasodilation
ELECT	Hypernatremia, hyperosmolarity, hypocalcemia, hypokalemia
MISC	Metabolic alkalosis, weight gain, water retention

Precautions:

- Ensure adequate ventilation because buffering action produces CO_2, which crosses blood-brain barrier and cell membranes more rapidly than HCO_3^-. If ventilation is inadequate, increased CO_2 may result in transient paradoxical CSF and intracellular acidosis.
- Drug may inactivate catecholamines.
- By increasing pH, will produce a decrease in serum potassium and ionized calcium concentrations.
- When combined with calcium salts, will precipitate into insoluble calcium carbonate crystals that may obstruct the IV catheter or tubing.
- Routine administration is not recommended in cardiac arrest.

Special Considerations:

- Drug should not be administered via the endotracheal route.
- Irrigate IV/IO tubing with NS before and after infusion.
- 4.2% concentration recommended for infants younger than 1 month.

Terbutaline

Classification: Selective β_2-adrenergic agonist, bronchodilator

Indications:

- Asthma (status asthmaticus)
- Hyperkalemia

Available Forms: Injection: 1 mg/mL

Dose and Administration:

Asthma (Status Asthmaticus), Hyperkalemia	
IV/IO	0.1 to 10 mcg/kg per minute infusion; consider 10 mcg/kg load over 5 minutes
Subcutaneous	10 mcg/kg subcutaneously every 10 to 15 minutes until IV/IO infusion is initiated (maximum dose 0.4 mg)

Action: Stimulates β_2-adrenergic receptors

- Causes bronchodilation
- Causes dilation of arterioles
- Causes potassium to move intracellularly (reducing serum potassium concentration)

Pharmacokinetics:

Absorption	(Not applicable with IV/IO route of administration)
Distribution	Extracellular fluid
Metabolism	Liver (partial)
Excretion	Primarily unchanged in urine
Half-life	3 to 16 hours

Pharmacodynamics:

IV/IO

- Onset—Rapid
- Peak—Unknown
- Duration—2 to 6 hours

Monitoring: Monitor ECG and SpO$_2$ continuously and blood pressure frequently.

Adverse Effects:

CNS	Tremors, anxiety, headache, dizziness, stimulation
CV	Palpitations, tachycardia, hypertension, hypotension, arrhythmias, myocardial ischemia
GI	Nausea, vomiting

Special Considerations: Like other β_2-adrenergic agonists, terbutaline can lower serum potassium concentration. The drug should be used cautiously in children with hypokalemia.

Vasopressin

Classification: Antidiuretic hormone analogue

Indications:

- Cardiac arrest
- Catecholamine-resistant hypotension (e.g., septic shock)

Available Forms: Injection: 20 units/mL

Dose and Administration:

Cardiac Arrest	
IO/IV	0.4 to 1 unit/kg bolus (maximum dose 40 units)
Catecholamine-Resistant Hypotension	
IV/IO	0.0002 to 0.002 unit/kg per minute (0.2 to 2 milliunits/kg per minute) continuous infusion

Actions:

- Mediated through actions at vasopressin receptors
- Direct vasoconstrictor at serum concentrations higher than those used for diuresis inhibition; also increases response to catecholamines
- Increases water permeability at renal tubule to increase urine osmolality, thus concentrating urine
- Stimulates gastrointestinal smooth muscle at large doses

Pharmacokinetics:

Absorption	(Not applicable with IV/IO route of administration)
Distribution	Extracellular fluid, wide
Excretion	Liver, kidneys
Half-life	10 to 20 minutes

Monitoring:

- Monitor blood pressure and distal pulses.
- Watch for signs of water intoxication (headaches, drowsiness).

Adverse Effects:

CNS	Fever, vertigo, water intoxication syndrome
RESP	Bronchial constriction
CV	Arrhythmia, hypertension
GI	Mesenteric ischemia, nausea, vomiting, abdominal cramps
GU	Uterine contraction
SKIN	Urticaria, skin necrosis

Precautions:

- Use with caution in patients with renal insufficiency or hyponatremia/free water overload.
- Vasoconstriction and tissue necrosis may occur if extravasation is present.
- Use with caution in patients with asthma or cardiovascular disease.

Special Considerations: Limited data available regarding use in children

Appendix

Appendix

BLS Competency Testing

BLS Skills Testing Sheets

The 1- and 2-Rescuer Child BLS With AED Skills Testing Sheet and the 1- and 2-Rescuer Infant BLS Skills Testing Sheet provide detailed descriptions of the CPR skills that you will be expected to perform. Your instructor will evaluate your CPR skills during the skills test on the basis of these descriptions.

If you perform a specific skill exactly as described in the critical performance criteria details, the instructor will check that specific skill as "passing." If you do not perform a specific skill exactly as it is described, the skill will not be checked off and you will require remediation in that skill.

Study the BLS skills testing sheets in this section so that you will be able to perform each skill correctly.

Remediation

Any student who does not pass both skills tests will practice and undergo remediation during the remediation lesson at the end of the course.

Students who require remediation and retesting will be tested in the entire skill.

BLS Skills Testing
1- and 2-Rescuer Child BLS With AED Skills Testing Sheet

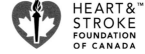

HEART&™
STROKE
FOUNDATION
OF CANADA

See 1- and 2-Rescuer Child BLS With AED Skills Testing Criteria and Descriptors on next page

Student Name: _____ Test Date: _____

1-Rescuer BLS and CPR Skills (circle one):	Pass	Needs Remediation
2-Rescuer CPR Skills		
Bag-Mask (circle one):	Pass	Needs Remediation
AED Skills (circle one):	Pass	Needs Remediation

Skill Step	Critical Performance Criteria	✓ if done correctly	
1-Rescuer Child BLS Skills Evaluation			
During this first phase, evaluate the first rescuer's ability to initiate BLS and deliver high-quality CPR for 5 cycles.			
1	ASSESSES: Checks for response and for no breathing or only gasping (at least 5 seconds but no more than 10 seconds)		
2	Sends someone to ACTIVATE emergency response system		
3	Checks for PULSE (no more than 10 seconds)		
4	GIVES HIGH-QUALITY CPR:		
	• Correct compression HAND PLACEMENT	Cycle 1:	
	• ADEQUATE RATE: At least 100/min (i.e., delivers each set of 30 chest compressions in 18 seconds or less), using 1 or 2 hands	Cycle 2:	Time:
	• ADEQUATE DEPTH: Delivers compressions at least one third the depth of the chest (approximately 5 cm [2 inches]) (at least 23 out of 30)	Cycle 3:	
	• ALLOWS COMPLETE CHEST RECOIL (at least 23 out of 30)	Cycle 4:	
	• MINIMIZES INTERRUPTIONS: Gives 2 breaths with pocket mask in less than 10 seconds	Cycle 5:	
Second Rescuer AED Skills Evaluation and SWITCH			
During this next phase, evaluate the second rescuer's ability to use the AED and both rescuers' abilities to switch roles.			
5	DURING FIFTH SET OF COMPRESSIONS: Second rescuer arrives with AED and bag-mask device, turns on AED, and applies pads		
6	First rescuer continues compressions while second rescuer turns on AED and applies pads		
7	Second rescuer clears victim, allowing AED to analyze—RESCUERS SWITCH		
8	If AED indicates a shockable rhythm, second rescuer clears victim again and delivers shock		
First Rescuer Bag-Mask Ventilation			
During this next phase, evaluate the first rescuer's ability to give breaths with a bag-mask device.			
9	Both rescuers RESUME HIGH-QUALITY CPR immediately after shock delivery:	Cycle 1	Cycle 2
	• SECOND RESCUER gives 15 compressions (in 9 seconds or less) immediately after shock delivery (for 2 cycles)	Time:	
	• FIRST RESCUER successfully delivers 2 breaths with bag-mask device (for 2 cycles)		
AFTER 2 CYCLES, STOP THE EVALUATION			

- If the student completes all steps successfully (a ✓ in each box to the right of Critical Performance Criteria), the student passed this scenario.
- If the student does not complete all steps successfully (as indicated by a blank box to the right of any of the Critical Performance Criteria), give the form to the student for review as part of the student's remediation.
- After reviewing the form, the student will give the form to the instructor who is reevaluating the student. The student will reperform the entire scenario, and the instructor will notate the reevaluation on this same form.
- If the reevaluation is to be done at a different time, the instructor should collect this sheet before the student leaves the classroom.

	Remediation (if needed):
Instructor Signature: _____	Instructor Signature: _____
Print Instructor Name: _____	Print Instructor Name: _____
Date: _____	Date: _____

BLS Skills Testing
1- and 2-Rescuer Child BLS With AED Skills Testing Criteria and Descriptors

1. **Assesses victim (Steps 1 and 2, assessment and activation, must be completed within 10 seconds of arrival at scene):**
   - Checks for unresponsiveness (this MUST precede starting compressions)
   - Checks for no breathing or only gasping
2. **Sends someone to activate emergency response system (Steps 1 and 2, assessment and activation, must be completed within 10 seconds of arrival at scene):**
   - Shouts for help/directs someone to call for help AND get AED/defibrillator
3. **Checks for pulse:**
   - Checks carotid or femoral pulse
   - This should take no more than 10 seconds
4. **Delivers high-quality CPR (initiates compressions within 10 seconds of identifying cardiac arrest):**
   - Correct placement of hand(s) in centre of chest
     - Child: 1 or 2 hands on lower half of breastbone
   - Compression rate of at least 100/min
     - Delivers 30 compressions in 18 seconds or less with 1 rescuer
     - Delivers 15 compressions in 9 seconds or less with 2 rescuers
   - Adequate depth for age
     - Child: at least one third the depth of the chest (approximately 5 cm [2 inches])
   - Complete chest recoil after each compression
   - Appropriate ratio for age and number of rescuers
     - 1 rescuer: 30 compressions to 2 breaths
   - Minimizes interruptions in compressions:
     - Less than 10 seconds between last compression of one cycle and first compression of next cycle
     - Compressions not interrupted until AED analyzing rhythm
     - Compressions resumed immediately after shock/no shock indicated
5-8. **Integrates prompt and proper use of AED with CPR:**
   - Turns AED on
   - Places proper-sized pads for victim's age in correct location; if available, uses child-sized pads/dose attenuator for victims younger than 8 years
   - Clears rescuers from victim for AED to analyze rhythm (pushes ANALYZE button if required by device)
   - Clears victim and delivers shock
   - Resumes chest compressions immediately after shock delivery
   - Does NOT turn off AED during CPR
   - Provides safe environment for rescuers during AED shock delivery:
     - Communicates clearly to all other rescuers to stop touching victim
     - Delivers shock to victim after all rescuers are clear of victim
   - Switches during analysis phase of AED
9. **Provides effective breaths with bag-mask device during 2-rescuer CPR:**
   - Provides effective breaths:
     - Opens airway adequately
     - Delivers each breath over 1 second
     - Delivers breaths that produce visible chest rise
     - Avoids excessive ventilation
10. **Provides high-quality chest compressions during 2-rescuer CPR:**
   - Correct placement of hand(s) in centre of chest
   - Compression rate of at least 100/min
     - Delivers 15 compressions in 9 seconds or less
   - Adequate depth for age
     - Child: at least one third the depth of the chest (approximately 5 cm [2 inches])
   - Complete chest recoil after each compression
   - Appropriate ratio for age and number of rescuers
     - 2 rescuers: 15 compressions to 2 breaths
   - Minimizes interruptions in compressions
     - Less than 10 seconds between last compression of one cycle and first compression of next cycle

BLS Skills Testing
1- and 2-Rescuer Infant BLS Skills Testing Sheet

HEART & ™
STROKE
FOUNDATION
OF CANADA

See 1- and 2-Rescuer Infant BLS Skills Testing Criteria and Descriptors on next page

Student Name: _____ Test Date: _____

1-Rescuer BLS and CPR Skills (circle one):	Pass	Needs Remediation
2-Rescuer CPR Skills		
Bag-Mask (circle one):	Pass	Needs Remediation
2 Thumb–Encircling Hands (circle one):	Pass	Needs Remediation

Skill Step	Critical Performance Criteria	✓ if done correctly	
1-Rescuer Infant BLS Skills Evaluation During this first phase, evaluate the first rescuer's ability to initiate BLS and deliver high-quality CPR for 5 cycles.			
1	ASSESSES: Checks for response and for no breathing or only gasping (at least 5 seconds but no more than 10 seconds)		
2	Sends someone to ACTIVATE emergency response system (no AED available)		
3	Checks for PULSE (no more than 10 seconds)		
4	GIVES HIGH-QUALITY CPR:		
	• Correct compression FINGER PLACEMENT	Cycle 1:	
	• ADEQUATE RATE: At least 100/min (i.e., delivers each set of 30 chest compressions in 18 seconds or less)	Cycle 2:	Time:
	• ADEQUATE DEPTH: Delivers compressions at least one third the depth of the chest (approximately 4 cm [1½ inches]) (at least 23 out of 30)	Cycle 3:	
	• ALLOWS COMPLETE CHEST RECOIL (at least 23 out of 30)	Cycle 4:	
	• MINIMIZES INTERRUPTIONS: Gives 2 breaths with pocket mask in less than 10 seconds	Cycle 5:	
2-Rescuer CPR and SWITCH During this next phase, evaluate the FIRST RESCUER'S ability to give breaths with a bag-mask device and give compressions by using the 2 thumb–encircling hands technique. Also evaluate both rescuers' abilities to switch roles.			
5	DURING FIFTH SET OF COMPRESSIONS: Second rescuer arrives with bag-mask device. RESCUERS SWITCH ROLES.		
6	Both rescuers RESUME HIGH-QUALITY CPR:	Cycle 1	Cycle 2
	• SECOND RESCUER gives 15 compressions in 9 seconds or less by using 2 thumb–encircling hands technique (for 2 cycles)	X	X
	• FIRST RESCUER successfully delivers 2 breaths with bag-mask device (for 2 cycles)		
	AFTER 2 CYCLES, PROMPT RESCUERS TO SWITCH ROLES		
7	Both rescuers RESUME HIGH-QUALITY CPR:	Cycle 1	Cycle 2
	• FIRST RESCUER gives 15 compressions in 9 seconds or less by using 2 thumb–encircling hands technique (for 2 cycles)	Time:	Time:
	• SECOND RESCUER successfully delivers 2 breaths with bag-mask device (for 2 cycles)	X	X
AFTER 2 CYCLES, STOP THE EVALUATION			

- If the student completes all steps successfully (a ✓ in each box to the right of Critical Performance Criteria), the student passed this scenario.
- If the student does not complete all steps successfully (as indicated by a blank box to the right of any of the Critical Performance Criteria), give the form to the student for review as part of the student's remediation.
- After reviewing the form, the student will give the form to the instructor who is reevaluating the student. The student will reperform the entire scenario, and the instructor will notate the reevaluation on this same form.
- If the reevaluation is to be done at a different time, the instructor should collect this sheet before the student leaves the classroom.

	Remediation (if needed):
Instructor Signature: _____	Instructor Signature: _____
Print Instructor Name: _____	Print Instructor Name: _____
Date: _____	Date: _____

BLS Skills Testing
1- and 2-Rescuer Infant BLS
Skills Testing Criteria and Descriptors

1. **Assesses victim (Steps 1 and 2, assessment and activation, must be completed within 10 seconds of arrival at scene):**
   - Checks for unresponsiveness (this MUST precede starting compressions)
   - Checks for no breathing or only gasping

2. **Sends someone to activate emergency response system (Steps 1 and 2, assessment and activation, must be completed within 10 seconds of arrival at scene):**
   - Shouts for help/directs someone to call for help AND get AED/defibrillator
   - If alone, remains with infant to provide 2 minutes of CPR before activating emergency response system

3. **Checks for pulse:**
   - Checks brachial pulse
   - This should take no more than 10 seconds

4. **Delivers high-quality 1-rescuer CPR (initiates compressions within 10 seconds of identifying cardiac arrest):**
   - Correct placement of fingers in centre of chest
     - 1 rescuer: 2 fingers just below the nipple line
   - Compression rate of at least 100/min
     - Delivers 30 compressions in 18 seconds or less
   - Adequate depth for age
     - Infant: at least one third the depth of the chest (approximately 4 cm [1½ inches])
   - Complete chest recoil after each compression
   - Appropriate ratio for age and number of rescuers
     - 1 rescuer: 30 compressions to 2 breaths
   - Minimizes interruptions in compressions:
     - Less than 10 seconds between last compression of one cycle and first compression of next cycle

5. **Switches at appropriate intervals as prompted by the instructor (for purposes of this evaluation)**

6. **Provides effective breaths with bag-mask device during 2-rescuer CPR:**
   - Provides effective breaths:
     - Opens airway adequately
     - Delivers each breath over 1 second
     - Delivers breaths that produce visible chest rise
     - Avoids excessive ventilation

7. **Provides high-quality chest compressions during 2-rescuer CPR:**
   - Correct placement of hands/fingers in centre of chest
     - 2 rescuers: 2 thumb–encircling hands just below the nipple line
   - Compression rate of at least 100/min
     - Delivers 15 compressions in 9 seconds or less
   - Adequate depth for age
     - Infant: at least one third the depth of the chest (approximately 4 cm [1½ inches])
   - Complete chest recoil after each compression
   - Appropriate ratio for age and number of rescuers
     - 2 rescuers: 15 compressions to 2 breaths
   - Minimizes interruptions in compressions:
     - Less than 10 seconds between last compression of one cycle and first compression of next cycle

Skills Station Competency Checklists
Management of Respiratory Emergencies Skills Station Competency Checklist

Critical Performance Steps	For more information, see
Verbalizes difference between high-flow and low-flow O₂ delivery systems • High flow (>10 L/min): O₂ flow exceeds patient inspiratory flow, preventing entrainment of room air if system is tight-fitting; delivers nearly 1.00 FIO₂, e.g., nonrebreathing mask with reservoir • Low flow (≤10 L/min): patient inspiratory flow exceeds O₂ flow, allowing entrainment of room air; typically delivers 0.23 to 0.50 FIO₂, e.g., nasal cannula, simple O₂ mask	
Verbalizes maximum nasal cannula flow rate (4 L/min)	
Opens airway by using head tilt–chin lift maneuver while keeping mouth open (jaw thrust for trauma victim)	Instructor demonstration
Verbalizes different indications for OPA and NPA • OPA only for unconscious victim without a gag reflex • NPA for conscious or semiconscious victim	
Selects correctly sized airway by measuring • OPA from corner of mouth to angle of mandible	
Inserts OPA correctly	
Verbalizes assessment for adequate breathing after insertion of OPA	
Suctions with OPA in place; states suctioning not to exceed 10 seconds	
Selects correct mask size for ventilations	"Bag-Mask Ventilation" at the end of Part 5, "Resources for Management of Respiratory Emergencies
Assembles bag-mask device, opens airway, and creates seal by using E-C clamp technique	
With bag-mask device gives 1 breath every 3 to 5 seconds for about 30 seconds. Gives each breath in approximately 1 second; each breath should cause chest rise	
States equipment needed for endotracheal (ET) tube intubation procedure	"Pre-Event Equipment Checklist for Endotracheal Intubation" at the end of Part 5, "Resources for Management of Respiratory Emergencies"
Demonstrates technique to confirm proper ET tube placement by physical examination and use of an exhaled CO₂ detector device	
Secures ET tube	
Suctions with ET tube in place	
The following steps are optional. They are demonstrated and evaluated only when the student's scope of practice involves endotracheal intubation.	
Prepares equipment for ET intubation	
Inserts ET tube correctly	

Rhythm Disturbances/Electrical Therapy Skills Station Competency Checklist

Critical Performance Steps	For more information, see
Applies ECG leads correctly • Negative (white) lead: to right shoulder • Positive (red) lead: to left ribs • Ground (black, green, brown) lead: to left shoulder	Instructor demonstration
Demonstrates correct operation of monitor • Turns monitor on • Adjusts device to manual mode (not AED mode) to display rhythm in standard limb leads (I, II, III) or paddles/electrode pads	Instructor demonstration
Verbalizes correct electrical therapy for appropriate core rhythms • Synchronized cardioversion for unstable SVT, VT with pulses • Defibrillation for pulseless VT, VF	Part 9: "Recognition and Management of Tachycardia"; Part 10: "Recognition and Management of Cardiac Arrest"
Selects correct paddle/electrode pad for infant or child; places paddles/electrode pads in correct position	Part 10: "Recognition and Management of Cardiac Arrest"
Demonstrates correct and safe synchronized cardioversion • Places device in synchronized mode • Selects appropriate energy (0.5 to 1.0 J/kg for initial shock) • Charges, clears, delivers current	Part 9: "Recognition and Management of Tachycardia"
Demonstrates correct and safe manual defibrillation • Places device in unsynchronized mode • Selects energy (2 to 4 J/kg for initial shock) • Charges, clears, delivers current	Part 10: "Recognition and Management of Cardiac Arrest"

Vascular Access Skills Station Competency Checklist

Critical Performance Steps	For more information, see
Verbalizes indications for IO insertion	"Intraosseous Access" at the end of Part 7, "Resources for Management of Circulatory Emergencies"
Verbalizes sites for IO insertion (anterior tibia, distal femur, medial malleolus, anterior-superior iliac spine)	
Verbalizes contraindications for IO placement • Fracture in extremity • Previous insertion attempt in the same bone • Infection overlying bone	
Inserts IO catheter safely	
Verbalizes how to confirm IO catheter is in correct position; verbalizes how to secure IO catheter	
Attaches IV line to IO catheter; demonstrates giving IO fluid bolus by using 3-way stopcock and syringe	Instructor demonstration
Shows how to determine correct drug doses by using a colour-coded length-based tape or other resource	"Colour-Coded Length-Based Resuscitation Tape" at the end of Part 7, "Resources for Management of Circulatory Emergencies"
The following is optional:	
Verbalizes correct procedure for establishing IV access	

Rhythm Recognition Review

Rhythm Strip 1

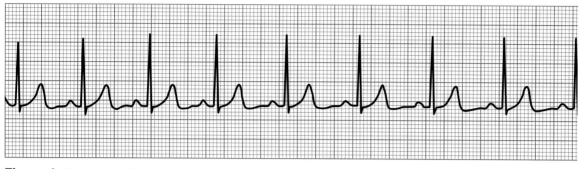

Figure 1. Normal sinus rhythm, rate 100/min.

Note that every P wave conducts to the ventricle, resulting in a QRS complex. Be aware that normal heart rates are age dependent in the pediatric population. For example, a heart rate of 75/min would be normal for a 10 year old but bradycardic for a neonate. Likewise, a rate of 140/min would be normal for an infant but tachycardic for an adolescent.

Rhythm Strip 2

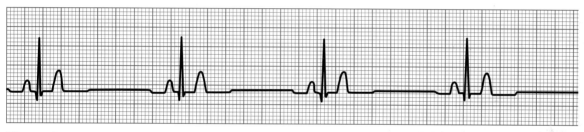

Figure 2. Sinus bradycardia.

Note that the P waves result in a QRS complex (conducted to the ventricle). The rate is very slow (approximately 45/min). Sinus bradycardia is often a manifestation of hypoxemia and acidosis. It may be seen in healthy children, particularly during sleep.

Rhythm Strip 3

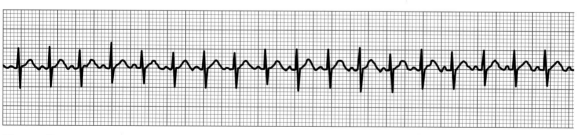

Figure 3. Sinus tachycardia, 180/min.

Note that P waves are visible preceding every QRS. The rate for sinus tachycardia may vary according to age. In an infant, sinus tachycardia could be as high as 220/min.

Rhythm Strip 4

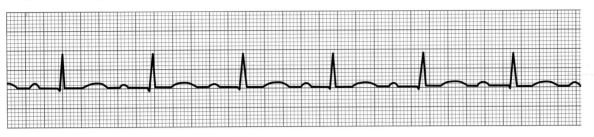

Figure 4. Sinus rhythm with first-degree heart block.

Note that the PR interval is prolonged (0.3 second). This is often a reflection of increased vagal tone and may be seen in healthy children. Less often, it can be a sign of intrinsic AV node disease, myocarditis, electrolyte disturbances (such as hyperkalemia), hypoxemia, drug toxicity (such as digoxin, β-blocker, or calcium channel blocker), or acute rheumatic fever.

Rhythm Strip 5

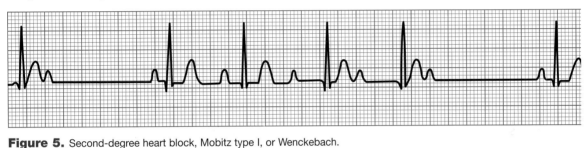

Figure 5. Second-degree heart block, Mobitz type I, or Wenckebach.

Note that the PR interval progressively prolongs until a P wave fails to conduct to the ventricle. Like first-degree heart block, this is often seen in healthy children, especially during sleep. It may also be a manifestation of drug toxicity, such as digoxin, β-blocker, or calcium channel blocker.

Rhythm Strip 6

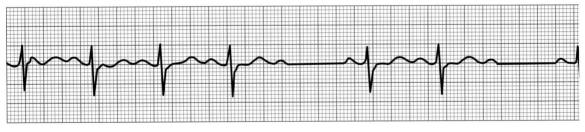

Figure 6. Second-degree heart block, Mobitz type II.

Note that some but not all of the P waves do not conduct to the ventricle. There is no progressive prolongation of the PR interval. This is a sign of intrinsic conduction system disease, typically related to cardiac surgery or myocardial inflammation or infarction.

Rhythm Strip 7

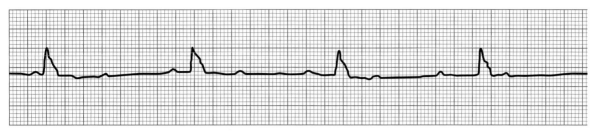

Figure 7. Third-degree (complete) heart block with ventricular escape rhythm.

Note that none of the P wave conducts to the ventricle. Often the QRS complex "marches" at a constant interval because of junctional or ventricular escape rhythm. There is no relation between P waves and QRS complexes. Occasionally this is a result of severe hypoxemia and acidosis. This may also be a manifestation of damage to the AV node or extensive conduction system disease, such as that seen following cardiac surgery, or myocarditis, or with congenital complete heart block.

Rhythm Strip 8

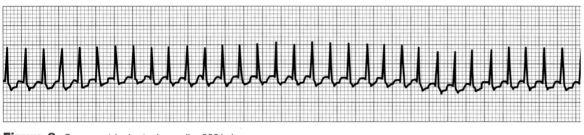

Figure 8. Supraventricular tachycardia, 230/min.

Note that the QRS complexes are narrow and regular, the rate is very fast (>200/min), and P waves are not obvious.

Rhythm Strip 9

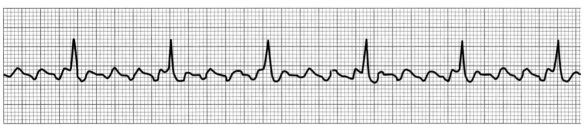

Figure 9. Atrial flutter.

Note that there is a "sawtooth" pattern to the P waves, reflecting an extremely rapid atrial rate. Conduction of the P waves to the ventricle may be variable, resulting in an irregular QRS rate.

Rhythm Strip 10

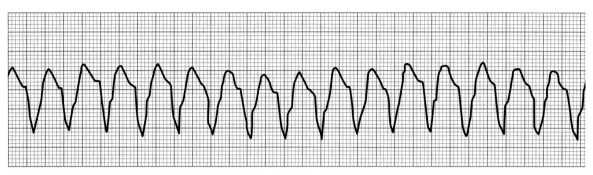

Figure 10. Ventricular tachycardia, 150/min.

Note that the QRS complexes are wide (>0.09 second), regular, and fast. The QRS morphologies are all identical, characterizing it as monomorphic ventricular tachycardia. P waves are not identifiable.

Rhythm Strip 11

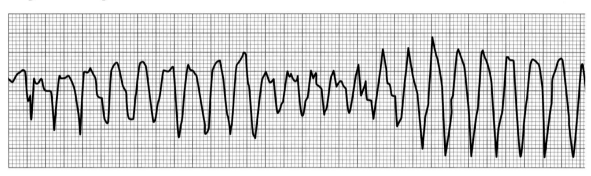

Figure 11. Polymorphic ventricular tachycardia.

Note that the QRS complexes are wide, irregular, and very fast (>200/min). The QRS complexes vary in appearance, characterizing it as polymorphic. In fact, there is a phase change during this recording where the QRS complexes are initially positive and then become negative before returning to positive polarity. This is torsades de pointes ("turning of points") type of polymorphic ventricular tachycardia, seen most often in states where the QT interval is prolonged during the baseline.

Rhythm Strip 12

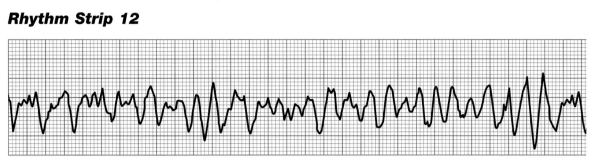

Figure 12. Ventricular fibrillation.

Note that there are no definable QRS complexes, just irregular disorganized electrical activity.

Rhythm Strip 13

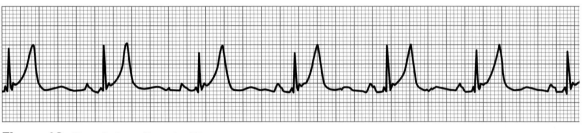

Figure 13. Sinus rhythm with peaked T waves.

Note how the T waves have increased amplitude and are even larger than the QRS complexes. This may be indicative of hyperkalemia.

Learning Station Competency Checklists
Respiratory Learning Station Competency Checklists

Core Case 1
Upper Airway Obstruction

Use this checklist during the PALS core case simulations and tests to check off the performance of the team leader.

Critical Performance Steps	Details	✓ if done correctly
Team Leader		
Assigns team member roles	Team leader identifies self and assigns team roles	
Uses effective communication throughout	Closed-loop communication Clear messages Clear roles and responsibilities Knowing limitations Knowledge sharing Constructive intervention Reevaluation and summarizing Mutual respect	
Patient Management		
Directs assessment of airway, breathing, circulation, disability, and exposure, including vital signs	Team leader directs or performs assessment to determine responsiveness, breathing, and pulse	
Directs manual airway maneuver with administration of 100% oxygen	Team leader directs manual airway maneuver and administration of 100% oxygen	
Directs placement of pads/leads and pulse oximetry	Team leader directs that pads/leads be properly placed and that the monitor be turned on to an appropriate lead; requests use of pulse oximetry	
Recognizes signs and symptoms of upper airway obstruction	Team leader verbalizes features of history and exam that indicate upper airway obstruction	
Categorizes as respiratory distress or failure	Team leader verbalizes whether patient is in respiratory distress or failure	
Verbalizes indications for assisted ventilations or CPAP	Team leader verbalizes that for patient with ineffective ventilations or poor oxygenation, assisted ventilations are required	
Directs IV or IO access	Team leader directs team member to place IV (or IO) access, if appropriate; placement simulated properly	
Directs reassessment of patient in response to treatment	Team leader directs team member to reassess airway, breathing, and circulation	
Case Conclusion		
Summarizes specific treatments for upper airway obstruction	Team leader summarizes specific treatments for upper airway obstruction (e.g., IM epinephrine, racemic epinephrine, CPAP)	
***If scope of practice applies:* Verbalizes indications for endotracheal intubation and special considerations when intubation is anticipated**	*If scope of practice applies:* Verbalizes indications for endotracheal intubation (child unable to maintain adequate airway, oxygenation, or ventilation despite initial intervention). Notes need to anticipate use of an ET tube smaller than predicted for age, especially if subglottic narrowing is suspected.	

Core Case 2
Lower Airway Obstruction

Use this checklist during the PALS core case simulations and tests to check off the performance of the team leader.

Critical Performance Steps	Details	✓ if done correctly
Team Leader		
Assigns team member roles	Team leader identifies self and assigns team roles	
Uses effective communication throughout	Closed-loop communication Clear messages Clear roles and responsibilities Knowing limitations Knowledge sharing Constructive intervention Reevaluation and summarizing Mutual respect	
Patient Management		
Directs assessment of airway, breathing, circulation, disability, and exposure, including vital signs	Team leader directs or performs assessment to determine airway patency, adequacy of breathing and circulation, level of responsiveness, temperature, and vital signs	
Directs administration of 100% oxygen	Team leader instructs team member to provide 100% oxygen	
Directs placement of pads/leads and pulse oximetry	Team leader directs that pads/leads be properly placed and that the monitor be turned on to an appropriate lead; requests use of pulse oximetry	
Recognizes signs and symptoms of lower airway obstruction	Team leader verbalizes features of history and exam that indicate lower airway obstruction	
Categorizes as respiratory distress or failure	Team leader verbalizes whether patient has respiratory distress or failure	
Verbalizes indications for assisted ventilations	Team leader verbalizes that for patient with ineffective ventilations or poor oxygenation, assisted ventilations are required	
Directs IV or IO access	Team leader directs team member to place IV (or IO) access, if appropriate; placement simulated properly	
Directs reassessment of patient in response to treatment	Team leader directs team members to reassess airway, breathing, and circulation	
Case Conclusion		
Summarizes specific treatments for lower airway obstruction	Team leader summarizes specific treatments for lower airway obstruction (e.g., nebulized salbutamol)	
***If scope of practice applies:* Verbalizes indications for endotracheal intubation**	*If scope of practice applies:* Verbalizes indications for endotracheal intubation (child unable to maintain adequate airway, oxygenation, or ventilation despite initial intervention)	

Core Case 3
Lung Tissue Disease

Use this checklist during the PALS core case simulations and tests to check off the performance of the team leader.

Critical Performance Steps	Details	✓ if done correctly
Team Leader		
Assigns team member roles	Team leader identifies self and assigns team roles	
Uses effective communication throughout	Closed-loop communication Clear messages Clear roles and responsibilities Knowing limitations Knowledge sharing Constructive intervention Reevaluation and summarizing Mutual respect	
Patient Management		
Directs assessment of airway, breathing, circulation, disability, and exposure, including vital signs	Team leader directs or performs assessment to determine airway patency, adequacy of breathing and circulation, level of responsiveness, temperature, and vital signs	
Directs assisted ventilations with administration of 100% oxygen	Team leader directs assisted ventilations with 100% oxygen	
Ensures that bag-mask ventilations are effective	Team leader observes or directs team member to observe for chest rise and breath sounds	
Directs placement of pads/leads and pulse oximetry	Team leader directs that pads/leads be properly placed and that the monitor be turned on to an appropriate lead; requests use of pulse oximetry	
Recognizes signs and symptoms of lung tissue disease	Team leader verbalizes features of history and exam that indicate lung tissue disease	
Categorizes as respiratory distress or failure	Team leader verbalizes whether patient has respiratory distress or failure	
Directs IV or IO access	Team leader directs team member to place IV (or IO) access, if appropriate; placement simulated properly	
Directs reassessment of patient in response to treatment	Team leader directs team members to reassess airway, breathing, and circulation	
Case Conclusion		
Summarizes specific treatments for lung tissue disease	Team leader summarizes specific treatments for lung tissue disease (e.g., antibiotics for suspected pneumonia)	
***If scope of practice applies:* Verbalizes indications for endotracheal intubation**	*If scope of practice applies:* Verbalizes indications for endotracheal intubation (child unable to maintain adequate airway, oxygenation, or ventilation despite initial intervention)	

Core Case 4
Disordered Control of Breathing

Use this checklist during the PALS core case simulations and tests to check off the performance of the team leader.

Critical Performance Steps	Details	✓ if done correctly
Team Leader		
Assigns team member roles	Team leader identifies self and assigns team roles	
Uses effective communication throughout	Closed-loop communication Clear messages Clear roles and responsibilities Knowing limitations Knowledge sharing Constructive intervention Reevaluation and summarizing Mutual respect	
Patient Management		
Directs assessment of airway, breathing, circulation, disability, and exposure, including vital signs	Team leader directs or performs assessment to determine airway patency, adequacy of breathing and circulation, level of responsiveness, temperature, and vital signs	
Directs assisted ventilations with administration of 100% oxygen	Team leader directs assisted ventilations with 100% oxygen	
Ensures that bag-mask ventilations are effective	Team leader ensures that there is chest rise with assisted ventilations	
Directs placement of pads/leads and pulse oximetry	Team leader directs that pads/leads be properly placed and that the monitor be turned on to an appropriate lead; requests use of pulse oximetry	
Recognizes signs and symptoms of disordered control of breathing	Team leader verbalizes features of history and exam that indicate disordered control of breathing	
Categorizes as respiratory distress or failure	Team leader verbalizes whether patient is in respiratory distress or failure (note that respiratory failure can occur without distress in this setting)	
Directs IV or IO access	Team leader directs team member to place IV (or IO) access, if appropriate; placement simulated properly	
Directs reassessment of patient in response to treatment	Team leader observes or directs team members to reassess airway, breathing, and circulation	
Case Conclusion		
Summarizes specific treatments for disordered control of breathing	Team leader summarizes specific treatments for disordered control of breathing (e.g., sedation reversal agents)	
If scope of practice applies: **Verbalizes indications for endotracheal intubation**	*If scope of practice applies:* Verbalizes indications for endotracheal intubation (child unable to maintain adequate airway, oxygenation, or ventilation despite initial intervention)	

Shock Learning Station Competency Checklists

Core Case 5
Hypovolemic Shock

Use this checklist during the PALS core case simulations and tests to check off the performance of the team leader.

Critical Performance Steps	Details	✓ if done correctly
Team Leader		
Assigns team member roles	Team leader identifies self and assigns team roles	
Uses effective communication throughout	Closed-loop communication Clear messages Clear roles and responsibilities Knowing limitations Knowledge sharing Constructive intervention Reevaluation and summarizing Mutual respect	
Patient Management		
Directs assessment of airway, breathing, circulation, disability, and exposure, including vital signs	Team leader directs or performs assessment to determine airway patency, adequacy of breathing and circulation, level of responsiveness, temperature, and vital signs	
Directs administration of 100% oxygen	Team leader directs administration of 100% oxygen	
Directs placement of pads/leads and pulse oximetry	Team leader directs that pads/leads be properly placed and that the monitor be turned on to an appropriate lead; requests use of pulse oximetry	
Recognizes signs and symptoms of hypovolemic shock	Team leader verbalizes features of history and exam that indicate hypovolemic shock	
Categorizes as compensated or hypotensive shock	Team leader verbalizes whether patient is compensated or hypotensive	
Directs IV or IO access	Team leader directs team member to place IV (or IO) access; placement simulated properly	
Directs rapid administration of a fluid bolus of isotonic crystalloid	Team leader directs administration of isotonic crystalloid, 20 mL/kg rapidly (over 5 to 20 minutes) IV or IO	
Directs reassessment of patient in response to treatment	Team leader directs team members to reassess airway, breathing, and circulation	
Case Conclusion		
Verbalizes therapeutic end points during shock management	Team leader identifies parameters that indicate response to therapy (heart rate, blood pressure, distal pulses and capillary refill, urine output, mental status)	

Core Case 6
Obstructive Shock

Use this checklist during the PALS core case simulations and tests to check off the performance of the team leader.

Critical Performance Steps	Details	✓ if done correctly
Team Leader		
Assigns team member roles	Team leader identifies self and assigns team roles	
Uses effective communication throughout	Closed-loop communication Clear messages Clear roles and responsibilities Knowing limitations Knowledge sharing Constructive intervention Reevaluation and summarizing Mutual respect	
Patient Management		
Directs assessment of airway, breathing, circulation, disability, and exposure, including vital signs	Team leader directs or performs assessment to determine airway patency, adequacy of breathing and circulation, level of responsiveness, temperature, and vital signs	
Directs placement of pads/leads and pulse oximetry	Team leader directs that pads/leads be properly placed and that the monitor be turned on to an appropriate lead; requests use of pulse oximetry	
Verbalizes DOPE mnemonic for intubated patient who deteriorates	Team leader reviews elements of DOPE mnemonic (displacement, obstruction, pneumothorax, equipment failure)	
Recognizes signs and symptoms of obstructive shock	Team leader verbalizes features of history and exam that indicate obstructive shock	
States at least 2 causes of obstructive shock	Team leader states at least 2 common causes of obstructive shock (tension pneumothorax, cardiac tamponade, pulmonary embolus)	
Categorizes as compensated or hypotensive shock	Team leader verbalizes whether patient is compensated or hypotensive	
Directs IV or IO access	Team leader directs team member to place IV (or IO) access; placement simulated properly	
Directs rapid administration of a fluid bolus of isotonic crystalloid	Team leader directs administration of isotonic crystalloid, 10 to 20 mL/kg rapidly (over 5 to 20 minutes) IV or IO	
Directs reassessment of patient in response to treatment	Team leader directs team member to reassess airway, breathing, and circulation	
Case Conclusion		
Summarizes the treatment for a tension pneumothorax	Team leader describes use of emergency pleural decompression (second intercostal space, midclavicular line)	
Verbalizes therapeutic end points during shock management	Team leader identifies parameters that indicate response to therapy (heart rate, blood pressure, perfusion, urine output, mental status)	

Core Case 7
Distributive Shock

Use this checklist during the PALS core case simulations and tests to check off the performance of the team leader.

Critical Performance Steps	Details	✓ if done correctly
Team Leader		
Assigns team member roles	Team leader identifies self and assigns team roles	
Uses effective communication throughout	Closed-loop communication Clear messages Clear roles and responsibilities Knowing limitations Knowledge sharing Constructive intervention Reevaluation and summarizing Mutual respect	
Patient Management		
Directs assessment of airway, breathing, circulation, disability, and exposure, including vital signs	Team leader directs or performs assessment to determine airway patency, adequacy of breathing and circulation, level of responsiveness, temperature, and vital signs	
Directs administration of 100% oxygen	Team leader directs team member to provide 100% oxygen	
Directs placement of pads/leads and pulse oximetry	Team leader directs that pads/leads be properly placed and that the monitor be turned on to an appropriate lead; requests use of pulse oximetry	
Recognizes signs and symptoms of distributive (septic) shock	Team leader verbalizes features of history and exam that indicate distributive shock	
Categorizes as compensated or hypotensive shock	Team leader verbalizes whether patient is compensated or hypotensive	
Directs IV or IO access	Team leader directs team member to place IV (or IO) access; placement simulated properly	
Directs rapid administration of a fluid bolus of isotonic crystalloid	Team leader directs administration of isotonic crystalloid, 20 mL/kg rapidly (over 5 to 20 minutes) IV or IO	
Directs reassessment of patient in response to treatment	Team leader directs team member to reassess airway, breathing, and circulation	
If scope of practice applies: **Recalls that early administration of antibiotics is essential in septic shock**	*If scope of practice applies:* Team leader directs administration of antibiotics	
Case Conclusion		
Summarizes indications for vasoactive drug support	Team leader verbalizes that vasoactive medications are indicated for fluid-refractory septic shock	
Verbalizes therapeutic end points during shock management	Team leader identifies parameters that indicate response to therapy (heart rate, blood pressure, perfusion, urine output, mental status)	

Core Case 8
Cardiogenic Shock

Use this checklist during the PALS core case simulations and tests to check off the performance of the team leader.

Critical Performance Steps	Details	✓ if done correctly
Team Leader		
Assigns team member roles	Team leader identifies self and assigns team roles	
Uses effective communication throughout	Closed-loop communication Clear messages Clear roles and responsibilities Knowing limitations Knowledge sharing Constructive intervention Reevaluation and summarizing Mutual respect	
Patient Management		
Directs assessment of airway, breathing, circulation, disability, and exposure, including vital signs	Team leader directs or performs assessment to determine responsiveness, breathing, and pulse	
Directs administration of 100% oxygen	Team leader directs administration of 100% oxygen by high-flow device	
Directs placement of pads/leads and pulse oximetry	Team leader directs that pads/leads be properly placed and that the monitor be turned on to an appropriate lead; requests use of pulse oximetry	
Recognizes signs and symptoms of cardiogenic shock	Team leader verbalizes features of history and exam that indicate cardiogenic shock	
Categorizes as compensated or hypotensive shock	Team leader verbalizes whether patient's shock is compensated or hypotensive	
Directs IV or IO access	Team leader directs team member to place IV (or IO) access; placement simulated properly	
Directs slow administration of 5 to 10 mL/kg fluid bolus of isotonic crystalloid	Team leader directs administration of isotonic crystalloid, 5 to 10 mL/kg IV or IO (over 10 to 20 minutes), while carefully monitoring patient for signs of pulmonary edema or worsening heart failure	
Directs reassessment of the patient in response to treatment	Team leader directs team member to reassess airway, breathing, and circulation	
Recalls indications for use of vasoactive drugs during cardiogenic shock	Team leader verbalizes indications for initiation of vaso-active drugs (persistent signs of shock despite fluid therapy)	
Case Conclusion		
Verbalizes therapeutic end points during shock management	Team leader identifies parameters that indicate response to therapy (heart rate, blood pressure, perfusion, urine output, mental status). In cardiogenic shock, team leader recognizes importance of reducing metabolic demand by reducing work of breathing and temperature.	

Cardiac Learning Station Competency Checklists

Core Case 9
Supraventricular Tachycardia

Use this checklist during the PALS core case simulations and tests to check off the performance of the team leader.

Critical Performance Steps	Details	✓ if done correctly
Team Leader		
Assigns team member roles	Team leader identifies self and assigns team roles	
Uses effective communication throughout	Closed-loop communication Clear messages Clear roles and responsibilities Knowing limitations Knowledge sharing Constructive intervention Reevaluation and summarizing Mutual respect	
Patient Management		
Directs assessment of airway, breathing, circulation, disability, and exposure, including vital signs	Team leader directs or performs assessment to determine airway patency, adequacy of breathing and circulation, level of responsiveness, temperature, and vital signs	
Directs administration of supplementary oxygen	Team leader directs administration of supplementary oxygen by high-flow device	
Directs placement of pads/leads and pulse oximetry	Team leader directs that pads/leads be properly placed and that the monitor be turned on to an appropriate lead; requests use of pulse oximetry	
Recognizes narrow-complex tachycardia and verbalizes how to distinguish between ST and SVT	Team leader recognizes narrow-complex tachycardia and verbalizes reasons for identification as SVT versus ST	
Categorizes as compensated or hypotensive	Team leader verbalizes whether patient is compensated or hypotensive	
Directs performance of appropriate vagal maneuvers	Team leader directs team member to perform appropriate vagal maneuvers (e.g., Valsalva, blowing through straw, ice to face)	
Directs IV or IO access	Team leader directs team member to place IV (or IO) access; placement simulated properly	
Directs preparation and administration of appropriate dose of adenosine	Team leader directs team member to prepare correct dose of adenosine (first dose: 0.1 mg/kg, maximum: 6 mg; second dose: 0.2 mg/kg, maximum: 12 mg), uses drug dose resource if needed; states need for rapid administration with use of saline flush	
Directs reassessment of patient in response to treatment	Team leader directs team member to reassess airway, breathing, and circulation	
Case Conclusion		
Verbalizes indications and appropriate energy doses for synchronized cardioversion	Team leader verbalizes indications and correct energy dose for synchronized cardioversion (0.5 to 1 J/kg for initial dose)	

Core Case 10
Bradycardia

Use this checklist during the PALS core case simulations and tests to check off the performance of the team leader.

Critical Performance Steps	Details	✓ if done correctly
Team Leader		
Assigns team member roles	Team leader identifies self and assigns team roles	
Uses effective communication throughout	Closed-loop communication Clear messages Clear roles and responsibilities Knowing limitations Knowledge sharing Constructive intervention Reevaluation and summarizing Mutual respect	
Patient Management		
Directs assessment of airway, breathing, circulation, disability, and exposure, including vital signs	Team leader directs or performs assessment to determine airway patency, adequacy of breathing and circulation, level of responsiveness, temperature, and vital signs	
Directs initiation of assisted ventilations with 100% oxygen	Team leader instructs team member to provide assisted ventilations with 100% oxygen	
Directs placement of pads/leads and activation of monitor and requests pulse oximetry	Team leader directs that pads/leads be properly placed and that monitor be turned on to an appropriate lead; requests use of pulse oximetry	
Recognizes bradycardia with cardiorespiratory compromise	Team leader recognizes rhythm and verbalizes presence of bradycardia to team members	
Characterizes as compensated or hypotensive	Team leader communicates that patient has cardiorespiratory compromise and is hypotensive	
Recalls indications for chest compressions in a bradycardic patient	Team leader verbalizes indications for chest compressions (may or may not perform)	
Directs IV or IO access	Team leader directs team member to place IV (or IO) access; placement simulated properly	
Directs preparation and administration of appropriate dose of epinephrine	Team leader directs team member to prepare initial dose of epinephrine (0.01 mg/kg or 0.1 mL/kg of 1:10 000 dilution IV/IO), uses drug dose resource if needed; directs team member to administer epinephrine dose and saline flush	
Directs reassessment of patient in response to treatment	Team leader directs team members to reassess airway, breathing, and circulation	
Case Conclusion		
Verbalizes consideration of at least 3 underlying causes of bradycardia	Team leader verbalizes potentially reversible causes of bradycardia (e.g., toxins, hypothermia, increased ICP)	

Core Case 11
Asystole/PEA

Use this checklist during the PALS core case simulations and tests to check off the performance of the team leader.

Critical Performance Steps	Details	✓ if done correctly
Team Leader		
Assigns team member roles	Team leader identifies self and assigns team roles	
Uses effective communication throughout	Closed-loop communication Clear messages Clear roles and responsibilities Knowing limitations Knowledge sharing Constructive intervention Reevaluation and summarizing Mutual respect	
Patient Management		
Recognizes cardiopulmonary arrest	Team leader directs or performs assessment to determine absence of responsiveness, breathing, and pulse	
Directs initiation of CPR by using the C-A-B sequence and ensures performance of high-quality CPR at all times	Team leader monitors quality of CPR (e.g., adequate rate, adequate depth, chest recoil) and provides feedback to team member providing compressions; directs resuscitation so as to minimize interruptions in CPR; directs team members to rotate role of chest compressor approximately every 2 minutes	
Directs placement of pads/leads and activation of monitor	Team leader directs that pads/leads be properly placed and that the monitor be turned on to an appropriate lead	
Recognizes asystole or PEA	Team leader recognizes rhythm and verbalizes presence of asystole or PEA to team members	
Directs IO or IV access	Team leader directs team member to place IO (or IV) access; placement simulated properly	
Directs preparation of appropriate dose of epinephrine	Team leader directs team member to prepare initial dose of epinephrine (0.01 mg/kg or 0.1 mL/kg of 1:10 000 dilution IO/IV), uses drug dose resource if needed	
Directs administration of epinephrine at appropriate intervals	Team leader directs team member to administer epinephrine dose with saline flush and prepare to administer again every 3 to 5 minutes	
Directs checking rhythm on the monitor approximately every 2 minutes	Team leader directs team members to stop compressions and checks rhythm on monitor approximately every 2 minutes	
Case Conclusion		
Verbalizes consideration of at least 3 reversible causes of PEA or asystole	Team leader verbalizes at least 3 potentially reversible causes of PEA or asystole (e.g., hypovolemia, tamponade)	

Core Case 12
VF/Pulseless VT

Use this checklist during the PALS core case simulations and tests to check off the performance of the team leader.

Critical Performance Steps	Details	✓ if done correctly
Team Leader		
Assigns team member roles	Team leader identifies self and assigns team roles	
Uses effective communication throughout	Closed-loop communication Clear messages Clear roles and responsibilities Knowing limitations Knowledge sharing Constructive intervention Reevaluation and summarizing Mutual respect	
Patient Management		
Recognizes cardiopulmonary arrest	Team leader directs or performs assessment to determine absence of responsiveness, breathing, and pulse	
Directs initiation of CPR by using the C-A-B sequence and ensures performance of high-quality CPR at all times	Team leader monitors quality of CPR (e.g., adequate rate, adequate depth, chest recoil) and provides feedback to team member providing compressions; directs resuscitation so as to minimize interruptions in CPR; directs team members to rotate role of chest compressor approximately every 2 minutes	
Directs placement of pads/leads and activation of monitor	Team leader directs that the pads/leads be properly placed and that the monitor be turned on to an appropriate lead	
Recognizes VF or pulseless VT	Team leader recognizes rhythm and verbalizes presence of VF/VT to team members	
Directs attempted defibrillation at 2 to 4 J/kg safely	Team leader directs team member to set proper energy and attempt defibrillation; observes for safe performance	
Directs immediate resumption of CPR by using the C-A-B sequence	Team leader directs team member to resume CPR immediately after shock (no pulse or rhythm check)	
Directs IO or IV access	Team leader directs team member to place IO (or IV) access; placement simulated properly	
Directs preparation of appropriate dose of epinephrine	Team leader directs team member to prepare initial dose of epinephrine (0.01 mg/kg or 0.1 mL/kg of 1:10 000 dilution IO/IV), uses drug dose resource if needed	
Directs attempted defibrillation at 4 J/kg or higher (not to exceed 10 J/kg or standard adult dose) safely	Team leader directs team member to set proper energy and attempt defibrillation; observes for safe performance	
Directs immediate resumption of CPR by using the C-A-B sequence	Team leader directs team member to resume CPR immediately after shock (no pulse or rhythm check)	
Directs administration of epinephrine	Team leader directs team member to administer epinephrine dose followed by saline flush	
Case Conclusion		
Verbalizes consideration of anti-arrhythmic (amiodarone or lidocaine), using appropriate dose	Team leader indicates consideration of appropriate antiarrhythmic in proper dose	

PALS Systematic Approach Summary

Initial Impression	*Your first quick (in a few seconds) "from the doorway" observation*

Consciousness	Level of consciousness (e.g., unresponsive, irritable, alert)
Breathing	Increased work of breathing, absent or decreased respiratory effort, or abnormal sounds heard without auscultation
Colour	Abnormal skin colour, such as cyanosis, pallor, or mottling
	The purpose is to quickly identify a life-threatening problem.

Is the child unresponsive with no breathing or only gasping?	
If YES:	
• Shout for help.	• Check for a pulse.
• Activate emergency response as appropriate for setting.	• Begin lifesaving interventions as needed.
If NO:	
• Continue the evaluate-identify-intervene sequence.	

Use the **evaluate-identify-intervene** sequence when caring for a seriously ill or injured child.

- *Evaluate* the child to gather information about the child's condition or status.
- *Identify* any problem by type and severity.
- *Intervene* with appropriate actions to treat the problem.

Then repeat the sequence; this process is ongoing.

Evaluate
- Primary assessment
- Secondary assessment
- Diagnostic tests

Intervene

Identify

If at any time you identify a life-threatening problem, immediately begin appropriate interventions. Activate emergency response as indicated in your practice setting.

Evaluate	*"Evaluate" consists of the primary assessment (ABCDE), secondary assessment, and diagnostic tests.*

Primary Assessment	A rapid, hands-on ABCDE approach to evaluate respiratory, cardiac, and neurologic function; this step includes assessment of vital signs and pulse oximetry

Airway

Clear	Maintainable	Not maintainable

Breathing

Respiratory Rate and Pattern	**Respiratory Effort**	**Chest Expansion and Air Movement**	**Abnormal Lung and Airway Sounds**	**Oxygen Saturation by Pulse Oximetry**
Normal Irregular Fast Slow Apnea	Normal Increased • Nasal flaring • Retractions • Head bobbing • Seesaw respirations Inadequate • Apnea • Weak cry or cough	Normal Decreased Unequal Prolonged expiration	Stridor Snoring Barking cough Hoarseness Grunting Gurgling Wheezing Crackles Unequal	Normal oxygen saturation (≥94%) Hypoxemia (<94%)

Circulation

Heart Rate and Rhythm	**Pulses**		**Capillary Refill Time**	**Skin Colour and Temperature**	**Blood Pressure**
Normal Fast (tachycardia) Slow (bradycardia)	***Central*** Normal Weak Absent	***Peripheral*** Normal Weak Absent	Normal: ≤2 seconds Delayed: >2 seconds	Pallor Mottling Cyanosis Warm skin Cool skin	Normal Hypotensive

Disability

AVPU Pediatric Response Scale				**Pupil Size Reaction to Light**		**Blood Glucose**	
Alert	Responds to **V**oice	Responds to **P**ain	**U**nresponsive	Normal	Abnormal	Normal	Low

Exposure

Temperature			**Skin**	
Normal	High	Low	Rash (e.g., purpura)	Trauma (e.g., injury, bleeding)

Secondary Assessment	A focused medical history (SAMPLE) and a focused physical exam
Diagnostic Tests	Laboratory, radiographic, and other advanced tests that help to identify the child's physiologic condition and diagnosis

Identify	*Identify the child's problem as respiratory, circulatory, or both. Determine the type and severity of the problem(s). The table below lists common clinical signs that typically correlate with a specific type of problem and its severity.*

Type		Severity	
Respiratory	• Upper airway obstruction • Lower airway obstruction • Lung tissue disease • Disordered control of breathing	• Respiratory distress • Respiratory failure	
Circulatory	• Hypovolemic shock • Distributive (e.g., septic, anaphylactic) shock • Obstructive shock • Cardiogenic shock	• Compensated shock • Hypotensive shock	
Cardiac Arrest			

Respiratory

Signs	Type of Problem	Severity
• Increased respiratory rate and effort (e.g., retractions, nasal flaring) • Decreased air movement • Stridor (typically inspiratory) • Barking cough • Snoring or gurgling • Hoarseness	**Upper airway obstruction**	**Respiratory distress** • Some abnormal signs but no signs of respiratory failure **Respiratory failure** *One or more of the following:* • Very rapid or inadequate respiratory rate • Significant or inadequate respiratory effort • Low oxygen saturation despite high-flow oxygen • Bradycardia (ominous) • Cyanosis • Decreased level of consciousness
• Increased respiratory rate and effort (e.g., retractions, nasal flaring) • Decreased air movement • Prolonged expiration • Wheezing	**Lower airway obstruction**	
• Increased respiratory rate and effort • Decreased air movement • Grunting • Crackles	**Lung tissue disease**	
• Irregular respiratory pattern • Inadequate or irregular respiratory depth and effort • Normal or decreased air movement • Signs of upper airway obstruction (see above)	**Disordered control of breathing**	

Circulatory

• Tachycardia • Weak peripheral pulses • Delayed capillary refill time • Changes in skin colour (pallor, mottling, cyanosis)	• Cool skin • Changes in level of consciousness • Decreased urine output	Signs of poor perfusion

Signs	Type of Problem	Severity
• Signs of poor perfusion (see above)	**Hypovolemic shock** **Obstructive shock**	**Compensated shock** • Signs of poor perfusion and *normal* blood pressure **Hypotensive shock** • Signs of poor perfusion and *low* blood pressure
• Possible signs of poor perfusion (see above) *or* • Warm, flushed skin with brisk capillary refill (warm shock) • Peripheral pulses may be bounding • Possible crackles • Possible petechial or purpuric rash (septic shock)	**Distributive shock**	
• Signs of poor perfusion (see above) • Signs of CHF	**Cardiogenic shock**	

Intervene	*On the basis of your identification of the problem, intervene with appropriate actions. Your actions will be determined by your scope of practice and local protocol.*

Index